AF689458

HIGH-FREQUENCY VENTILATION IN INTENSIVE CARE AND DURING SURGERY

LUNG BIOLOGY IN HEALTH AND DISEASE

Executive Editor: **Claude Lenfant**

Director, National Heart, Lung, and Blood Institute
National Institutes of Health
Bethesda, Maryland

Volume 1 IMMUNOLOGIC AND INFECTIOUS REACTIONS IN THE LUNG, *edited by Charles H. Kirkpatrick and Herbert Y. Reynolds*

Volume 2 THE BIOCHEMICAL BASIS OF PULMONARY FUNCTION, *edited by Ronald G. Crystal*

Volume 3 BIOENGINEERING ASPECTS OF THE LUNG, *edited by John B. West*

Volume 4 METABOLIC FUNCTIONS OF THE LUNG, *edited by Y. S. Bakhle and John R. Vane*

Volume 5 RESPIRATORY DEFENSE MECHANISMS (in two parts), *edited by Joseph D. Brain, Donald F. Proctor, and Lynne M. Reid*

Volume 6 DEVELOPMENT OF THE LUNG, *edited by W. Alan Hodson*

Volume 7 LUNG WATER AND SOLUTE EXCHANGE, *edited by Norman C. Staub*

Volume 8 EXTRAPULMONARY MANIFESTATIONS OF RESPIRATORY DISEASE, *edited by Eugene Debs Robin*

Volume 9 CHRONIC OBSTRUCTIVE PULMONARY DISEASE, *edited by Thomas L. Petty*

Volume 10 PATHOGENESIS AND THERAPY OF LUNG CANCER, *edited by Curtis C. Harris*

Volume 11 GENETIC DETERMINANTS OF PULMONARY DISEASE, *edited by Stephen D. Litwin*

Volume 12 THE LUNG IN THE TRANSITION BETWEEN HEALTH AND DISEASE, *edited by Peter T. Macklem and Solbert Permutt*

Volume 13 EVOLUTION OF RESPIRATORY PROCESSES: A COMPARATIVE APPROACH, *edited by Stephen C. Wood and Claude Lenfant*

Volume 14 PULMONARY VASCULAR DISEASES, *edited by Kenneth M. Moser*

Volume 15 PHYSIOLOGY AND PHARMACOLOGY OF THE AIRWAYS, *edited by Jay A. Nadel*

Volume 16 DIAGNOSTIC TECHNIQUES IN PULMONARY DISEASE (in two parts), *edited by Marvin A. Sackner*

Volume 17 REGULATION OF BREATHING (in two parts), *edited by Thomas F. Hornbein*

Volume 18 OCCUPATIONAL LUNG DISEASES: RESEARCH APPROACHES AND METHODS, *edited by Hans Weill and Margaret Turner-Warwick*

Volume 19 IMMUNOPHARMACOLOGY OF THE LUNG, *edited by Harold H. Newball*

Volume 20 SARCOIDOSIS AND OTHER GRANULOMATOUS DISEASES OF THE LUNG, *edited by Barry L. Fanburg*

Volume 21 SLEEP AND BREATHING, *edited by Nicholas A. Saunders and Colin E. Sullivan*

Volume 22 *PNEUMOCYSTIS CARINII* PNEUMONIA: PATHOGENESIS, DIAGNOSIS, AND TREATMENT, *edited by Lowell S. Young*

Volume 23 PULMONARY NUCLEAR MEDICINE: TECHNIQUES IN DIAGNOSIS OF LUNG DISEASE, *edited by Harold L. Atkins*

Volume 24 ACUTE RESPIRATORY FAILURE, *edited by Warren M. Zapol and Konrad J. Falke*

Volume 25 GAS MIXING AND DISTRIBUTION IN THE LUNG *edited by Ludwig A. Engel and Manuel Paiva*

Volume 26 HIGH-FREQUENCY VENTILATION IN INTENSIVE CARE AND DURING SURGERY, *edited by Graziano C. Carlon and William S. Howland*

Other volumes in preparation

THE THORAX (in two parts),
edited by Charis Roussos and Peter T. Macklem

THE PLEURA IN HEALTH AND DISEASE,
edited by Jacques Chretien, Jean Bignon, Albert Hirsch, and Gerard Huchon

HIGH-FREQUENCY VENTILATION IN INTENSIVE CARE AND DURING SURGERY

Edited by
Graziano C. Carlon
William S. Howland
Memorial Sloan-Kettering Cancer Center
New York, New York

MARCEL DEKKER, INC. New York • Basel

Library of Congress Cataloging in Publication Data

Main entry under title:

High-frequency ventilation in intensive care and during
surgery.

(Lung biology in health and disease ; v. 26)
Includes Bibliographies and indexes.
1. Pressure breathing. 2. Artificial respiration.
3. Critical care medicine. 4. Therapeutics, Surgical.
I. Carlon, Graziano C. II. Howland, William S.
III. Series. [DNLM: 1. Critical Care–methods.
2. Intraoperative Care–methods. 3. Positive Pressure
Respiration. W1 LU62 v.26 / WF 145 H6383]
RM161.H54 1985 615.8'36 85-4411
ISBN 0-8247-7364-0

Copyright © 1985 by Marcel Dekker, Inc. All Rights Reserved

Neither this book nor any part may be reproduced or transmitted in any form or by any means, electronic or mechanical, including photocopying, microfilming, and recording, or by any information storage and retrieval system, without permission in writing from the publisher.

Marcel Dekker, Inc.
270 Madison Avenue, New York, New York 10016

Current printing (last digit):
10 9 8 7 6 5 4 3 2 1

Printed in the United States of America

CONTRIBUTORS

Neel B. Ackerman, Jr., M.D.* Assistant Director, Newborn Nurseries, Department of Pediatrics, Wilford Hall U.S. Air Force Medical Center, San Antonio, Texas

Michael J. Banner, Ph.D. Professor, Department of Engineering Science, University of Florida, Gainesville, Florida

Marcel L. Baum, M.S. Chief Technician, Research Center for Intensive Medicine, University of Vienna, Vienna, Austria

Herbert R. Benzer, M.D. Professor of Anesthesiology and Surgery, Research Center for Intensive Medicine, University of Vienna, Vienna, Austria

Jerry Milan Calkins, Ph.D., M.D. Associate Professor, Department of Anesthesiology, University of North Carolina School of Medicine, Chapel Hill, North Carolina

Graziano C. Carlon, M.D. Clinical Chief, Department of Critical Care, Memorial Sloan-Kettering Cancer Center, New York, New York

Robert A. de Lemos, M.D. Chairman, Division of Maternal-Child Health, Wilford Hall U.S. Air Force Medical Center, San Antonio, Texas

Nabil M. I. El-Baz, M.D. Assistant Professor, Department of Anesthesiology, Rush Medical College, Rush Presbyterian-St. Luke's Medical Center, Chicago, Illinois

T. James Gallagher, M.D. Associate Professor of Anesthesiology and Surgery, and Chief, Division of Critical Care Medicine, University of Florida College of Medicine, Gainesville, Florida

---

Present affiliation:
*Research Director, Aeromedical Evacuation Group, U.S. Air Force School of Aerospace Medicine, Brooks Air Force Base, San Antonio, Texas

Andrew Gettinger, M.D. Assistant Professor of Surgery (Anesthesiology), Department of Surgery-Anesthesiology Section, Dartmouth-Hitchcock Medical Center, Dartmouth Medical School, Hanover, New Hampshire

Anton Michael Geyer Research Center for Intensive Care, Clinic of Anesthesia, University of Vienna, Vienna, Austria

D. David Glass, M.D. Professor of Surgery (Anesthesiology) and Medicine, Chairman, Department of Anesthesiology, and Director, Critical Care Medicine, Dartmouth-Hitchcock Medical Center, Dartmouth Medical School, Hanover, New Hampshire

William S. Howland, M.D. Chairman, Department of Critical Care, Memorial Sloan-Kettering Cancer Center, New York, New York

Marc J. Jaeger, M.D. Professor, Department of Physiology, University of Florida Gainesville, Florida

Hugo Keszler, M.D., F.R.C.P.(C) Professor, Departments of Anesthesiology and Critical Care Medicine, University of Pittsburgh School of Medicine, Pittsburgh, Pennsylvania

Robert R. Kirby, M.D. Chairman, Department of Anesthesiology, Wilford Hall U.S. Air Force Medical Center, San Antonio, Texas

Miroslav Klain, M.D. Professor, Department of Anesthesiology and Critical Care Medicine, University of Pittsburgh School of Medicine, Pittsburgh, Pennsylvania

Ulrich H. Kurzweg, M.A., Ph.D. Professor, Department of Engineering Sciences, University of Florida, Gainesville, Florida

C. Philip Larson, Jr., M.D. Professor, Departments of Anesthesia and Surgery, Stanford University School of Medicine, Stanford, California

R. Douglas McEvoy, B.Med.Sc., M.B.B.S., F.R.A.C.P. Staff Specialist, Thoracic Medicine Unit, Royal Adelaide Hospital, Adelaide, South Australia

Saul Miodownik, M.E.E. Senior Biomedical Engineer, Department of Medical Physics, Memorial Sloan-Kettering Cancer Center, New York, New York

Wayne Mitzner, Ph.D. Associate Professor, Department of Environmental Health Sciences, The Johns Hopkins Medical Institutions, Baltimore, Maryland

Norbert J. Mutz, M.D. Associate Professor, Research Center for Intensive Medicine, University of Vienna, Vienna, Austria

Solbert Permutt, M.D. Professor, Departments of Medicine, Environmental Health Sciences, Anesthesia, and Critical Care Medicine, The Johns Hopkins Medical Institutions, Baltimore, Maryland

Cole Ray, Jr., R.R.T. Technical Director, Respiratory Therapy/Critical Care Services, Respiratory Therapy Department, Memorial Sloan-Kettering Cancer Center, New York, New York

Paul A. Scheck, M.D. Vice Chairman, Institute of Anesthesiology, Erasmus University, Academic Hospital, Rotterdam, The Netherlands

Edith R. Schmid, M.D. Privatdozent, Institute of Anesthesiology, University Hospital, Zurich, Switzerland

Peter M. Suter, M.D. Professor, Division des Soins Intensifs Chirsurgicaux, Departments of Anesthesiology and Surgery, Hôpital Cantonal Universitaire, Geneva, Switzerland

PREFACE

The decision to compile a summary of existing knowledge on the subject of high-frequency ventilation in book form was a controversial issue. Some of the leading investigators in the field believe that basic understanding of the physiologic basis of high-frequency ventilation is still inadequate. A major concern of theirs is that the very availability of a book may encourage empiric use of high-frequency ventilation, based on anecdotal reports billed as firmly established principles of management. Indeed, the printed word often acquires the mystical characteristics of absolute truth, impossible to deny or contradict.

On the other hand, it must be acknowledged that high-frequency ventilation is now widely used in clinical practice, not only in large academic centers but also in smaller hospitals, often with positive results. There is little doubt that some patients who cannot be supported with conventional mechanical modalities benefit from high-frequency ventilation. In recent years a substantial amount of basic investigative work has been performed on the subject and several theoretical models to explain gas exchange have been developed.

Several chapters of this volume describe rigorous mathematical evaluations of high-frequency ventilation, which provide a valid balance to clinical and laboratory reports. Although caution should always be exercised when theoretical models are used to describe physiologic events, the papers presented in this book lucidly define the mechanisms by which CO_2 is cleared from the lungs on high-frequency ventilation. Many misunderstandings and prejudices are satisfactorily dispelled by the scientific explanations provided.

A well-recognized problem when interpreting studies with high-frequency ventilation is the differences between the devices used by each investigative group, which often preclude valid comparisons. In this volume, the standardization of ventilators and the relationships between mechanical characteristics and physiologic consequences are specifically addressed, providing a rational basis for evaluating different devices.

We have included an extensive review of existing clinical experience with high-frequency ventilation techniques. The advantages of high-frequency positive pressure ventilation in the operating room, for laryngoscopies, bronchoscopies, and surgical procedures involving the upper airway, are authoritatively confirmed. The benefits of high-frequency jet ventilation in some forms of acute respiratory failure, with or without airway disruption, are discussed in depth.

Two chapters written by highly respected investigators who have been involved for many years with research on conventional mechanical support of respiratory failure offer the necessary counterpoint to overenthusiastic evaluations of the new technique. These chapters should prove quite helpful to any reader attempting to form an opinion on the applicability of high-frequency ventilation in patient management.

In conclusion, despite the valid reservations of some investigators, we believe that a comprehensive volume on high-frequency ventilation is justified and the information provided herein is reasonably complete and well balanced. Future investigation may well expand, revise, perhaps contradict some of the principles and statements presented. This risk is inherent to the imprecise nature of biological sciences.

At this time, the expansion of clinical utilization of high-frequency ventilation and the recognized need for a new form of mechanical support for the many patients who still fail to improve on conventional ventilation justify, in our opinion, the publication of this book.

Graziano C. Carlon
William S. Howland

INTRODUCTION

The means used to provide respiratory support have been a subject of research for centuries. Although there are indirect references to respiratory assistance in the Yellow Emperor's *Classic of Internal Medicine* (about 1000 B.C.), it is probably in Vesalius' *Pulmonis Motuum* (1543) that we find the first description of rhythmic artificial ventilation (in a pig). This description was repeated again in 1667, this time by Hooke. By the eighteenth century there were new efforts to find ways to maintain life in individuals succumbing from asphyxia. In 1774, for instance, Gardane published, under order of his government, the most unexpected means to prevent and remedy asphyxia or sudden death (Fig. 1).

In the nineteenth century, with the advent of surgery, there were new thrusts to develop means to provide respiratory support. Tracheotomy was introduced in 1893 to provide "forced respiration" to patients with opium poisoning.

Since World War II, we have witnessed an explosion of knowledge in respiratory physiology, especially with regard to respiratory mechanics and gas exchange. This knowledge has provided the foundation on which a great number of approaches to respiratory support have been developed and successfully pursued. During the last 10 years, high-frequency ventilation has attracted the interest of the scientific and clinical communities, but despite numerous studies of its theory and application, its case has not yet been completely made.

Thus, this book edited by Drs. Carlon and Howland is timely and important. It may well be the first comprehensive review of high-frequency ventilation. It addressed all the important questions. The editors have selected distinguished authors who have contributed a great deal to our current state of knowledge about high-frequency ventilation. It is a great privilege to add this volume to the series "Lung Biology in Health and Disease."

Claude Lenfant, M.D.
Bethesda, Maryland

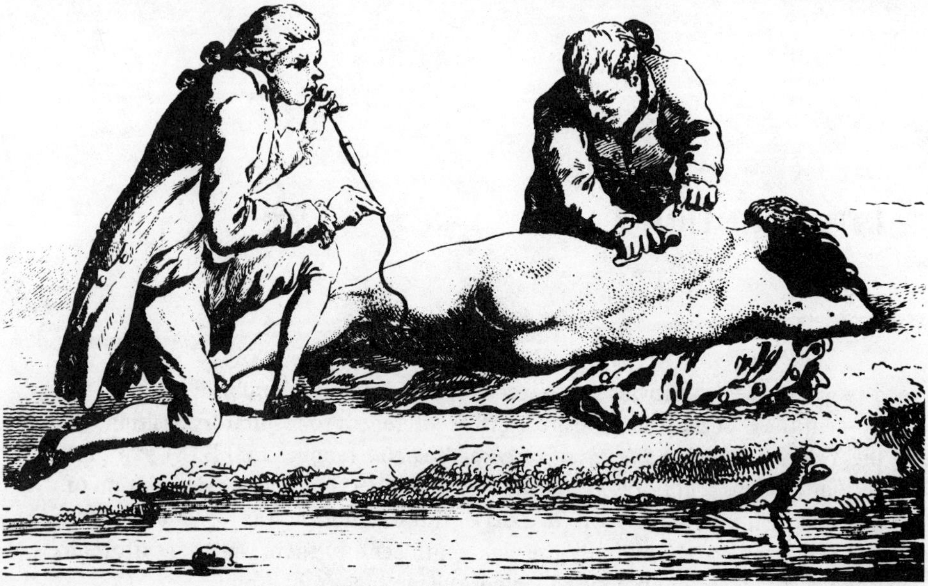

Figure 1 From *Avis au Peuple sur les Asphyxies ou Morts Apparents et Subites,* by J. J. Gardane (1774) Ruault, Paris.

CONTENTS

HIGH-FREQUENCY VENTILATION IN INTENSIVE CARE AND DURING SURGERY

1

Historical Development of High-Frequency Ventilation Techniques

WILLIAM S. HOWLAND
GRAZIANO C. CARLON

Memorial Sloan-Kettering Cancer Center
New York, New York

Considerable interest surrounds high-frequency ventilation, which is a generic term describing very diverse modalities of ventilation at supraphysiological rates. There continues to be considerable confusion about the exact scope and precise definition of each technique. A review of the development of high-frequency ventilation modalities may prove useful to place this support method properly among those used in the management of patients with acute respiratory failure.

Although reports of investigations with high-frequency ventilators date as far back as 1915 (Henderson et al., 1915), this review is restricted to studies of the last 20 years, which still have clinical or experimental relevance.

Four distinct methods of delivery of high-frequency ventilation can be recognized:

1. High-frequency positive-pressure ventilation (HFPPV), which was initially studied by Oberg and Sjostrand (1969).
2. High-frequency oscillation (HFO), first experimentally considered by Lunkenheimer et al. (1972). The earliest clinical applications were described by Butler and co-workers in 1980.

3. High-frequency jet ventilation (HFJV) has been extensively studied in bench models and animals by Klain and Brian Smith (1977). The first reports of successful clinical applications and the first large patient series were published by Carlon et al. (1980, 1981a, 1982).
4. High-frequency chest wall compression (HFCWC), a strictly experimental technique described by Zidulka et al. (1983). This modality was used only to improve gas exchange in animals and not for total respiratory report.

High-frequency positive-pressure ventilation (HFPPV) requires a ventilator with negligible compressible volume. Gas flow is controlled by a pneumatic valve. Tidal volume is usually small (3-4 ml/kg) and peak inspiratory pressure proportionally low. Respiratory rate is usually 60-100 breaths/min (Sjostrand, 1977).

High-frequency oscillation (HFO) occurs when a piston pump or a diaphragm, such as a loudspeaker, imparts an oscillating motion to the column of gases present in the airway. At the rate of 900-3000/min, minimal gas exchange (50-100 ml/breath) occurs. Fresh gas supply is provided by a bias flow. Airway pressure is usually low, but when the rate approaches the natural frequency of the lungs, a paradoxical elevation of alveolar pressure above airway pressure has been noted.

High-frequency jet ventilation (HFJV) is based upon the physical principle of the jet injector. A high-pressure source (500-2000 mmHg) is used to overcome the resistance of a narrow cannula to deliver short bursts (100-200 msec) into the upper airways. A gating mechanism, which may consist of a fluid (Klain and Brian Smith, 1977; Calkins et al., 1982), pneumatic (Sjostrand, 1980), or solenoid valve (Carlon et al., 1981b), controls gas flow from the pressure source to the patient. Tidal volume is 3-5 ml/kg, although no intrinsic restrictions are posed by the apparatus. Peak inspiratory pressure is a function of flow rate. Respiratory rates in the range of 100-200 breaths/min and higher can be used.

High-frequency chest wall compression (HFCWC) is delivered with an inflatable harness, which surrounds the chest wall and is inflated to a pressure of 30-230 cmH_2O. A piston pump, operating at frequencies of 3-11 Hz, induces oscillations of the chest wall, favoring alveolar mixing. This technique has only been used in animals.

High-frequency ventilation developed serendipitously from two sources. The first occurred in Sweden in 1967 when, during studies on the carotid sinus reflex, Oberg and Sjostrand (1969) anticipated that experimental conditions would improve if respiratory synchronous variations in blood pressure (Traube-Hering waves) could be abolished. To obviate this condition a ventilatory technique was developed that did not have this effect on the blood pressure. This technique, soon to be called high-frequency positive pressure ventilation (HFPPV), resulted in low tidal volumes that gave adequate alveolar ventilation with no negative effects on the circulation and exerted low maximal intratracheal pressures (Sjostrand and Eriksson, 1980).

In 1972 in Germany, Lunkenheimer et al. (1972) developed a means of measuring cardiac performance based on myocardial reaction to pericardial pressure oscillations. The application of intrathoracic pressure oscillations by transtracheal vibrations to measure transmyocardial pressure transmission was accompanied by cessation of ventilation because the experiments required complete muscle relaxation. Thus the problem of gas exchange arose. Since blood gas measurements demonstrated that gas exchange did indeed occur, further studies were undertaken which demonstrated that in apneic dogs adequate oxygenation and ventilation could occur with high-frequency oscillations. By experimentation they found the optimal vibration frequency to be 23-40 Hz (1380-2400 counts/sec). This technique evolved into HFO.

The next stage in the evolution of high-frequency ventilators was the development of better methods to control gas delivery. Tidal volume, ratio of entrained to directly delivered gases, bias flow, respiratory rate, and inspiratory/expiratory ratio are either ignored on volume-cycled ventilation or have considerably different physiological implications than in HFJV. Efficient controls and alarms for each variables monitored, as well as airway pressure, must be available, before the ventilator is used in clinical practice. Advances in this field are still limited. Reliable tidal volume control is restricted to a few models of HFPPV and HFJV. Separate computation of entrained and direct flow is not present in any system. In general, high-frequency ventilators have very few and relatively unsophisticated alarms and controls compared to conventional devices.

Early investigations demonstrated that alternative techniques to humidify gases delivered on HFV were necessary (Carlon et al., 1981a). Two major techniques have since been developed and extensively described.

With the first, a continuous infusion of 25-30 mg of an electrolyte solution/liter (0.30-0.90% NaCl) of jet flow is delivered, in small droplets, in front of the distal opening of the cannula. Pressurized gases exiting from the jet injector fragment and distribute the water particles to the lower airway. Entrained gases are humidified by conventional methods (Carlon et al., 1981b). Chatburn and McClellan (1982) devised a second method of humidification, applicable to pediatric patients. A heat exchanger, surrounding the inspiratory line which delivers the jet flow, provides a high relative humidity, and little or no particulate water reaches the patient. A commercially available humidifier in Europe also delivers *heated* humidified air directly in the jet. This might be the optimal type of humidification.

HFPPV as used by Sjostrand and his colleagues initially included endotracheal insufflation via a catheter positioned within the endotracheal tube, with expiration through an expiratory valve connected to the outer orifice. However, technology continued to develop and in 1973 a pneumatic valve, based on the Coanda or wall effect, was developed in which a conditioned gas mixture was intermittently delivered via a large-diameter sidearm branching off the main channel of the pneumatic valve connector. This main channel remained open and could be used for the insertion of bronchoscopic or laryngoscopic equipment. Even though both techniques utilize "open systems," gas entrainment does not occur. Because of their "open character," these low-compression ventilator systems and techniques lacked the capacity to provide volume-controlled ventilation.

Clinical demonstrations of the efficacy of high frequency ventilation followed. Heijman et al. (1972) used HFPPV during routine surgery in humans. Smith and co-workers (1976) employed jet during fiberoptic bronchoscopy. Borg (1977) used HFPPV with PEEP. Carlon and associates (1980) reported the first successful treatment of bronchopleural fistula and also (1983) the first randomized comparison of HFJV and conventional ventilation.

In 1981, Rossing et al. ventilated six patients at a frequency of 30-900 breaths and a tidal volume of 20-120 ml with a piston-generated sinusoidal wave form. They found that at 200 breaths/min, CO_2 elimination is mainly a function of tidal volume and independent of frequency.

In 1980, Butler et al. ventilated 12 patients for periods up to 1 hr using very-high-frequency (15 Hz) sinusoidal oscillation with a volume less than half of the physiological dead space. This resulted in improvement in shunt fraction and cardiac output.

In 1981, Goldstein et al. used a sine wave generator, amplifier, and 30.5-cm loudspeaker at a frequency of 4-10 Hz to achieve adequate ventilation in eight normal subjects.

It should be noted, however, that 90% of the presently used high-frequency ventilation employs the jet technique because it allows easy adjustment and control. There is limited clinical experience with short-term oscillations and only very few experimental trials of modifying alveolar gas exchange by external vibrations.

Carlon et al. (1982) provided the first extensive comparison of HFJV and conventional volume-cycled ventilation in acute respiratory insufficiency. A prospective randomized study of more than 300 patients demonstrated that HFJV was safe, predictable, reliable, and effective. No obvious advantages over conventional ventilation could be identified in the population studied (Carlon et al., 1983b).

Several international meetings on high-frequency ventilation have been sponsored in Europe (Scheck et al., 1983) and the United States (Carlon et al., 1983a; Workshop, 1982). The consensus of the experts indicates that additional extensive investigations are necessary, employing sophisticated physiological monitoring techniques (CO_2 waveform analysis, lung-volume measurements) to identify which patients may benefit most from each modality of mechanical ventilatory support.

References

Bjerager, K., Sjostrand, U., and Wattwil, W. (1977). Long term treatment of two patients with respiratory insufficiency with IPPV/PEEP and HFPPV/PEEP. *Acta Anaesth. Scand. (Suppl.)* **64**:55.

Butler, W. J., Bohn, D. J., Bryan, A. C., and Froese, A. B. (1980). Ventilation by high frequency oscillation in humans. *Anesth. Analg.* **59**:577.

Calkins, J. M., Waterson, C. K., Hameroff, S. R., Harris, T. R., and Jones, J. F. (1982). A single flueric high frequency jet ventilator. *Anesth. Analg.* **61**:138.

Carlon, G. C., Ray, C., Klain, M., and McCormack, P. M. (1980). High frequency positive pressure ventilation in a patient with broncho-pleural fistula. *Anesthesiology* **52**:160.

Carlon, G. C., Kahn, R. C., Howland, W. S., Ray, C., and Turnbull, A. D. (1981a). Clinical experience with high frequency jet ventilation. *Crit. Care Med.* **9**:1.

Carlon, G. C., Miodownik, S., Ray, C., Jr., Kahn, R. C. (1981b). Technical aspects and clinical implications of high frequency jet ventilation with a solenoid valve. *Crit. Care Med.* **9**:47.

Carlon, G. C., Ray, C., Jr., Pierri, M. K., Groeger, J. S., and Howland, W. S. (1982). High frequency ventilation: theoretical considerations and clinical observations. *Chest* **81**:350.

Carlon, G. C., and Howland, W. S. (Editors). (1983a). International Symposium on High Frequency Ventilation. New York, Memorial Sloan-Kettering Cancer Center

Carlon, G. C., Howland, W. S., Ray, C., Miodownik, S., Griffin, J. P., and Groeger, J. S. (1983b). High frequency jet ventilation. A prospective randomized evaluation. *Chest* **84**:551.

Chatburn, R. L., and McClellan, L. D. (1982). A heat and humidification system for high frequency jet ventilation. *Respir. Care* **9**:158.

Eriksson, I., Heijman, L., and Sjostrand, U. (1974). High frequency positive pressure ventilation (HFPPV) in bronchoscopy during anesthesia. *Opusc. Med.* **19**:14.

Goldstein, D., Slutsky, A. S., Ingram, R. H., Jr., Westerman, P., Venegas, J., and Drazen, J. M. (1981). CO_2 eliminations by high frequency ventilation (4 to 10 Hz) in normal subjects. *Am. Rev. Respir. Dis.* **123**:251.

Heijman, K., Heijman, L., Jonzon, A., Sedin, U., Sjostrand, U., and Widman, B. (1972). High frequency positive-pressure ventilation during anesthesia and routine surgery in man. *Acta Anaesth. Scand.* **16**:176.

Henderson, Y., Chillingworth, F. P., and Whitney, J. L. (1915). The respiratory dead space. *Am. J. Physiol.* **38**:1.

Jonzon, A. (1977). Phrenic and vagal nerve activities during spontaneous respiration and positive pressure ventilation. *Acta Anaesth. Scand. (Suppl.)* **64**: 29.

Klain, M., and Brian Smith, R. (1977). High frequency percutaneous transtracheal jet ventilation. *Crit. Care Med.* **5**:280.

Lunkenheimer, P. P., Rafflenbeul, W., Keller, H., Frank, I., Dickhut, H. H., and Fuhrmann, C. (1972). Application of transtracheal pressure oscillations as modification of "diffusion respiration." *Br. J. Anaesth.* **44**:627.

Oberg, P. A., and Sjostrand, U. (1969). Studies of blood pressure regulation. Common carotid artery clamping in studies of the carotid-sinus baroreceptor control of the systemic blood pressure. *Acta Physiol. Scand.* **75**:276.

Rossing, T. H., Slutsky, A. S., Lehr, J. L., Drinker, P. A., Kamm, R., and Drazen J. M. (1981). Tidal volume and frequency dependence of carbon dioxide elimination by high frequency ventilation. *N. Engl. J. Med.* **305**:1375.

Scheck, P. A., Sjostrand, U. H., and Smith, R. B. (Editors) (1983). *Perspectives in High Frequency Ventilation.* Boston, Martinus Nijhoff.

Sjostrand, U. (1977). Review of the physiological rationale for and development of high-frequency positive-pressure ventilation (HFPPV). *Acta Anaesth. Scand. (Suppl.)* **64**:7.

Sjostrand, U. (1980). High frequency positive pressure ventilation. A review. *Crit. Care Med.* **8**:354.

Sjostrand, U., and Eriksson, I. (1980). High rates and low volumes in mechanical ventilation: not just a matter of ventilatory frequency. *Anesth. Analg.* **59**: 567.

Smith, R. B., Lindholm, C. E., and Klain, M. (1976). Jet ventilation for fiberoptic bronchoscopy under general anesthesia. *Acta Anaesth. Scand.* **20**: 111.

Workshop on High Frequency Ventilation. (1982). National Institutes of Health, New Orleans, Dec. 5.

Zidulka, A., Gross, D., Minami, H., Vartian, V., and Chang, H. K. (1983). Ventilation by high frequency chest wall compression in dogs with normal lungs. *Am. Rev. Respir. Dis.* **127**:709.

2

Practical and Ethical Considerations

ROBERT R. KIRBY

Wilford Hall U.S. Air Force
Medical Center
San Antonio, Texas

C. PHILIP LARSON, Jr.

Stanford University School of Medicine
Stanford, California

I. Is there a Need to Develop New Modalities of Mechanical Ventilatory Support?

Robert R. Kirby

Few, if any, techniques for ventilatory support have excited the minds and imaginations of laboratory and clinical investigators as much as high-frequency ventilation (HFV). In recent years so much has been written in scientific journals and presented at national meetings that objective evaluation of the subject has been difficult. Despite the voluminous outpouring of reference material, very little clinical use has been documented thus far. Furthermore, if one peruses the literature carefully, many studies appear repetitious, while the amount of pertinent new information seems scanty. Much money is being spent in support of HFV research, yet some individuals have suggested waggishly, that HFV represents a treatment in search of a disease. Clearly, some perspective must be brought to focus on the subject, and the enthusiasm of most investigators must be balanced by a "sober" appraisal of efforts to date. Some attempts have been made to do so, but they have been few (Butler et al., 1980; Froese and Bryan, 1951; Gillespie, 1983; Ackerman et al., 1984).

II. Problems with Conventional Mechanical Ventilation

Three basic reasons may justify the development of new therapy: a desire for an increase in knowledge, per se; problems or complications with other established techniques used to treat the same disease(s); evidence that the proposed therapy will be superior to any already existing.

HFV has stimulated an interest in respiratory physiology unmatched since the reintroduction of positive end-expiratory pressure (PEEP) and continuous positive airway pressure (CPCP) in the late 1960s. Whether we can state that our *knowledge* has greatly increased is perhaps debatable. However, theories concerning the mechanisms by which HFV exerts its effects are numerous (Eriksson and Sjöstrand, 1980; Carlon et al., 1981; Lunkenheimer et al., 1977; Goldstein et al., 1981; Slutsky, 1981; Scherer and Haselton, 1982; Lehr et al., 1981; Keszler and Klain, 1982) and we have little doubt that our understanding of both conventional ventilation and high-frequency techniques will ultimately be enhanced as a result.

Established modes of ventilatory support leave much to be desired. Nevertheless, it is not a lack of efficacy of intermittent positive-pressure ventilation (IPPV) that suggests the need for new support techniques. Most patients, even with advanced or fulminant respiratory failure, can be treated adequately with IPPV and/or PEEP/CPAP to maintain levels of PaO_2 and $PaCO_2$ compatible with life (Kirby et al., 1975a,b). The cost, however, in terms of complications such as cardiovascular depression and pulmonary barotrauma, may be prohibitive. Alternative forms of ventilator therapy are desirable, if they can maintain similar (or even better) arterial blood gas values with a decreased incidence of complications. Indeed, a reduction of complications has been one of the major advantages cited for various techniques of HFV (Sjöstrand and Eriksson, 1980; Sladen et al., 1982; Eriksson, 1982; Fletcher and Epstein, 1982; Armengo et al., 1981; Kolton et al., 1982).

At present, the available evidence does not establish the superiority of HFV in the clinical support of patients with serious or life-threatening respiratory failure. Although HFV in one form or another has been studied since 1967, a paucity of well-designed clinical studies is available for review. Few prospective, randomized trials comparing HFV to conventional ventilatory support have been published. Perhaps this fact should not surprise us, since there is no agreement on what constitutes "conventional" therapy. The same problem occurred approximately a decade earlier following the introduction of extracorporeal membrane oxygenation (ECMO). Then, as now, clinicians were frustrated by their frequent inability to deal with the ravages of acute pulmonary decompensation. ECMO appeared to offer an attractive alternative to traditional ventilator therapy. An expensive, and apparently well-designed, prospective multi-institutional study carried out in the mid-1970s failed to demonstrate any improvement in survival for patients receiving ECMO compared to conventional treatment (Zapol et al.,

1979). One of the problems of this undertaking was a failure to define "conventional" adequately. Since the total number of patients was small (only 90 in 9 centers), the inability to prescribe absolute uniformity of conventional care doomed the study before it was ever started, and ECMO, for practical purposes, was discarded for long-term ventilatory support. The possibility that HFV might suffer a similar fate is real, but appears to have been reduced significantly following a recent NIH conference in which participants agreed to proceed slowly with widespread clinical application, but to continue gathering additional laboratory information (Workshop, 1982). They also determined that the only collaborative multi-institutional study of HFV warranted at this time should be in the treatment of respiratory distress syndrome (RDS) of the newborn. The lessons from ECMO appear to have been well-learned.

Pulmonary barotrauma associated with IPPV (with or without PEEP) occurs in about 10% of the cases treated (Kumar et al., 1973), although an occasional report has suggested a much lower incidence (Cullen and Caldera, 1979). The generally accepted mechanism, elucidated by Macklin and Macklin (1944), involves alveolar rupture into adjacent perivascular sheaths, with subsequent dissection to the mediastinum over the pleural reflections of the great vessels, then along the fascial plains of the head and neck (subcutaneous emphysema); into the mediastinum or pericardium (pneumomediastinum and pneumopericardium, respectively); the peritoneal or retroperitoneal areas; rupture into the free pleural space (tension pneumothorax); or into the vascular system (arterial or venous air embolization). Whether high airway pressure or large tidal volume is primarily responsible for barotrauma is unclear. Since both are increased during IPPV treatment of respiratory failure, the exact cause may be largely of academic interest. Furthermore, since high pressure and large tidal volumes decrease venous return, and perhaps also affect ventricular interdependence through shifts of the interventricular septum (Laver et al., 1979), reduction of ventilator pressure and volume is desirable.

III. Does HFV Reduce the Incidence of Ventilator-Related Complications?

This question has yet to be answered. Some complications of IPPV are due to inappropriate ventilator use. For example, acute respiratory insufficiency often responds well to PEEP/CPAP, with minimal or even no adjunctive ventilator support. However, if a clinician does not use PEEP/CPAP, or fails to use such treatment at a sufficiently high level, choosing instead to attempt therapy with IPPV, the incidence of complications may be expected to increase. Here the fault lies in the attempt to use a ventilator for treatment of a problem which it is poorly designed to handle. That this is true is suggested by numerous reports which have shown that modification of IPPV through the use of intermittent mandatory ventilation (IMV) is associated with a decreased incidence of complications (Kirby et al., 1975a,b; Kirby and Graybar, 1980; Downs et al., 1973).

In assessing the effect of HFV on the incidence of ventilator-related complications, investigators must be careful not to repeat previous mistakes. When Cournand et al. (1948) reported the adverse cardiovascular effects of IPPV, they inadvertently became responsible for impeding the development of ventilator therapy over the next 30 years. The problem was in the failure of clinicians who read their reports to recognize that observations made in normal experimental subjects cannot always be extrapolated to sick patients. In particular, the amount of pressure transmitted to the intrapleural space is reduced significantly in patients with decreased pulmonary compliance, and the circulatory effects of this pressure are likewise decreased. However, many years elapsed before clinicians recognized this and were willing to employ increased levels of inspiratory and expiratory positive pressure.

Perhaps the same phenomenon has occurred with HFV, although the clinical extrapolations have been somewhat different. Initial studies by Sjöstrand (1977) and Sjöstrand and Eriksson (1950) emphasized the lack of adverse circulatory effects of high-frequency positive-pressure ventilation (HFPPV) compared to conventional controlled mechanical ventilation (CMV). These investigators used experimental animals with normal lungs in whom pressure transmission to the intrapleural space was maximal. Hence, a technique of mechanical ventilation which employed generally small tidal volume and low airway pressure would be expected to have less impact on hemodynamic function. Despite these investigators' demonstration of the circulatory-sparing effects of HFPPV, there was almost no application to acute respiratory failure in the years following its introduction; no more than a handful of such patients were reported to have been treated (Bjerager et al., 1977). Subsequently, when experimental studies were published in which induced respiratory failure was treated with HFV, the alleged benefit of low airway pressure often was not seen. In order to provide adequate oxygenation, investigators had to employ proximal mean airway pressures equal to those found with conventional mechanical ventilation (Froese and Bryan, 1981; Thompson et al., 1982). *Mean* distal airway pressures with HFO were found sometimes to be higher than those in the proximal airway (Ackerman et al., 1983; Allen et al., 1983). Since the direct correlation of PaO_2 with mean airway pressure had been documented previously, these findings were not altogether unexpected. What was unusual is that no one seems to have anticipated such a finding. Many investigators and clinicians were so caught up in their enthusiasm for HFV that they initially were unable to accept the possibility that it might not be a panacea for all forms of respiratory insufficiency.

Another problem that has plagued the development and clinical application of HFV is that "it" is not really a single modality. Currently, three distinct categories have been defined: HFPPV, high-frequency jet ventilation (HFJV), and high-frequency oscillation (HFO). The only common attributes of these techniques are a higher frequency and lower tidal volume than customarily employed with IPPV; "higher" in the case of HFPPV generally means 60-150 breaths/min, whereas it may be up to 3000/min (or even more) with HFO. Although tidal volume is around that of calculated physiological deadspace for HFPPV, it is usually significantly less with HFO. The physiological effects of these therapeutic approaches may well differ from each other as much as IPPV does from spontaneous breathing. Often, the characteristics of the system employed in a given study or clinical report have been defined poorly, if at all, so that the reader and even experts in the field are left in the dark as to what occurred and why.

The differences between the various types of HFV extend beyond rates and tidal volume. Although the precise mechanisms by which gas is transferred through the airway and alveolar ventilation occurs are not fully delineated, the available evidence suggests that they differ substantially from one to another. Thus, HFPPV is very similar to conventional IPPV, with convection playing the major role in gas movement, while with HFO enhanced diffusivity, internal circulating currents (Lehr et al., 1981), and other proposed mechanisms (Slutsky, 1981; Scherer and Haselton, 1982) probably predominate.

Finally, those who use HFV must realize that experimental results reported from one technique may not be found with another. Perhaps this explains in part the apparent discrepancies between the lack of impaired cardiovascular function originally described with HFPPV (Sjöstrand, 1977) and the significant effects (essentially identical to those of IPPV) reported during HFO (Thompson et al., 1982). Similarly, although one would anticipate that techniques of ventilation characterized by low tidal volumes and airway pressure should decrease the incidence of pulmonary barotrauma associated with IPPV, evidence for this is not yet established. When HFJV is used with dry gas, the airway mucosa may be disrupted by the high-velocity jet stream distal to the cannula tip (Nordin et al., 1982; Ophoven et al., 1983). In contrast, "inadvertent PEEP" occurring with HFO (presumably associated with air trapping) may lead to airway disruption and/or aneurysmal dilatation of the distal bronchioles (Ackerman et al., 1983). In the latter cases, mean distal airway pressure, as mentioned previously, may actually be *higher* than the mean pressure measured within the ventilator circuit (Ackerman et al., 1983).

IV. Documented and Proposed Uses for HFV

At the time of this writing, only one area of care is clearly enhanced by HFV, and that involves the use of HFPPV (Borg et al., 1980) and HFJV (Babinski et al., 1980) for diagnostic or therapeutic laryngotracheal surgery. Case reports in which

HFJV has been used to treat persons with open bronchopleural cutaneous fistulas have been published (Carlon et al., 1980), and this area of therapy appears very promising. However, very few patients have been managed in this way; obviously the difficulty in obtaining a large series is a major impediment to placing such therapy in perspective with other, previously reported, treatment modalities.

If HFV could be shown to improve the outcome of acute respiratory failure in neonates (RDS) or adults (adult respiratory distress syndrome, ARDS) when compared to other forms of ventilator management, no other justification for its use would be necessary. However, such evidence is not yet available. Few clinical studies have been published in which HFV has been used to treat RDS (Bland et al., 1980). Since conventional techniques are associated with a survival rate of 80-90% or better in babies born weighing more than 1,000 g, documentation of the superiority of HFV will require very large numbers of patients. Perhaps for this reason the previously mentioned, multi-institutional NIH-supported study has been proposed (Workshop, 1982).

With ARDS, the evidence is even less conclusive. Prior to 1977 only two patients with ARDS were reported to have been treated with HFV (HFPPV) (Bjerager et al., 1977). Since that time, relatively few additional patients with ARDS have been treated with any form of HFV and the results published. Following the introduction of IMV, investigators were frequently criticized for the lack of prospective randomized studies which compared it with other forms of IPPV (Luce et al., 1981; Weisman et al., 1983). Similar criticism can be leveled against HFV. No studies have demonstrated the superiority of HFV in terms of a reduction in mortality of ARDS; whether the morbidity can be decreased remains to be seen.

Many other areas of respiratory support *potentially* can be enhanced by one or more forms of HFV. In the operating room, a reduction of lung and brain movement associated with IPPV reasonably may be expected to improve operating conditions in thoracic, abdominal, and neurological surgical procedures. Experimental studies in these areas are promising; however, published clinical studies are limited.

A specific disease state which has proven refractory to all techniques of conventional ventilator support is diaphragmatic hernia of the newborn. In those infants who require ventilation, mortality exceeds 80%. Any technique that decreases airway pressure and tidal volume, while maintaining satisfactory alveolar ventilation, is obviously desirable. A large percentage of the ventilator-related deaths in diaphragmatic hernia are caused by barotrauma and cardiovascular compromise. Thus far, little clinical experience has been accumulated to support these concepts, but further research is certainly indicated.

Another area of potential usefulness for HFV is in aeromedical transportation and evacuation. No conventional ventilator meets all requirements for support in helicopters, fixed-wing aircraft, or even surface ambulances. Limitations include size, power sources, oxygen requirements, and inability to operate efficiently at altitude or in unusual positions that might occur in flight. Most high-frequency ventilators are compact, and many overcome some of the other difficulties encountered with standard machines. Hence, their application in patient transport, into or out of the hospital setting, is an attractive consideration.

In a related area, the use of HFJV with either endotracheal or tracheostomy tubes or through a cannula inserted by cricothyrotomy has been proposed for certain emergency conditions (Klain et al., 1981a,b). These may include massive head and neck trauma, when the usual methods of tracheal intubation are dangerous and/or impossible, or selected mass casualty situations when airway and ventilatory support with HFV by paramedical personnel is envisioned. Once again, little or no clinical experience is available to support or refute this concept; however, further study is probably warranted.

V. Summary

A recent review on HFV summarizes our current knowledge (Gillespie, 1983). Unfortunately, although the answer to the question, "Is there a need to develop new modalities of mechanical ventilatory support?," appears to be "yes," it is not yet clear that HFV provides all of the answers being sought. Most of the work to date has been experimental, with a minimal amount of clinical correlation. We lack satisfactory understanding of the mechanisms by which HFV may work. Most clinicians also have little knowledge of the mechanics of specific ventilators which they will ultimately be called upon to operate. Operational problems include poor humidification, high gas consumption, lack of satisfactory alarms, and even the capability to monitor what is happening with the ventilator and to the patient.

Nevertheless, the interest and research accorded HFV is certainly justified. No other "discovery" in recent times has awakened a similar interest in classic respiratory physiology and few have been proposed for as wide a range of pathological conditions. Perhaps the slow development of the field is more apparent than real. Although the roots of HFV can be traced at least to 1915 (Henderson et al., 1915), widespread research and attempted clinical application in the United States has been undertaken only since about 1978.

Finally, other comparisons are pertinent. PEEP/CPAP in one form or another has been with us since 1912, was reintroduced in the 1930s, again in 1967 to 1971, and is still a topic for debate about its indications, overall clinical efficacy, complications, and other aspects. The same is true, probably on a greater scale, for IMV (Luce et al., 1981; Weisman et al., 1983). Yet, despite disagreement among clinical scientists, each of these support modes has proven useful and is firmly entrenched in our clinical armamentarium. We have no reason to expect that HFV will be any different.

Indeed, the greatest value of HFV may be that it provides a viable alternative to conventional ventilation support (Carlon et al., 1983). Although overall morbidity and mortality from respiratory insufficiency may not be reduced one can easily envision selected parients in that HFV works when other methods will not. Our overall therapeutic armamentarium is thereby enhanced, and the patient ultimately benefits.

VI. The Future Role of HFV in Respiratory Care

C. Philip Larson, Jr.

The future role of high-frequency ventilation in respiratory care is virtually impossible to predict with confidence at this time, for several reasons. First, there is incomplete knowledge or understanding of how high-frequency ventilation works to produce gas exchange. Admittedly, while it is not always necessary to understand the mechanism(s) whereby a new technology produces its salutary effects to apply it in clinical practice, it is highly desirable, if that new technology is to receive the broadest application. Without a clear understanding of how high-frequency ventilation works, clinicians will be reluctant to use it except in cases where there are no other more favorable alternatives.

Second, there is incomplete knowledge or understanding of the physiological effects or potential complications of high-frequency ventilation. Just as with the need to understand how high-frequency ventilation produces gas exchange, before they will be comfortable with its use clinicians must know what physiological effects it induces on various organ systems, and whether any of those effects are hazardous to the patient.

Third, the optimal design of equipment for high-frequency ventilation has not yet been established. There are almost as many different systems for delivery of high-frequency ventilation as there are investigators working in the field, which is one of the factors that make comparisons of various studies difficult. However, this problem is readily surmountable, and with time and experience, the ideal systems will emerge and become conventional.

Fourth, the need for the development of high-frequency ventilation is not readily apparent. Most clinical conditions that require respiratory care are adequately managed by existing forms of mechanical ventilation. While there are some exceptions, they occur infrequently or are conditions for which high-frequency ventilation has not proven to be substantially superior to conventional mechanical ventilation. Without a clear and compelling demand for a new form of ventilation to resolve existing problems, the development of new technology is slowed. In the minds of some, high-frequency ventilation is still a technique in search of an application.

Despite these reservations, some applications for high-frequency ventilation have emerged and others will likely do so in the future. We will summarize these applications and consider future progress in this fascinating field.

VII. Applications in Surgical Anesthesia

A. Surgery of the Airway

The clearest and most attractive indication for the use of high-frequency ventilation is to provide ventilation during anesthesia for laryngeal or tracheal surgery. In any surgical procedure involving the upper airway, the anesthesiologist must compete with the surgeon for the limited space available within the airway. The anesthesiologist must ensure that the airway is patent and that ventilation is adequate during the surgical procedure, while the surgeon must obtain the essential surgical exposure and airway manipulations that will make the operation technically feasible. To facilitate the surgeon's work, a number of techniques have evolved to minimize the intra-airway space occupied by the anesthesiologist's equipment. For short airway operations, most anesthesiologists use apneic oxygenation: the lungs are filled with oxygen and no ventilation occurs for periods of 5-10 min while the surgeon performs the operation. For longer operations on the airway, most anesthesiologists have resorted to the use of an endotracheal tube. A variety of tubes and techniques have evolved to meet this challenge. However, all of them take up space, and none are ideal, and hence the attractiveness of high-frequency ventilation for upper-airway surgery.

High-frequency jet ventilation (HFJV) has proven to be the ideal method for maintaining ventilation during reconstructive surgery of the upper airway. The catheter required for ventilation is much smaller than any endotracheal tube, and it can be inserted through the airway and positioned below the level of the surgical site. When this technique is used, excellent gas exchange can be assured during longer operative procedures. HFJV has the additional advantage over other techniques for microlaryngeal surgery that it minimizes the excursions of the larynx during ventilation. Any movement of the larynx during ventilation is exaggerated for the surgeon who is working through a microscope, and hence is to be minimized as much as possible. The principal disadvantage of this technique is the risk of sudden pulmonary hyperinflation and subsequent tension pneumothorax if outflow obstruction occurs. The jet ventilation catheter can be placed above the level of the glottis, but the technique then depends upon a patent glottis for gas exchange to occur. Placement of the catheter above the glottis has the additional disadvantage of blowing oropharyngeal debris such as secretions, blood, or smoke from a laser down the airway.

HFJV is also highly satisfactory for providing ventilation during anesthesia for laryngoscopy or bronchoscopy, particularly in children in whom the airway is small. Extraction of foreign bodies from the airway can be especially tedious and time-consuming in children, making HFJV an ideal method for ventilation during the procedure. Placement of the jet catheter into the noninvolved bronchus permits vigorous ventilation of that lung with oxygen while the surgeon explores the involved bronchus. With the increased use of fiberoptic techniques for bronchoscopy in adults, during which the bronchoscope is inserted through the endotracheal tube, the competition between surgeon and anesthesiologist for airway space is greatly diminished and with it the advantages of HFJV.

B. Surgery of the Lung

High-frequency ventilation has been advocated for maintenance of ventilation during surgical procedures on the lung to minimize ventilatory excursions. Vigorous excursions of the lungs can be disruptive while the surgeon is dissecting lung tissue, or during dissection of the heart or thoracic wall. However, two alternative techniques, either of which is satisfactory in selected instances, obviate the need for reliance on high-frequency ventilation. The first is the use of endobronchial intubation, in which one bronchus is selectively intubated and ventilated, while the other lung is allowed to collapse. The development of reliable, disposable endobroncheal tubes, the use of pure oxygen for ventilation, and the development of reliable devices for continuous monitoring of arterial oxygen saturation make this an attractive technique for lung or other forms of intrathoracic surgery.

Even if endobronchial intubation is not possible, high-frequency ventilation is not the only alternative. For years anesthesiologists have used ventilatory patterns that involve smaller-than-normal tidal volumes and higher-than-normal ventilatory frequencies during pulmonary or other types of thoracic surgery. Tidal volume values of 3-5 ml/kg and breathing frequencies of 30-50/min will generally provide adequate gas exchange and yet not interfere with the surgeon's need for a relatively quiet field. There is no evidence that higher frequencies and smaller tidal volumes are needed or that they further improve operating conditions.

Because existing technology is satisfactory, it is doubtful that high-frequency ventilation will become the primary mode of ventilation for surgery of the lung or thorax. However, it is certainly an acceptable technique and one that will be preferred by some.

C. Microvascular Surgery of the Brain

High-frequency ventilation has been advocated for ventilatory management during anesthesia for microvascular surgery of the brain to diminish the brain excursions that accompany changes in intrathoracic pressure during conventional ventilation. Experimental studies in cats demonstrate that brain excursions are less when frequencies of 100/min and tidal volumes of 3.3 ml/kg are used, compared to frequencies of 11/min and tidal volume values of 15 ml/kg (Todd et al., 1981). While this study is interesting, its clinical relevance remains untested. No comparison of high-frequency ventilation with conventional mechanical ventilation during microvascular surgery of the brain in humans has been made to determine if the former is preferred. As in lung surgery, breathing frequencies and tidal volume values somewhere between slow conventional mechanical ventilation and high-frequency ventilation may be quite satisfactory.

D. Miscellaneous Applications

High-frequency jet ventilation has been used in more than 300 patients undergoing a wide variety of surgical procedures at the University of Pittsburgh hospitals (Marquez et al., 1982). Although it has been suggested that high-frequency ventilation may provide greater circulatory stability than conventional mechanical ventilation because of the lower peak and mean airway pressures used, this was not observed in this study. Cardiac and stroke index, mean arterial blood pressure, and heart rate values were not significantly different when high-frequency jet ventilation was compared to conventional intermittent positive-pressure ventilation. The investigators suggest that HFJV was particularly useful during upper abdominal operations because of the lack of diaphragmatic movement, but this was not documented by any comparative analysis with conventional ventilation, nor was it determined that intermediate modes of ventilation were not just as satisfactory. Further studies of this nature are needed before the value of high-frequency ventilation in anesthesia for abdominal surgery can be stated.

VIII. Applications in Critical Care Medicine

A. Disruptions of the Airway

An increasing body of clinical evidence indicates that high-frequency ventilation is the most effective, and in fact may be the only form of ventilation that provides adequate gas exchange in patients with disruptions of the airway. Although the total experience with high-frequency ventilation of the lungs of patients with such disruptions is limited, this method appears to have distinct advantages over conventional mechanical ventilation. For example, when conventional mechanical ventilation is applied to the lungs of patients with a bronchopleural fistula, much of the inflation volume is transferred through the fistula to the chest cavity and out the chest tube. Increasing either tidal volume or airway pressure may only serve to drive more gas out of the fistulous tract. As a consequence, the fistulous lung receives little or no effective ventilation and the other lung is inadequately ventilated. In contrast, when high-frequency ventilation is used, the time constants for inflation of the lungs are so much shorter than the time constant for leak of gas through the fistula that much less gas is exhausted through the fistula and more of it participates in gas exchange. Comparative studies using the two modes of ventilation in the same patient document the superiority of high-frequency ventilation with this disease (Carlon et al., 1960). In addition to providing more effective ventilation, high-frequency ventilation would presumably hasten the healing of the fistula since the fistula would be less of a conduit for gas.

B. Infant Respiratory Distress Syndrome

High-frequency ventilation has been shown in selected centers to be an effective mode of ventilation of infants with respiratory distress syndrome. When used in combination with positive end-expiratory pressure (PEEP) or continuous positive airway pressure (CPAP), high-frequency ventilation will maintain adequate oxygenation and carbon dioxide removal, while permitting lower peak and mean airway pressures than does conventional mechanical ventilation (Carlon et al., 1984). The need for lower peak and mean airway pressures will lessen the impact of ventilation on cardiac output, and may decrease the incidence of pulmonary barotrauma. The incidence of bronchopulmonary dysplasia in infants following conventional mechanical ventilation for respiratory distress syndrome is variable but generally exceeds 15%. Studies in animals suggest that the incidence of bronchopulmonary dysplasia is less when high-frequency ventilation is used compared to conventional mechanical ventilation. If these findings are confirmed in humans, it is likely that high-frequency ventilation will supplant conventional mechanical ventilation in the early management of infant respiratory distress syndrome.

C. Adult Respiratory Disease

High-frequency ventilation has been applied for relatively brief periods of time in a wide variety of human lung diseases with mixed results. Clearly, high-frequency ventilation will provide good gas exchange in some adult patients with lung disease while not in others. The reasons for these differences are not always apparent, and they do not seem to be related to the type of lung disease. For example, while it might be predicted that high-frequency ventilation would be more effective in lung diseases that are traditionally associated with a low compliance (atelectasis, pneumonia, pulmonary fibrosis, etc.) than those traditionally associated with a high compliance (pulmonary emphysema), this has not proven to be the case. In some patients with lung disease, high-frequency ventilation improves the underlying ventilation/perfusion disorder, perhaps through augmented dispersion (Butler et al., 1980).

Unfortunately, to date there are few prospective, randomized studies that compare the effectiveness of high-frequency ventilation with conventional mechanical ventilation when each has been used for prolonged periods. Recently, Carlon and colleagues (1983) reported the results of a randomized comparison of conventional mechanical ventilation with high-frequency jet ventilation in 309 patients requiring ventilatory support. The principal finding was that oxygenation and ventilation were maintained at lower peak inspiratory pressures and smaller tidal volumes with HFJV than when conventional ventilation was used. While this study did not demonstrate that HFJV was superior to conventional mechanical ventilation, it did document that HFJV could be used safely for prolonged periods. Additional comparative evaluations of the use of high-frequency ventilation in the care of adults with respiratory disorders are needed. However, even if large comparative clinical trials are undertaken, they may not be capable of determining whether high-frequency ventilation or conventional mechanical ventilation is more efficacious. Adult respiratory disorders requiring ventilatory support have multiple causes and are associated with a variety of serious systemic complications, all of which will likely have a profound impact on respiratory function and outcome, and will overshadow any differences associated with the mode of ventilation being used.

Preliminary studies suggest that high-frequency ventilation, specifically jet ventilation, may be helpful in weaning patients from prolonged mechanical ventilatory support (Klain et al., 1982). After 3 or more weeks of mechanical ventilation in nine patients, HFJV facilitated weaning after trials of intermittent mandatory ventilation had failed. Additional studies are needed to substantiate this finding.

IX. Future Developments

The future of high-frequency ventilation will depend upon many factors including:

1. Identification of the optimal frequency, tidal volume, flow pattern and rate, and inspiratory and expiratory airway pressures
2. Development of reliable, easy-to-use devices for its implementation
3. Development of safety devices to prevent sudden increases in airway pressure or other system malfunctions that may cause catastrophic disasters for patients
4. Identification of the diseases in which it is the preferred mode of ventilation, and the potential complications associated with its use
5. Documentation that it can be used effectively for prolonged periods of time without system failure
6. Identification of reliable monitoring devices to assure that ventilation is adequate at all times
7. Increased experience and confidence with its use by nurses so that continual bedside attention by physicians will not be necessary

Depending on the outcome of these investigations, high-frequency ventilation may find wide application in respiratory care or only be of value in a few isolated, selected clinical conditions. Only through continued funding for research will the value of high-frequency ventilation ultimately be determined.

References

Ackerman, N. B., Kuehl, T. J., Coalson, J. J., Escobedo, M. B., Stoddard, R. A., Minnick, L. H., Null, D. M., Robotham, J. L., and de Lemos, R. A. (1983). Distal airway rupture during high frequency ventilation (HFV) in the premature baboon with hyaline membrane disease (abstr.). *Crit. Care Med.* **11**:223.

Ackerman, N. B., Null, D. M., and deLemos, R. A. (1984). High frequency ventilation: History, theory and practice. In *Mechanical Ventilation.* Edited by R. R. Kirby, R. A. Smith, and D. Desautels. New York, Churchill-Livingstone, pp. 307-325.

Allen, J. L., Keefe, D. H., and Fredberg, J. J. (1983). Alveolar pressures and pulmonary impedence during high frequency oscillation in excised rabbit lungs (abstr.). *Pediatr. Res.* **17**:370A.

Armengo, J. A., Man, S. F. P., Logus, J. W., Man, G. G., and King, E. G. (1981). Hemodynamic and blood gas effects of high frequency oscillatory ventilation. *Crit. Care Med.* **9**:192.

Babinski, M., Smith, R. B., and Klain, M. (1980). High frequency jet ventilation for laryngoscopy. *Anesthesiology* **52**:178.

Bjerager, K., Sjostrand, U., and Wattwil, M. (1977). Long term treatment of two patients with respiratory insufficiency with IPPV/PEEP and HFPPV/PEEP. *Acta Anesthesiol. Scand.* (*Suppl.*). **64**:55.

Bland, R. D., Kim, M. H., Light, M. J., and Woodson, J. L. (1980). High frequency mechanical ventilation in severe hyaline membrane disease: An alternative treatment? *Crit. Care Med.* **8**:275.

Borg, U., Eriksson, I., and Sjostrand, U. (1980). High frequency positive pressure ventilation (HFPPV): A review based upon its use during bronchoscopy and for laryngoscopy and microlaryngeal surgery under general anesthesia. *Anesth. Analg.* **59**:594.

Butler, W. J., Bohn, D. J., Bryan, A. C., and Froese, A. B. (1980). Ventilation by high frequency oscillation in humans. *Anesth. Analg.* **59**:577

Carlo, W. A., Chatburn, R. L., Martin, R. J., Lough, M. D., Shivpuri, C. R., Anderson, J. V., and Fanaroff, A. A. (1984). Decrease in airway pressure during high-frequency jet ventilation in infants with respiratory distress syndrome. *J. Pediatr.* **104**:101-107.

Carlon, G. C., Ray, C. Jr., Klain, M., and McCormack, P. M. (1980). High-frequency positive-pressure ventilation in management of a patient with bronchopleural fistula. *Anesthesiology* **52**:160-162.

Carlon, G. C., Miodownik, S., Ray, C. Jr., and Kahn, R. C. (1981). Technical aspects and clinical implications of high frequency jet ventilation with a solenoid valve. *Crit. Care Med.* **9**:47.

Carlon, G. L., Howland, W. S., Ray, C., Miodownik, S., Griffin, J. P., and Groeger, B. (1983). Frequency jet ventilation. A prospective randomized evaluation. *Chest* **84**:551.

Cournand, A., Motley, H. L., Werko, L., and Dickinson, W. R. (1948). Physiologic studies of the effects of intermittent positive pressure breathing on cardiac output in man. *Am. J. Physiol.* **152**:162.

Cullen, D. J., and Caldera, D. L. (1979). The incidence of ventilator induced pulmonary barotrauma in critically ill patients. *Anesthesiology* **50**:185.

Downs, J. B., Klein, E. F., Desautels, D., Modell, J. H., and Kirby, R. R. (1973). Intermittent mandatory ventilation: A new approach to weaning patients from mechanical ventilators. *Chest* **64**:331.

Eriksson, I. (1982). The role of conducting airways in gas exchange during high frequency ventilation—a clinical and theoretical analysis. *Anesth. Analg.* **61**:483.

Eriksson, I., and Sjöstrand, U. (1980). Effects of high-frequency positive pressure ventilation (HFPPV) and general anesthesia on intrapulmonary gas distribution in patients undergoing diagnostic bronchoscopy. *Anesth. Analg.* **59**:585.

Fletcher, P. R., and Epstein, R. A. (1982). Constancy of physiologic dead space during high frequency ventilation. *Respir. Physiol.* **47**:39.

Froese, A. B., and Bryan, A. D. (1981). High-frequency ventilation (editorial). *Am. Rev. Respir. Dis.* **123**:249.

Gillespie, D. J. (1983). High frequency ventilation: A new concept in mechanical ventilation. *Mayo Clin. Proc.* **58**:187.

Goldstein, D., Slutsky, A. S., Ingram, R. H. Jr., Westerman, P., Venegas, J., and Drazen, J. M. (1981). CO_2 elimination by high frequency ventilation (4 to 10 Hz) in normal subjects. *Am. Rev. Respir. Dis.* **123**:251.

Henderson, Y., Chillingworth, F. P., and Whitney, J. L. (1915). The respiratory dead space. *Am. J. Physiol.* **38**:1.

Keszler, H., and Klain, M. (1982). Importance of position of jet orifice in high frequency jet ventilation. *Crit. Care Med.* **10**:234.

Kirby, R. R., and Graybar, G. B. (Editors) (1980). Intermittent mandatory ventilation. Boston, Little, Brown.

Kirby, R. R., Downs, J. B., Civetta, J. M., Modell, J. H., Dannemiller, F. J., Klein, E. F., and Hodges, M. (1975a). High level positive end-expiratory pressure (PEEP) in acute respiratory insufficiency. *Chest* **67**:156.

Kirby, R. R., Perry, J. C., Calderwood, H. W., Ruiz, B. C., and Lederman, D. S. (1975b). Cardiorespiratory effects of high positive end-expiratory pressure. *Anesthesiology* **43**:533.

Klain, M., Keszler, H., and Broder, E. (1981a). High frequency jet ventilation in CPR. *Crit. Care Med.* **9**:421.

Klain, M., Miller, J., and Kalla, R. (1981b). Emergency use of high frequency jet ventilation (abstr.). *Crit. Care Med.* **9**:160.

Klain, M., Kalla, R., Sladen, A., Guntupalli, K., and Wald, M. (1982). Weaning from respiratory support by high frequency jet ventilation. *Anesthesiology* **57**:A468.

Kolton, M., Cattran, C. R., Keng, G., Volgyesi, G., Froese, A. B., and Bryan, A. C. (1982). Oxygenation during high frequency ventilation compared with conventional mechanical ventilation in two models of lung injury. *Anesth. Analg.* **61**:323.

Kumar, A., Pontoppidan, H., and Falke, K. J. (1973). Pulmonary barotrauma during mechanical ventilation. *Crit. Care Med.* **1**:181.

Laver, M. B., Pohost, G. M., and Strauss, H. W. (1979). Right and left ventricular geometry: Adjustments during acute respiratory failure. *Crit. Care. Med.* **7**:509.

Lehr, J., Barkyoumb, J., and Drazen, J. M. (1981). Gas transport during high frequency ventilation. *Fed. Proc.* **40**:384.

Luce, J. M., Pierson, D. J., and Hudson, L. D. (1981). Intermittent mandatory ventilation. *Chest* **79**:678.

Lunkenheimer, P. P., Ising, H., Frank, I., Scharsick, M., Welham, K., and Dittrich, H. (1977). Enhancement of CO_2-elimination by intrapulmonary pressure alteration during "apnoeic oxygenation." *Adv. Exp. Med. Biol.* **94**:599.

Macklin, M. T., and Macklin, C. C. (1944). Malignant interstitial emphysema of the lungs and mediastinum as an important occult complication in many respiratory diseases and other conditions: An interpretation of the clinical literature in light of laboratory experiments. *Medicine* **23**:281.

Marquez, J. Jr., Fine, J., Klain, M., Bennett, R., and Freeman, J. (1982). Clinical applications of high frequency jet ventilation in the operating room. *Anesthesiology* **57**:A464.

Nordin, U., Klain, M., and Keszler, H. (1982). Electron microscopic studies of tracheal mucosa after high frequency jet ventilation (abstr.). *Crit. Care Med.* **10**:211.

Ophoven, J. P., Mammel, M. C., Gordon, M. J., and Boros, S. J. (1983). High frequency jet ventilation: Tracheobronchial histopathology (abstr.). *Pediatr. Res.* **17**:386A.

Scherer, P. W., and Haselton, F. R. (1982). Convective exchange in oscillatory flow through bronchial tree models. *J. Appl. Physiol.* **53**:1023.

Sjöstrand, U. (1977). Summary of experimental and clinical features of high frequency positive-pressure ventilation–HFPPV. *Acta Anesthesiol. Scand.* (*Suppl.*). **64**:165.

Sjöstrand, U., and Eriksson, I. A. (1980). High rates and low volumes in mechanical ventilation–not just a matter of ventilatory frequency. *Anesth. Analg.* **59**:567.

Sladen, A., Guntapalli, K. K., Klain, M., and Romano, R. (1982). High frequency jet ventilation and conventional ventilation: A comparison of cardiorespiratory parameters. *Crit. Care Med.* **10**:212.

Slutsky, A. S. (1981). Gas mixing by cardiogenic oscillations: A theoretical quantitative analysis. *J. Appl. Physiol.* **51**:1287.

Thompson, W. K., Marchak, B. E., Bryan, A. C., and Froese, A. B. (1982). High frequency oscillation compared with standard ventilation in pulmonary injury model. *J. Appl. Physiol.* **52**:543.

Todd, M. M., Toutant, S. M., and Shapiro, H. M. (1981). The effects of high-frequency positive-pressure ventilation on intracranial pressure and brain surface movement in cats. *Anesthesiology* **54**:496-504.

Weisman, I. M., Rinaldo, J. E., Rogers, R. M., and Sanders, M. H. (1983). Intermittent mandatory ventilation. *Am. Rev. Respir. Dis.* **127**:641.

Workshop on High Frequency Ventilation (1982). Sponsored by the American Thoracic Society; American College of Chest Physicians; and Division of Lung Diseases, National Heart, Lung, Blood Institute. New Orleans, Dec. 6-7.

Zapol, W. M., Snider, M. T., Hill, J. D., Fallet, R. J., Bartlett, R. H., Edmunds, H., Morris, A. H., Peirce, E. C., Thomas, A. N., Proctor, H. J., Drinker, P. A., Pratt, P. C., Bagniewski, A., and Miller R. G., (1979). Extracorporeal membrane oxygenation in severe acute respiratory failure: A randomized prospective study. *JAMA* **242**:2193.

3

Theoretical Evaluation of Gas Exchange Mechanisms

MARCEL L. BAUM,
HERBERT R. BENZER,
ANTON MICHAEL GEYER, and
NORBERT J. MUTZ

University of Vienna
Vienna, Austria

MARC J. JAEGER,
ULRICH H. KURZWEG,
and MICHAEL J. BANNER

University of Florida
Gainesville, Florida

I. Characteristics of Gas Flow and Factors Influencing CO_2 Elimination

Marcel L. Baum, Herbert R. Benzer, Anton Michael Geyer, and Norbert J. Mutz

Many different mechanical ventilators can deliver ventilatory rates exceeding the range usually considered "physiological." They operate with tidal volumes smaller or only slightly larger than dead space (Sjostrand, 1977; Klain and Smith, 1977; Lunkenheimer et al., 1973; Bohn et al., 1980; Baum et al., 1980). The exact mechanisms of gas transport involved are not understood, but are probably different for each type of high-frequency ventilation.

Mathematical models have been designed to analyze gas motion processes. Elsewhere in this book theoretical principles of gas exchange on high-frequency oscillation (HFO) are discussed (Fredberg, 1980; Slutsky et al., 1980; Ouwerkerk et al., 1983). Attempts to apply a similar inductive method to high-frequency jet ventilation are more complex and require excessive simplification to be amenable to mathematical interpretation.

Investigations using physical models of the lungs avoid these problems, by allowing comparison of different ventilators and different settings. An obvious limitation of all test lungs is that all the intricacies of the human pulmonary structure cannot be duplicated. The use of different models to test each physiological hypothesis may, to a degree, circumvent this problem.

In the present study, four different high-frequency ventilators were tested on two lung models. The first one was designed to deliver different pressures, flows, and volumes, measured in central and peripheral lung compartments. Gas transport efficiency was determined by CO_2 concentration gradients along the conductive airway in a CO_2-producing lung model. The investigation aimed to identify similarities and differences in gas transport, pressure, and flow properties of four different high-frequency ventilators.

II. Test Lungs

A. Pressure-Flow Model

This test lung consists of a glass flask of 25 or 50 liters, with a compliance of approximately 50 or 25 ml/millibar (Fig. 1). A 20-mm inlet to the flask can be intubated with a cuffed endotracheal tube. A hot-wire flow sensor, built into the inlet, and

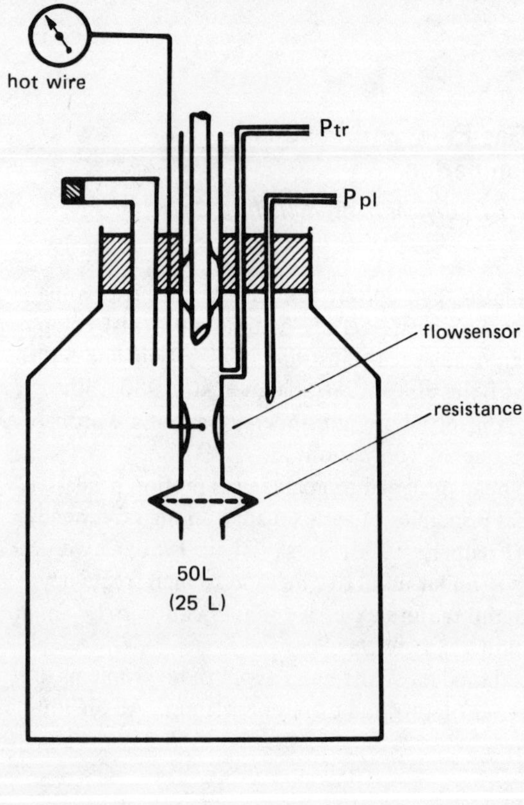

Figure 1 Lung model for pressure flow measurements.

placed approximately 15 cm distally to the tip of the endotracheal tube, measures total flow in and out of the flask. Volume is derived by integration of the flow signal. The flask has an adjustable resistance. Pressure can be measured at the inlet and inside the flask. Back pressure inside the flask can also be changed, when appropriate.

On HFJV, frequency response of measuring equipment is very important for accurate determinations. The hot-wire anemometer we used (Drager-Spirolog) is flat to 2 kHz, but does not recognize flow direction. Pressures were monitored by piezoresistive transducers (Honeywell 140 PC), connected with rigid, air-filled catheters. Frequency response was flat to 500 Hz.

B. Gas Transport Model

A rubber model of the bronchial tree was inserted in a rigid container of approximately 30 liters (Fig. 2). At the bottom of the container a diffusive plate delivered a stable, adjustable flow of 100-600 ml CO_2/min. A horizontal bar with multiple sampling ports can be positioned at variable distances from the diffusion

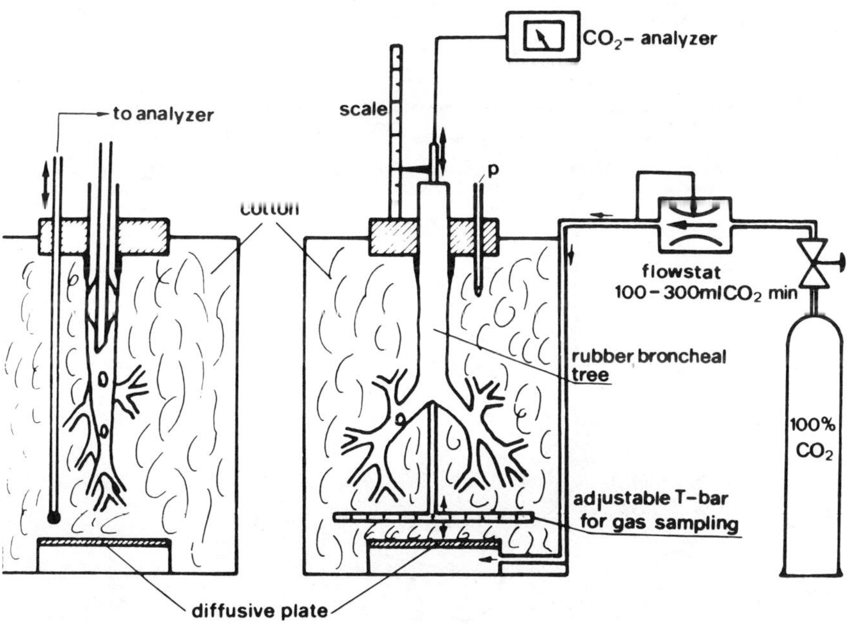

Figure 2 Lung model for gas transport studies. A constant flow of 100% CO_2 at rates between 100 and 600 ml/min enters the model via a large diffusive plate. Concentration gradiants in the model are measured at different locations from CO_2 inlet during various modes of HFV.

plate, to sample mean CO_2 concentration. The model is filled with cotton, to separate the gas streams originating from each of 21 distal openings of the model of the bronchial tree. The model is designed so that distances between carina and diffusive plate were similar to those occurring in vivo between carina and alveolar surface.

A very accurate infrared absorption analyzer (Binos Leybold-Heraeus) was used to measure CO_2 concentration. To prevent development of local convection currents, the gas sampling rate was maintained very low. For the same reason, CO_2 must be delivered through a wide surface.

III. Pressure-Flow Patterns of Different HFV Systems

A. High-Frequency Pulsation (HFP)

This system applies positive pressure pulses to the lungs (Fig. 3). An injector consisting of a nozzle and a Venturi entrainment port is attached to the top of the tube. The geometry of this patient adaptor governs the backpressure-flow ratio

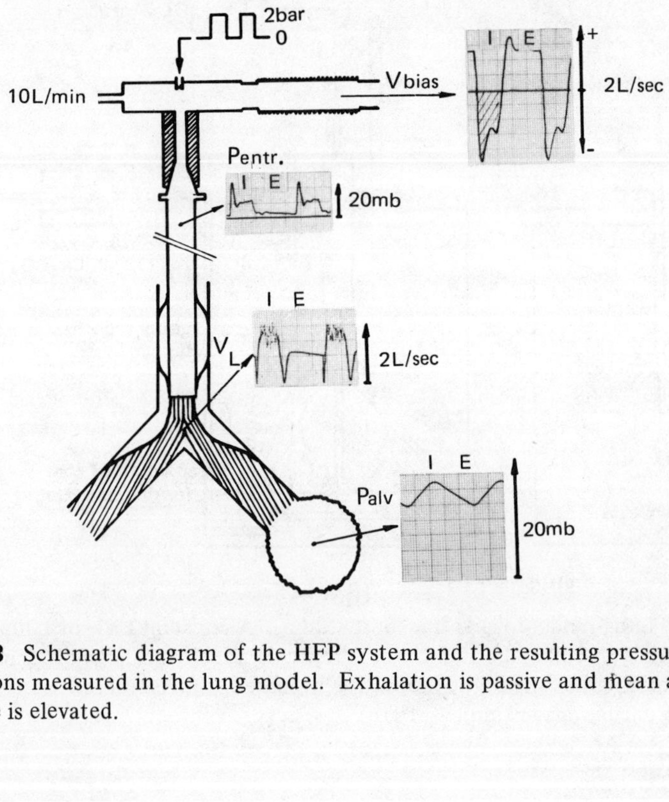

Figure 3 Schematic diagram of the HFP system and the resulting pressure flow conditions measured in the lung model. Exhalation is passive and mean alveolar pressure is elevated.

almost independently of the size of the endotracheal tube. In this system, the highest pressure amplitudes occur proximally in the tube ($P_{entr.}$). Depending on the response time of the solenoid valve gating gas flow, nearly rectangular inspiratory flows can be obtained ($\dot{V}_L$ [I] (Calkins et al., 1982). With this type of HFV, exhalation is passive, sustained only by the recoil of the lungs. Expiratory flow ($\dot{V}_L$ [E]) decays exponentially, with a time constant substantially longer than the actual duration of expiration. The resulting gas trapping generates an inadvertent PEEP at the alveolar level. Distal pressure amplitude is much smaller than proximal pressure. The degree of inadvertent PEEP is determined by I/E ratio and driving pressure, rather than frequency (Rouby, 1983).

Injector systems always tend to entrain gas; depending on the efficiency of the injector, the volume of gas entrained can substantially exceed the flow from the jet nozzle. This is demonstrated by observing tracings of the cross flow ($\dot{V}_{cross}$[I]). To avoid contaminating inspiratory gas with room air, a bias flow system must be provided. Simplified systems, such as those shown in Figure 3, will cause a certain degree of rebreathing.

B. High-Frequency Jet Oscillation (HFJO)

Some of the disadvantages of HFP can be overcome by adding a second nozzle, acting as ejector (Fig. 4). This nozzle is fed by counterphasic gas impulses. Inspiration and expiration are both supported, as evidenced by alternating positive-negative pressure pulses in the proximal section of the tracheal tube and the almost identical inspiratory and expiratory flow patterns ($\dot{V}_L$). With identical injector-ejector impulses, mean alveolar pressure (P_{alv}) can be kept near zero, independent of frequency and driving pressure. Gas entrainment is even more pronounced than with HFP. In contrast to the original HFO with constant tidal volume, this system acts as a constant minute volume ventilator. Changing frequency while keeping all other settings constant will alter tidal volumes in the opposite direction.

C. High-Frequency Oscillation (HFO)

This method is discussed at length elsewhere in this book (Fig. 5). It is mentioned here simply to compare it with other systems.

D. Forced Diffusion Ventilation (FDV)

Two jets of gases enter the airway at the carina level (Baum et al., 1980) (Fig. 6). A specially designed tracheal tube, with two pressure lines inside its walls, brings gas pulses to the desired location. The gas jets exiting from the tip of the tracheal tube remain coherent until they reach the inner edge of the carina. From this point, gas layers travel down the lungs without significant mixing. At the same

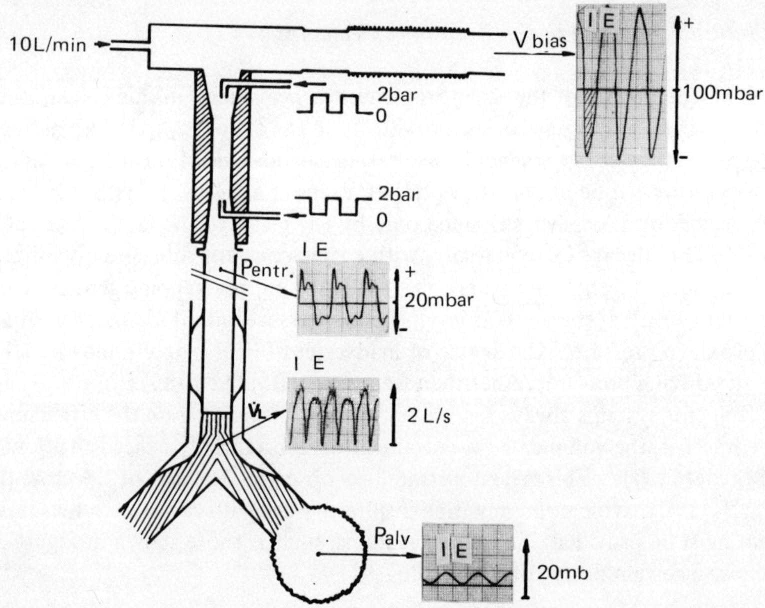

Figure 4 HFJO system: A second ejector nozzle allows active support of exhalation, mean alveolar pressure is close to zero.

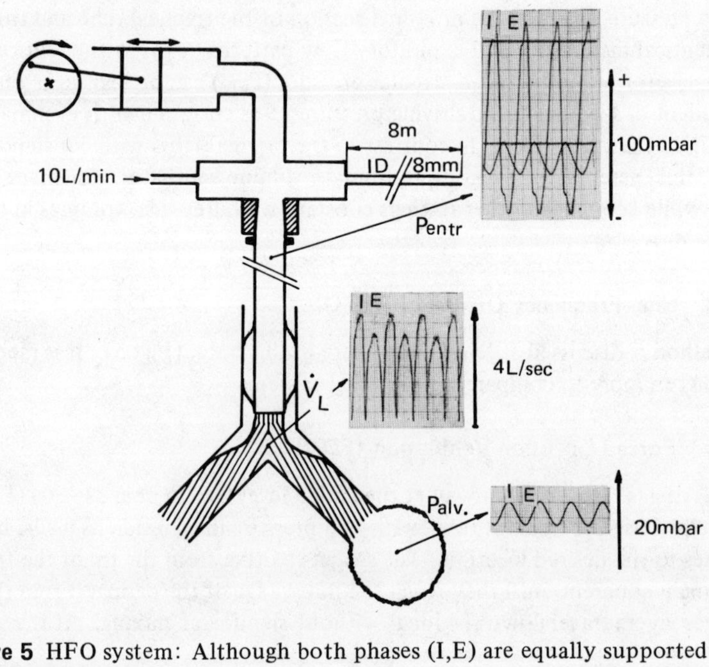

Figure 5 HFO system: Although both phases (I,E) are equally supported by the piston pump, mean alveolar pressure is elevated due to the pressure drop in the bias flow system.

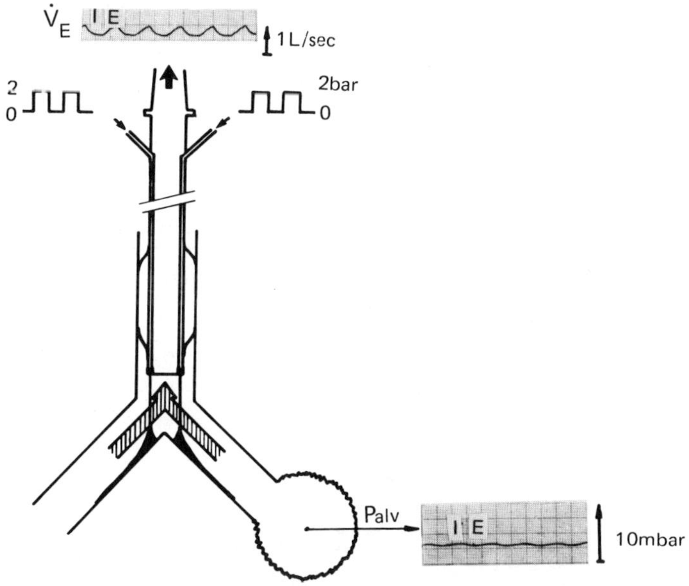

Figure 6 FDV system: Two jets are entering the lungs at the level of the carina. At the same time expired gas leaves the lungs via the main lumen of the tracheal tube. Mean alveolar pressure is low and there is almost no pressure swing in the lungs.

time, a retrograde flow of exhaled gases is established across the remaining bronchial cross-section, ultimately leaving the lungs through the main inlet. Thus, a continuous wash or washout process is responsible for gas transport on forced diffusion ventilation (FDV). With this type of HFV, no entrainment takes place ($\dot{V}_E$ is always positive) and alveolar pressure amplitude, as well as mean pressure, are very low. The major disadvantage of FDV lies in its dependence on tube position. If the tip of the tube is positioned more than 2 cm above the carina, the flow profile is lost and gas exchange for CO_2 becomes inadequate (Mutz, 1984).

IV. Results of Gas Transport Model

The CO_2 concentration gradients on HFJO, at three different frequencies—5, 10, and 20 Hz and constant volume-frequency-product ($\dot{V}_{OSC} = V_T \times F$) of 1.1 liters/sec—are shown in Figure 7. The sharpest decrease occurs within a few millimeters from the diffusive plate above that point; the lung model shows an almost uniform CO_2 concentration. There is no difference between 5 and 10 Hz,

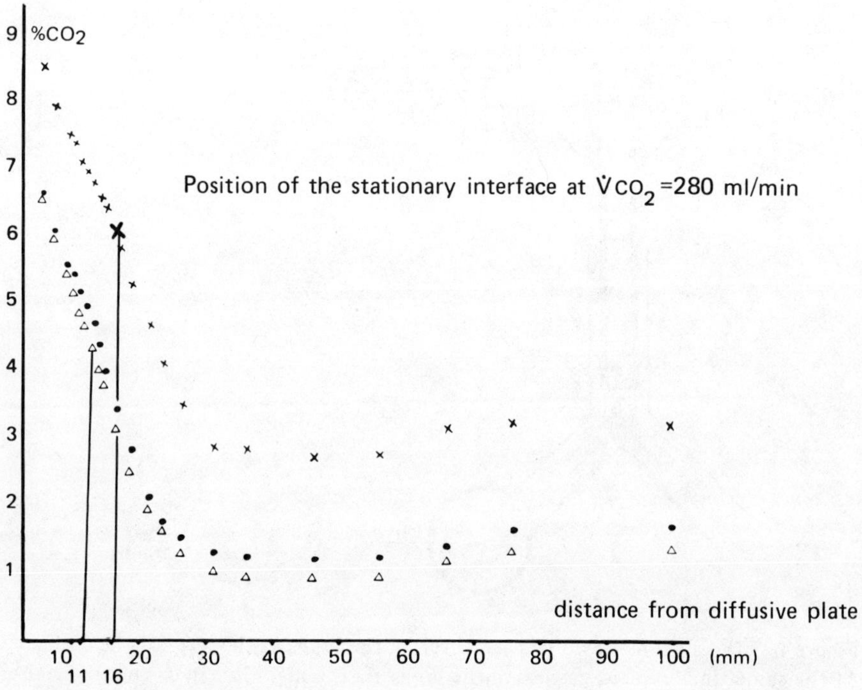

Figure 7 Gas transport model: HFJO $\dot{V}_{OSC}$ = 1.1 liters/sec △ 5Hz; ● 10 Hz; X 20 Hz. The interface is shifted away from the diffusive plate as frequency is increased.

but at 20 Hz CO_2 concentration in the lung model becomes more elevated, indicating a less-efficient CO_2 elimination.

At similar rates $\dot{V}CO_2$ with a $\dot{V}_{OSC}$ of only 0.4 liters/sec, FDV is much more efficient (Fig. 8). The CO_2 interface is closer to the diffusive plate and no influence of frequency on the interface position can be observed. Even an uninterrupted (continuous) jet inflow produces identical CO_2 concentrations. The only way to change the shape of the CO_2 gradient curve is to alter the total gas flow ($\dot{V}_{OSC}$)entering the lung model.

A comparison of HFP, HFJO, and HFO with a measured tidal volume of 100 ml and a frequency of 10 Hz ($V_{OSC}{}^{-1}$ liter/sec) is given in Figure 9. A high CO_2-production rate of 550 ml/min was adjusted as observed in septic patients to test the ultimate performance for each system. FDV was excluded in this figure because these settings are not relevant for this type of ventilation. Under these conditions, HFJO seems to be the most efficient mode of HFV. The inter-

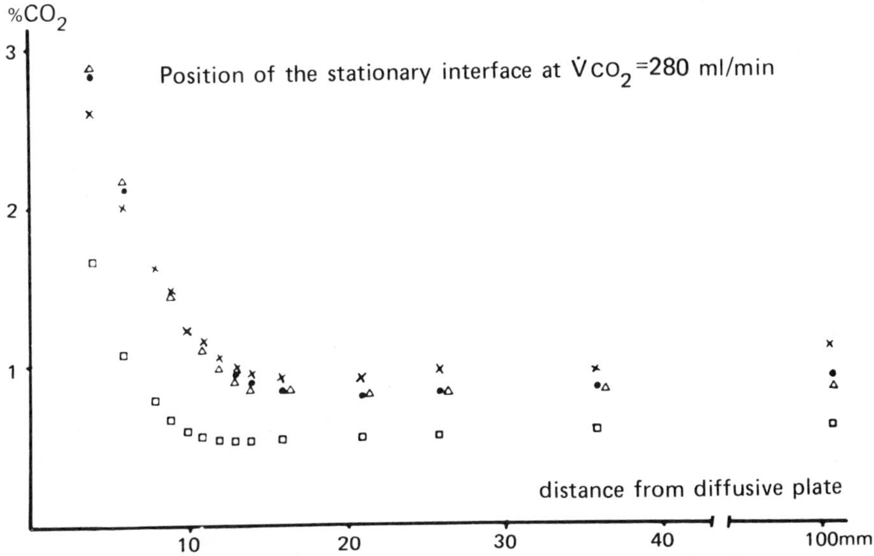

Figure 8 Gas transport model: FDV ($\dot{V}_{OSC}$ = 0.4 liter/sec) x 5 Hz; ● 10 Hz and 20 Hz; △ continuous jet; □ continuous jet ($\dot{V}_{OSC}$ = 0.55 liter/sec). The interface position is much closer to the CO_2 entrance compared to HFJO and does not respond to changes in frequency or even to a continuous jet flow. Only an increase in $\dot{V}_{OSC}$ further improves efficiency in this system.

face is shifted towards the upper airway during HFP and the total CO_2 concentration is higher. HFO was originally tested with a bias flow of 10 liters/min, to reproduce the conditions of other studies (Bohn et al., 1980). A uniformly high CO_2 concentration in the model indicated that these settings were inadequate to eliminate 550 ml CO_2/min. Bias flow was then increased to 22 liters/min, which neared the CO_2 interface to the same position observed with the other ventilation types. The baseline CO_2 concentration in the lung model still remained high (7%).

V. Discussion

Results from studies with HFV are often compared without consideration to the type of system used, assuming that different methods have more similarities than they actually do. Even simple variables, such as mean airway pressure and its correlation to upper airway pressure, depend on the HFV system used. In ventilators that provide assistance only during the inspiratory phase (HFJV, HFP),

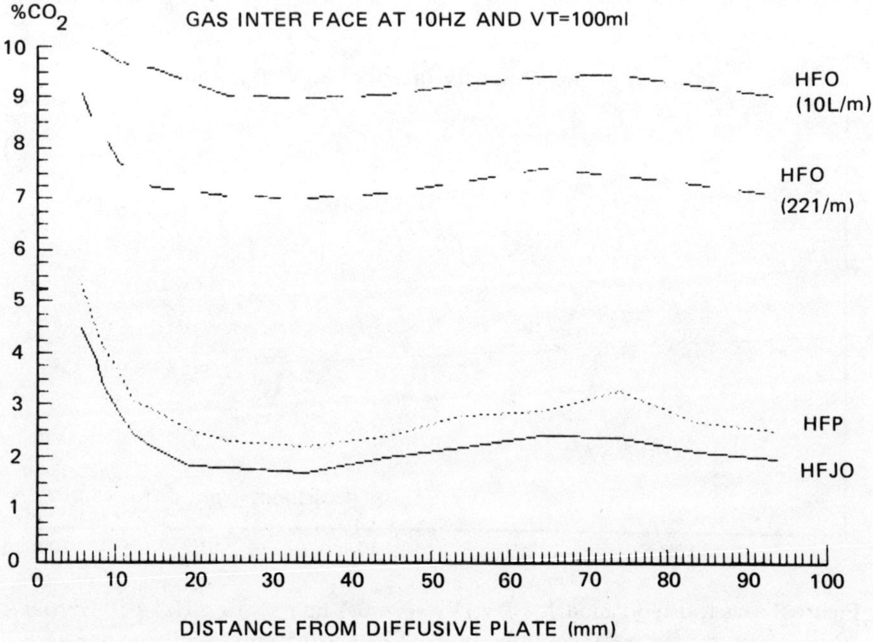

Figure 9 Comparison of different HFO systems at $\dot{V}_{OSC}$ = 1 liter/sec. HFO causes a very high baseline CO_2 concentration which can be reduced by an increase of bias flow from 10 to 22 liters/min.

mean airway pressure is primarily affected by I/E ratio and tidal volume. On FDV, this correlation no longer exists. In biphasic systems such as HFJO and HFO, a mean airway pressure of zero can theoretically be achieved, although the HFO circuit we used produced considerable mean airway pressures, related to the pressure drop of the bias flow along the impedance tube.

An additional source of confusion is the change in tidal volume caused by changes in settings or lung impedance. Systems using the injector principal generally deliver constant minute volume, rather than constant tidal volume, as is the case with certain HFO systems. Furthermore, the characteristics of the injector itself (nozzle diameter, diameter of the Venturi entrainment, tracheal tube size, relative positioning of the jet injector) may influence the response to changing lung impedance.

Flow changes at different back pressures of the injector we used for this study are reported in Figure 10. The solid lines indicate the correlation between pressure, measured proximally in the endotracheal tube (P_{entr}) and the corresponding flow. The dotted lines give the same correlation for the resulting back

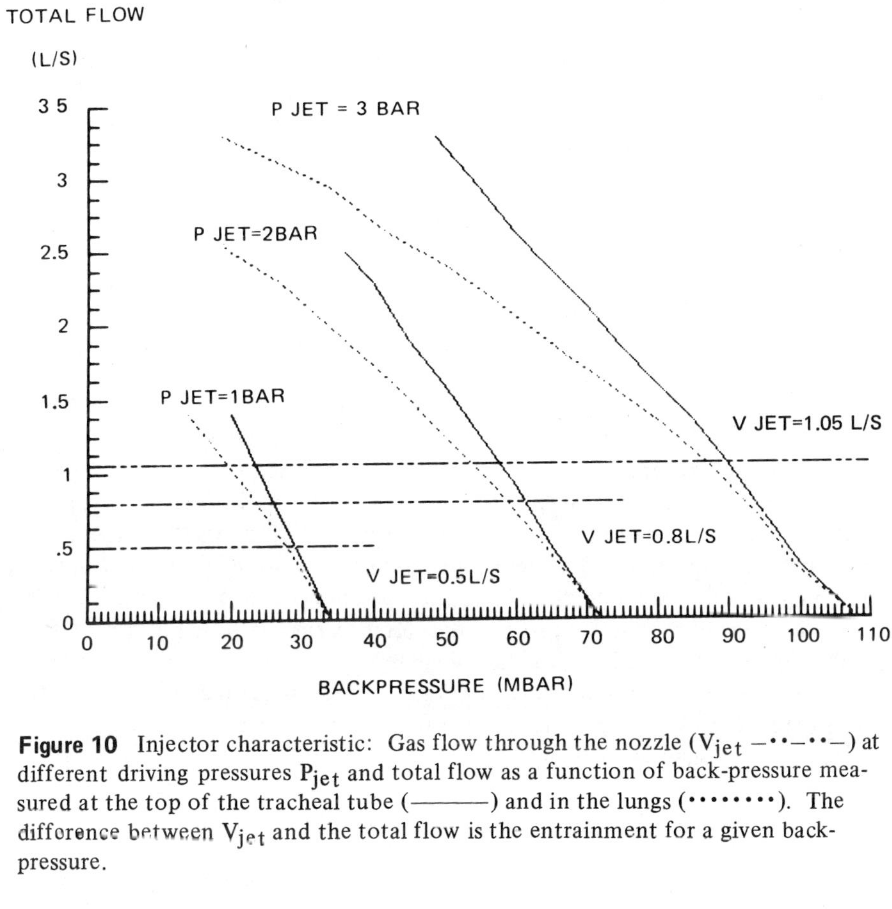

Figure 10 Injector characteristic: Gas flow through the nozzle (V_{jet} —••—••—) at different driving pressures P_{jet} and total flow as a function of back-pressure measured at the top of the tracheal tube (———) and in the lungs (••••••••). The difference between V_{jet} and the total flow is the entrainment for a given back-pressure.

pressure in the lungs (P_{alv}). The difference corresponds to the pressure drop through friction in the tracheal tube. At constant flow through the injector nozzle (V_{jet}, dotted horizontal lines) flow to the lungs decreases as downstream pressure increases. The difference between nozzle flow and flow to the lungs is the amount of gas entrained. When back pressure changes, either due to increased airway resistance or changes in I/E ratio, one shifts along the V-P line towards lower flow rates and tidal volume is reduced. For the same reason the ratio between nozzle flow and entrained flow will also vary according to lung impedance. In fact, this system is affected by so many variables that comparisons of patients' data are often problematic.

CO_2 elimination and shape of the gas interface indicated that in this model convective gas transport is much more important than should be predicted from mathematical models. Fresh gas seems to penetrate deeper into the airway without significant mixing because CO_2 concentration is nearly constant up to the most distal 10-20 mm. Nevertheless, HFJO seems to behave similarly to Slutsky's prediction (Slutsky et al., 1983), based on a mathematical model. The product of $V_T \times F$ determines CO_2 elimination efficiency with a strong tendency for improvements at higher tidal volumes.

During FDV this dependence on tidal volume no longer exists. Gas velocity upon entering into the lungs is much higher, close to the speed of sound. This physical characteristic favors convective gas transport mechanisms, such as eddy flows. Gating of the jet is no longer necessary to maintain gas exchange. The results have also been reproduced in dogs (Baum et al., 1980; Mutz, 1984; Lehnert et al., 1982). However, CO_2 elimination becomes poor as soon as the gas entry port is more than 2 cm above the carina.

A comparison of three different types of ventilation (HFP, HFJO, HFO), at predefined flow and volume conditions resulted in unexpectedly large differences in CO_2 concentration. A gas interface was established approximately at the same distance above a diffusive plate, indicating similar efficiency for all types for of HFV, but the baseline CO_2 concentration was much higher for HFO. There are two possible explanations for these observations: (1) with HFO, a significantly different amount of gas mixing always takes place in the larger airways; (2) fresh inspiratory gases already have a CO_2 concentration similar to that measured above the interface. Although many authors believe that HFO causes extensive gas mixing, the second assumption seems more valid because increasing bias flow significantly reduced CO_2 concentration. Bias flow should be matched to the metabolic rate and the magnitude of $\dot{V}_{OSC}$.

VI. Alveolar Gas Exchange and Deadspace in HFV

Marc J. Jaeger, Ulrich H. Kurzweg, and Michael J. Banner

The introduction into clinical medicine, of new techniques of ventilation which combine small tidal volume with high frequency (Carlon et al., 1983; Slutsky et al., 1980), has provided physicians with a new life support system which may prove very helpful in selected patients. The tidal volume delivered by such systems may be smaller than anatomical dead space. This challenges concepts of gas exchange mechanisms established more than 100 years ago. The function of the alveoli in gas transfer between the blood and the gas phase was first recognized in the middle of the 19th century. Researchers concluded that tidal volume (V_T) had to exceed the volume of the conducting airways (V_D) to achieve ventilation of the alveolar space ($V_A = V_T - V_D$). The term dead space was used for the first time by Zuntz in 1882 and the first measurements date back to 1894 (Loewy, 1894). Historical reviews of the evolution of these concepts are available (Otis, 1981).

Recent research into the principles of high-frequency jet ventilation (HFJV) and high-frequency oscillation (HFO) does not address the issue of gas exchange, when tidal volume is less than dead space. Some authors have suggested that the best explanation is enhancement of diffusion (Jaeger and Kurzweg, 1983; Fredberg, 1980). If this were true, the concept of alveolar ventilation must be reappraised, since there is no mass flow in diffusion processes and therefore no alveolar ventilation intended as delivery of fresh gas to replace the gas present in the alveoli.

This section discusses bench models of gas exchange which reproduce high-frequency ventilation (HFV). Equations derived from Fick's diffusion law are verified and applied to animal experiments. The results, which support diffusion as a mechanism of transport in HFV, are reconciled with accepted concepts of alveolar ventilation.

We have developed, in the last 2 years, a method to study gas transport in oscillating gas columns (Jaeger and Kurzweg, 1983). The experimental design measures the concentration gradient and the flow of gas between two sites (1 and 2) (Fig. 11). The coefficient D_{HFO} is determined, according to Fick's diffusion law as:

$$D_{HFO} = \frac{X}{A} \frac{\dot{V}}{F_1 - F_2} \tag{1}$$

where x is the distance between the two sites, $\dot{V}$ the gas flow due to diffusion, A the cross-section through which the diffusion occurs, and F_1 and F_2 the fractional concentration at the two sites. Note that in Fick's equation the diffusion coefficient has the dimension cm^2/sec. Details of the experiment have already been published (Jaeger and Kurzweg, 1983). One gas, O_2, diffuses through a second gas, N_2, while the mixture is oscillated at a given frequency (f) and amplitude (V_T).

Experiments were first performed in a straight tube, to keep the cross-section A constant. In branched tubes, such as the airway, the cross-section may vary and the Fick equation cannot be in applied directly. Figure 12 shows results obtained in a 62-cm-long tube with 1.98 cm^2 cross-section. This tube has approximately the same volume as the airways while having the same cross-section over its whole length. When diffusion coefficient D_{HFO}, computed with an equation analogous to Eq. (1), was plotted against V_T, a curvilinear relationship was obtained for each frequency (Fig. 12a). If tidal volume was squared (Fig. 12b), the relationship became linear with the slope proportional to frequency. Statistical analysis confirms that D_{HFO} is a function of $f \times V_T^2$ with a correlation coefficient of 0.95 and a slope 0.030, with 31 data points. Recently, similar results have been obtained independently by two other authors (Venegas, 1983; Dietz et al., 1983).

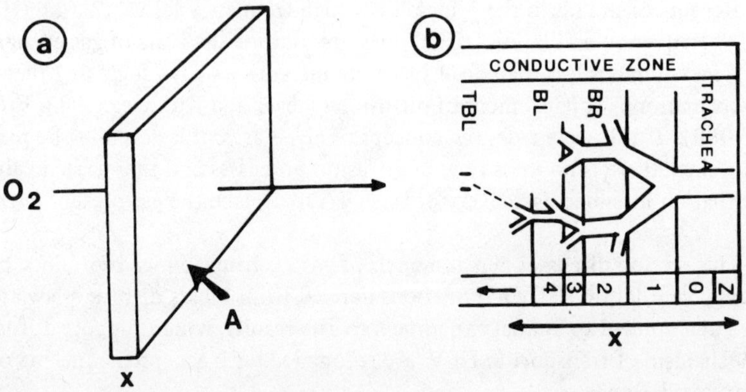

Figure 11 Schematic representation of gas diffusion. (a) Diffusion of O_2 through a membrane with area A and thickness x. Fick's diffusion law applies [Eq. (1)]. (b) Diffusion of O_2 through the airways. The distance is x; the cross-sectional area $\bar{A}$ varies with bronchial generation. The medium through which O_2 diffuses is assumed to be N_2.

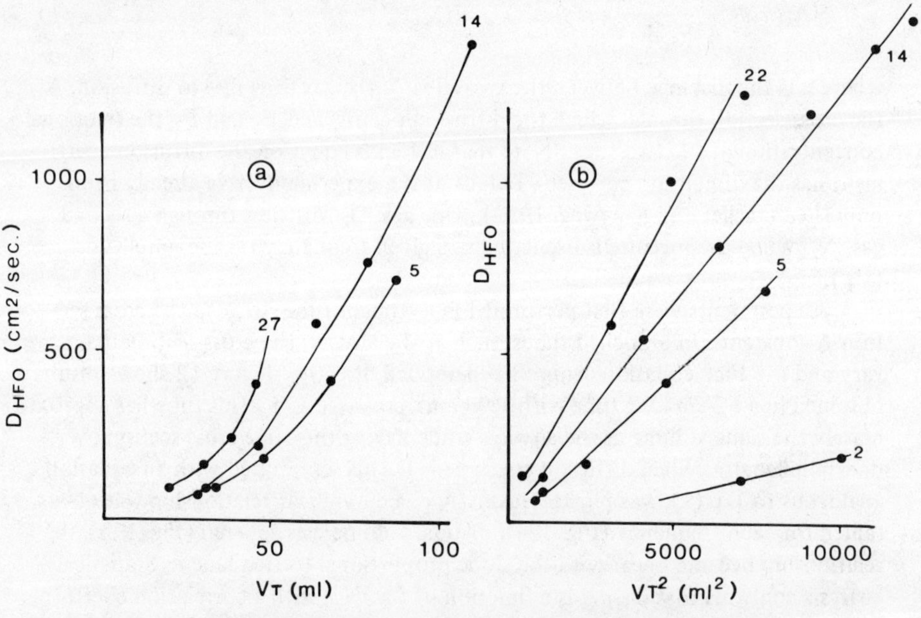

Figure 12 Results from a bench model. D_{HFO} values, computed with Eq. (1), are plotted against tidal volume V_T (a) and against the square of tidal volume (b) Frequencies were 2, 5, 14, 22, or 27 Hz. The relationship becomes linear when D_{HFO} is plotted against $V_T{}^2$. (Jaeger et al., 1984.)

The next series of experiments was designed to determine the effect of varying cross-sections in tubes varying from 0.007 to 5.07 cm^2, a 700-fold range. The results indicated that D_{HFO} was proportional to $1/A^2$. Statistical analysis of 141 data points obtained with four tubes of increasing cross-sections, (0.32, 1.27, 1.98, and 5.07 cm^2), yielded a correlation coefficient of 0.97 with a slope K = 0.031. In these experiments, f varied between 2 and 40 Hz and V_T between 10 and 100% of the volume of the pipes considered. Results in capillaries were almost identical, except that the slope was 0.077. By combining these findings with previous data, diffusion during HFV was computed as:

$$D_{HFO} = k\, f\, (V_T/A)^2 \qquad (2)$$

is expressed in cm^3 and A in cm^2. Thus, the gas transport is proportional to frequency and to the square of the linear oscillation amplitude, which may also be defined as "tidal length."

Data suggest very strongly that oscillatory gas transport follows Fick's diffusion law. Though the study is complex in mathematical terms (Jaeger and Kurzweg, 1983; Kurzweg et al., 1984), results are easy to illustrate. Transport is proportional to frequency and to the square of the tidal length. This relationship bears an interesting similarity to the molecular diffusion of gas, which depends on the brownian movement of molecules. In 1905, Einstein derived an equation which predicts that gas diffusion increases with the collision frequency of molecules and with the square of the mean free path length (Einstein, 1905). Eq. (2) is identical to Einstein's formula, if oscillation-frequency is analogous to collision frequency and tidal length analogous to mean free path length. The similarity may point to an analogous mechanism, as well, but the theory has not yet been developed.

Data from Figure 12 allow a quantitative evaluation of the efficiency of the diffusion process in oscillating gas columns. The values of D_{HFO} determined experimentally reach 1000 cm^2/sec; by comparison, molecular diffusion of O_2 into N_2 at room temperature is 0.2 cm^2/sec. Thus, oscillations may increase the transport up to 5,000 times. On the basis of these experimental models, it is tempting to hypothesize that this enhancement is sufficient to provide adequate alveolar gas exchange in patients and experimental animals subjected to respiratory oscillations with a V_T smaller than anatomical dead space.

We undertook two series of experiments in dogs, to determine the mathematical relationship between gas exchange and frequency and tidal volume. We assumed that, if gas exchange were a function of $f \times V_T^2$ [Eq. (2)], gas transport in the respiratory system would be similar to that of straight pipes.

To confirm the experiments with Fick's diffusion law, Eqs. (1) and (2) were combined and the term D_{HFO} was eliminated. The resulting relationship was solved for $(F_1 - F_2)$, assuming that F_1 is the fractional concentration of alveolar CO_2 (F_{ACO_2}) and that F_2 is zero (F_{ICO_2}); $\dot{V}$ indicated CO_2 elimination ($\dot{V}_{CO_2}$); the product xA, which represents the volume of the pipe, was replaced by V_D, the symbol for anatomical dead space. The result of these mathematical manipulations is:

$$F_{ACO_2} = x\,\dot{V}_{CO_2}\,A^2/A\,k\,f\,V_T{}^2 = V_D\,\dot{V}_{CO_2}/k\,f\,V_T{}^2 \tag{3}$$

It may be noted that the quotient $F_{ACO_2}/\dot{V}_{CO_2}$ represents the alveolar ventilation $\dot{V}_A$. The relationships may therefore be rewritten as:

$$\dot{V}_A = k\,f\,V_T{}^2/V_D \tag{4}$$

These formulas are similar to the classic alveolar gas equations yet, since they are modified for HFV, V_T is now squared. A relationship similar to Eq. (3) may be easily derived for O_2-gradient.

It may be useful to illustrate the relationship with a numerical example, considering a patient ventilated at 15 Hz (900 breaths/min) with a V_T of 100 ml. If V_D were 150 ml, $\dot{V}_{CO_2}$ = 250 ml/min, and k = 0.05 (all values expressed as ATPS units), solving Eqs. (3) and (4) yields F_{aCO_2} = 0.08, P_{aCO_2} = 59 mm Hg. and $\dot{V}_A$ = 3000 ml/min. The relationship provide quantitative guidelines for the evaluation of gas exchange in HFV. The value of k is discussed below.

Equations (3) and (4) were used to design two series of animal experiments. The first involved steady-state gas exchange measurements in eight dogs using HFJV (Carlon et al., 1983).

Alveolar ventilation was determined from blood gas values ($\dot{V}_A = \dot{V}_{CO_2}$ $[P_B-47]/P_{aCO_2}$) and plotted against $f\,V_T{}^2/V_D$ from Eq. (4). The ventilator was set as follows: the driving pressure was maintained at 20 psig; the frequency was varied in seven steps from 100 to 900 beats/min with a solenoid valve (Healthdyne, Inc.). The I/E ratio was set at 20/80, 30/70, or 40/60. V_T increased with each setting of the I/E ratio and was measured with a body plethysmograph. Each dog was subjected to all 21 conditions obtained by the combination of the settings. Each ventilatory setting was maintained for 15 min, before a blood gas sample was collected. The treatments were separated by periods of conventional mechanical ventilation (CMV) to restore basal conditions (P_{aCO_2} = 40 mmHg ± 5 mmHg). Figure 14 shows that most data points, representing the average of measurements made in eight dogs, fall in a straight line. This confirms Eq. (4). Figure 13 also shows that $\dot{V}_A$ increases with increasing I/E ratio since V_T increases with the I/E ratio. By contrast, V_T and therefore $\dot{V}_A$, decrease sharply if f is augmented. The correlation is good (r = 0.96), and the slope (k) is 0.05, close to that of straight pipes. There is an intercept with the ordinate at $\dot{V}_A$ = 450 ml/min.

In the second series of experiments, $\dot{V}_A$ was determined on the basis of N_2-washouts. $\dot{V}_A$ is inversely related to the time constant of the washout by the equation $\dot{V}_A$ = FRC/T (Jaeger et al., 1983). Six dogs were ventilated with HFO using a protocol previously described (Slutsky et al., 1980). Frequency was varied between 2 and 40 Hz, and V_T between 10 and 100% of the estimated anatomical dead space. Figure 14 shows the data from one dog as an example.

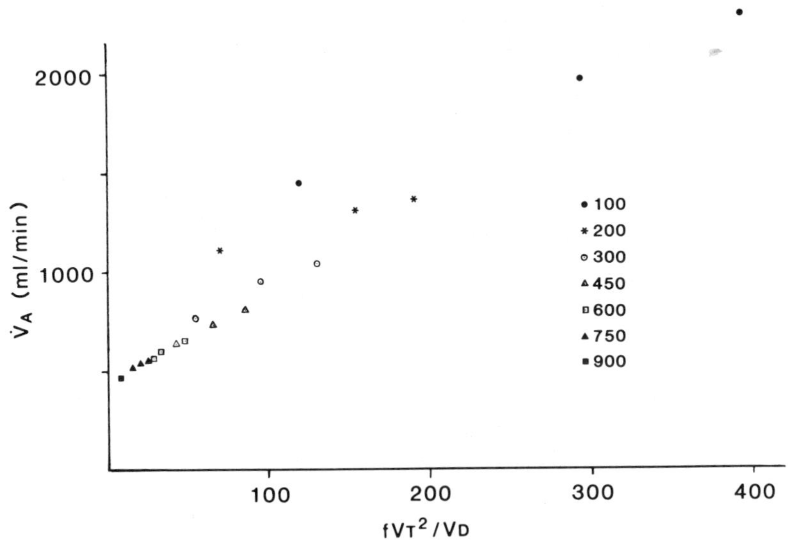

Figure 13 Results of steady-state dog experiments obtained with HFJV. $\dot{V}_A$ is computed from measurements of $PaCO_2$ and an assumed value of $\dot{V}CO_2$ (120 ml/min). V_T is measured with a body plethysmograph. V_D = 100 ml.

In the left panel $\dot{V}_A$ is plotted against V_T for a constant frequency. The curve looks very similar to the data obtained in the bench model (Fig. 12a). The right panel shows $\dot{V}_A$ as a function of f. The correlation coefficient obtained in this experiment was 0.95, the slope 0.04. The results obtained in the other five dogs were similar. They confirm the data obtained in the first series of dogs. They also show that N_2 is washed out of the lungs in HFO.

The animal experiments give solid support to the alveolar gas equation of HFV. Alveolar ventilation, determined with two techniques, is proportional to $f\,V_T{}^2/V_D$, as predicted on the basis of experiments performed on a very simple model, consisting only of a straight pipe. This equation bears similarity to the diffusion process described by Einstein, in which gas behavior is compared to that of a population of bounding balls. This may help us to understand the principles of operation of HFV, even though this mechanism has not yet been proved.

All experiments performed on animals indicate that measurable alveolar ventilation still exists, even when the total ventilation is zero. This value represented by the intercept of the y axis, is 380-500 ml/min (Figs. 13 and 14). Technical errors, such as incomplete steady state, may have contributed to this finding. Cardiac movements might also explain this observation, since they produce oscillations of gases in the respiratory tract so-called cardiogenic mixing.

It is important to consider that the theory presented here is very general; it applies to jet ventilation as well as to high-frequency oscillations. Its quantative application assumes, however, absence of rebreathing of expired gas, which would reduce alveolar ventilation.

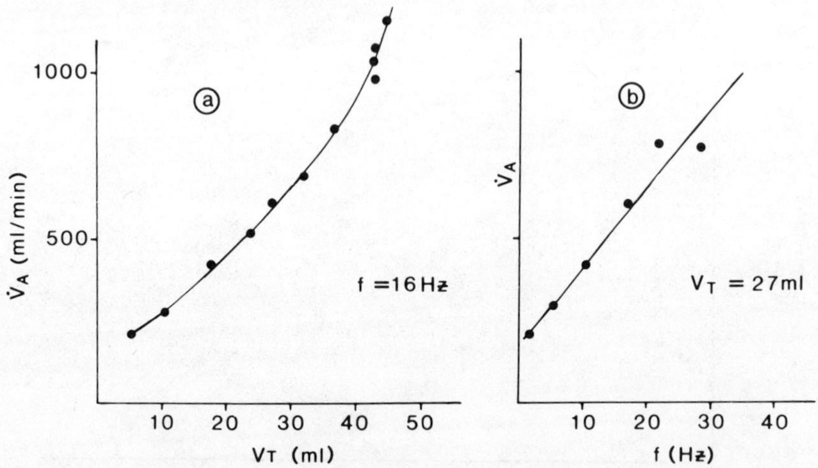

Figure 14 Results of N_2-washouts in dogs. $\dot{V}_A$ is computed as FRC/T plotted against V_T (a) and (b). (Jaeger et al., 1984.)

High-frequency ventilation is a relatively inefficient mode of ventilation. At an f of 15 Hz, with a V_T of 100 ml, total ventilation is 90 liters/min, while $\dot{V}_A$ is only 4.2 liters/min. The resulting $\dot{V}_A/\dot{V}_E$ ratio is 0.05 instead of 0.7 in normal breathing.

There is no reason to limit the gas transport principles presented in this section to very high frequencies. Excellent clinical results have been obtained at 100 breaths/min, a rate which lies at the borderline between "normal" and "high frequencies" (Carlon et al., 1983). The mechanism described probably works at any frequency. During CMV, when V_T exceeds anatomical dead space, $\dot{V}_A$ is presumably due to a combination of diffusion and mass transport.

The information obtained with the pipe experiment provides insight into gas transport at various levels of the respiratory tract. In human subjects ventilated with a V_T of 100 ml at an f of 15 Hz, D_{HFO} in the large airways is about 720 cm^2/sec. In the intermediate airways, the total cross-section rapidly increases from 2.5 to about 10 cm^2. D_{HFO} accordingly drops to 45 [Eq. (2)]. In the peripheral bronchi, where the cross-section is 200 cm^2, D_{HFO} is only 0.45 cm^2/sec. It appears from these figures, that D_{HFO} decreases with increasing bronchial cross-section, reaching a value barely higher than molecular diffusion. Even though the diffusion distance is proportionally reduced, the critical area, where gas transport requires a high concentration gradient, is probably located in the smaller airways. This observation may be important for the development of high-frequency ventilation techniques.

Chapter 3 has been written by two groups of authors working independently. It is remarkable that although different approaches and different methods of presentation were used, both groups came to similar findings. Baum et al. show that the CO_2 concentration at a given distance from the CO_2-diffusing plate declines to about 1/4 of its original value if frequency is reduced from 20 to 5 Hz (Figs. 7, 8). This implies, since $\dot{V}_{OSC}$ is constant, that the CO_2 concentration declines with increasing V_T, and that V_T is raised to a power higher than unity. This finding is in good agreement with the finding of Jaeger et al., who show that alveolar ventilation is proportional to V_{T2} [Figs. 13, 14; Eq. (4)]. By contrast, the two groups of authors seem to disagree on the efficiency of the different ventilators. Figure 9 demonstrates that different types of ventilators achieve different levels of CO_2 in a bottle while Figures 13 and 14 imply similar gas transport and similar mechanisms of two different modes of HFV if rebreathing is avoided.

No definitive solution to the question of the mechanism of gas transport in HFV is offered. However, an interesting idea is submitted by comparing the mixing in HFV with the Brownian movement. An analogy is drawn to Einstein's theory of diffusion. The comparison explains why, in HFV, not only O_2 and CO_2 are exchanged, but also inert N_2 molecules. This analogy gives new meaning to the term alveolar ventilation in HFV.

References

Baum, M., Benzer, H., Geyer, A., Haider, W., and Mutz, N. (1980). Forcierte Diffusionsventilation (FDV). *Anaesthesist* **29**:586.

Bohn, D. J., Miyasaka, K., Marchak, B. E., Thompson, W. K., Froese, A. B., and Bryan, A. C. (1980). Ventilation by high frequency oscillation. *J. Appl. Physiol.* **48**(4):710-716.

Calkins, J. M., Waterson, C. K., Hammeroff, S. R., and Kanel. J. (1982). Jet impulse characteristics for high-frequency jet ventilation in dogs. *Anaesth. Analg.* **61**:293.

Carlon, J. C., Howland, W. S., Ray, C., Miodownik, S., Griffin, J. P., and Groeger, J. S. (1983). High-frequency jet ventilation. A prospective standardized evaluation. *Chest* **84**:551.

Dietz, J., MacIntyre, N., and Leatherman, N. (1983). Gas transport and ventilation distribution as a function of tidal volume and breathing frequency in a mechanical lung model. In *International Symposium on High Frequency Ventilation.* Edited by C. G. Carlon. New York, Sloan Kettering, Cancer Center.

Einstein, A. (1905). Ueber die Theorie Der Warme. *Ann. Physik* **17**:549.

Fredberg, J. J. (1980). Augmented diffusion in the airway can support pulmonary gas exchange. *J. Appl. Physiol.* **48**:710-716.

Jaeger, M. J., and Kurzweg, U. H. (1983). Determination of the longitudinal dispersion coefficient in flows subjected to high frequency oscillations. *Phys. Fluids* **26**:1380.

Jaeger, M. J., Kurzweg, U. H., and Banner, M. J. (1984). Transport of gases in HFV. *Crit. Care* **12**:708-710.

Jaeger, M. J., Banner, M., and Kurzweg, U. (1983). Alveolar ventilation in high frequency studies. *Fed. Proc.* **42**:1351.

Klain, M., and Smith, R. B. (1977). High frequency percutaneous transtracheal jet ventilation. *Crit. Care Med.* **5**(6).

Kurzweg, U. H., Howell, G., and Jaeger, M. J. (1984). Enhanced dispersion in oscillatory flows. *Phys. Fluids* **27**:1046.

Lehnert, B. E., Oberdörster, G., and Slutsky, A. S. (1982). Constant-flow ventilation of apneic dogs. *J. Appl. Physiol.* **53**(2):483-489.

Loewy, A. (1894). Ueber die Bestimmung der Grosse des schadlichen Luftraumes. *Pflugers Arch. Physiol.* **58**(416.

Lunkenheimer, P. P., Frank, I., Ising, H., Keller, H., and Dickhut, H. H. (1973). Intrapulmonaler Gaswechsel unter simultaner Apnoe durch transtrachealen, periodischen intrathorakalen Druckwechsel. *Anaesthesist* **22**:232-238.

Mutz, N. (1984). Hochfrequenzbeatmung. Entwicklung neuer Beatmungssysteme—experimentelle und klinische Ergebnisse. *Wien. Klin. Wochenschr.* **96**: (Suppl. 146).

Otis, A. B. (1981). History of pulmonary gas exchange in the 19th century. *Progr. Respir. Res.* **16**:1-9.

Ouwerkerk, H. J. van, Gieles, P., and Bogaard, J. M. (1983). Convective diffusion in oscillatory flow as a gas transport mechanism during high frequency ventilation. In *Perspectives in High Frequency Ventilation.* Edited by P. A. Schenck, U. H. Sjöstrand, and R. B. Smith. Boston, Martinus Nijhoff.

Rouby, J. J. (1983). Jet ventilation à haute frequence: Aspects techniques et mechanisme des échanges gazeux dans les insuffisances respiratoires aigües. In *Ventilation A Haute Frequence.* Edited by J. L. Bourgain, A. Lienhart, and P. Viars. Paris, Libraire Arnette.

Sjöstrand, U. (1977). Review on the physiologic rationale for and development of high frequency positive pressure ventilation. *Acta Anaesth. Scand. Suppl.* **64**:4

Slutsky, A. S., Drazen, J. M., Ingram, R. H. Jr., Kamm, R. D., Shapiro, A. H., Fredberg, J. J., Loring, S. H., and Lehr, J. (1980). Effective pulmonary ventilation with small volume oscillation at high frequency. *Science* **209**: 609-611.

Slutsky, A. S., Kamm, R. D., and Drazen, J. M. (1983). A review of experimental and theoretical studies of high frequency ventilation. In *Perspectives in High Frequency Ventilation.* Edited by P. A. Scheck, U. H. Sjöstrand, R. B. Smith. Boston, Martinus Nijhoff.

Venegas, J. G. (1983). Efficiency and regional distribution of high frequency ventilation. Thesis, Massachusetts Institute of Technology.

Zuntz, N. (1882). Physiologie der blutgase. In *Hermann's Handbuch der Physiologie,* Leipzig, Vogel, Vol. 4, II.

4

High-Frequency Positive Pressure Ventilation

Utilization in the Operating Room

PAUL A. SCHECK

Erasmus University
Academic Hospital
Rotterdam, The Netherlands

Ventilation of the lungs using low tidal volumes was considered 70 years ago by Henderson and co-workers (1915). They stated that: "there may easily be gaseous exchange sufficient to support life even when tidal volume is considerably less than dead space." Briscoe et al. (1954) studied alveolar ventilation at very low tidal volumes. A group of Swedish investigators (Öberg and Sjöstrand, 1969) performed experimental studies on the carotid sinus reflex. Their experiments were disturbed by pressure variations during respiration. To overcome the problem, they designed a mechanical ventilator with negligible internal compliance, which employed lower tidal volumes and higher frequencies than those used for conventional ventilation. This technique, defined as high-frequency positive pressure ventilation (HFPPV) (Jonzon et al., 1973, 1980; Heijman et al., 1972) proved adequate to maintain ventilation in animals (Öberg and Sjostrand, 1969). Additional experimental studies demonstrated that intratracheal and intrapleural pressures were also lower with this ventilatory modality (Eriksson and Sjöstrand, 1977). HFPPV can be characterized by:

1. Ventilatory frequency of 60-110 breaths/min (1-1.8 Hz)
2. Small tidal volume, usually approaching calculated dead space
3. Inspiratory/expiratory ratio < 0.3

4. Low airway pressures
5. Fewer adverse circulatory effects than intermittent positive-pressure ventilation (IPPV).

I. Development

A. Models

Several physiological parameters such as circulation, alveolar gas exchange, and organ blood flow, have been experimentally evaluated.

Gas distribution was similar to that observed with spontaneous ventilation and lung compliance did not change after short periods of HFPPV (9 hr) (Borg et al., 1981). Adequate alveolar ventilation was achieved with minimal variations in intrathoracic and transpulmonary pressure. Inhibition of antidiuretic hormone secretion, with increased free water clearance is also observed on HFPPV. This finding may suggest that HFPPV induces less nonspecific stress than IPPV (Borg et al., 1981).

In deeply anesthetized dogs, total peripheral resistance was lower while cardiac output and stroke volume were higher with HFPPV than with IPPV (Eriksson et al., 1977). Hemodynamic effects of HFPPV and IPPV were compared during acute hemorrhage in dogs (Mankikar et al., 1982). Results suggested that in rapidly developing hypovolemic states, HFPPV improves cardiac output and blood pressure, possibly because transpulmonary pressure is lower. Elevated transpulmonary pressure during IPPV induces phasic variations of systemic arterial pressure. These are potentially detrimental to organ perfusion, and not observed on HFPPV. Organ blood flow was studied in dogs with normal or elevated intracranial pressure during HFPPV (Bunegin et al., 1982) and compared with IPPV. No significant differences were found in cerebral, pulmonary, renal, or cardiac circulation.

Todd et al. (1981) reported on measurements of brain movement in cats. They found significantly reduced brain surface movement during HFPPV, which greatly facilitated microscopic observation compared to IPPV.

Other investigators (Borg et al., 1982) confirmed that ventilator-synchronous changes in intracranial pressure could be eliminated by HFPPV. Changes in pulmonary tissue of dogs supported with HFPPV for 2-5 hr were investigated (Frank et al., 1975) using both light and electron microscopy. No significant difference was observed between experimental animals and controls.

B. Technique

For clinical applications of HFPPV, Sjöstrand and Eriksson (1980) developed a volume-controlled ventilator, which can deliver small tidal volumes at low pressure. Ventilation is provided through an insufflation catheter positioned either in an endotracheal tube or directly into the trachea, preferably through the nasal route. A pneumatic valve, based on the Coanda or wall effect, was also developed and proved especially advantageous for bronchoscopic procedures. The gas mixture is delivered through a side arm into the pneumatic valve connector. The main channel of the connector remains open and can be used for the insertion of the bronchoscope. The system is open, without air entrainment. A commercial version of the device (Bronchovent) was manufactured in Sweden by the AGA Company. The ventilator had a fixed frequency of 60 cycles/min (1 Hz) and an insufflation time of 22% (Borg et al., 1980). The parameters were derived from the ventilatory patterns Oberg and Sjöstrand (1969) had considered optimal during their earlier experimental studies. This ventilatory system was called "System H" (Sjöstrand, 1980). It delivers a biphasic flow profile during inspiration. An early accelerating flow is rapidly followed by a decelerating flow. Volume is the primary and pressure the secondary variable. In system H, the internal compressible gas volume is 50 ml and the internal compliance 0.06 ml/cm H_2O, a negligible value compared to most conventional ventilators (Sjöstrand, 1982). The Bronchovent has been extensively studied in clinical use. Nomograms were derived from the experience obtained with 800 bronchoscopies and 500 laryngoscopies (Borg et al., 1980) (Figs. 1, 2). They are adjusted for different models of rigid bronchoscopes and for insufflation catheters of different internal diameters, providing reliable safety margins for the use of HFPPV in clinical practice (Sjöstrand and Eriksson, 1980; Eriksson and Sjöstrand, 1980).

The Bronchovent also includes optical and acoustical alarms and safety features. Ventilation stops automatically when airway pressures exceed 20 cm H_2O. Leakage from the main valve is measured to deliver conditioned gas intermittently. When ventilation is automatically interrupted, the expiratory valve remains open. Ventilation is resumed as soon as both conditions are restored.

The prototype version of the Bronchovent was not equipped with a humidifier. Recently, a larger company has acquired production rights for the Bronchovent (Siemens Elema, Solna, Sweden). New models of the ventilator will have adjustable frequencies, inspiration/expiration ratios, and a humidifying device.

The inspiratory line consists of a rigid polyethylene hose, fitted at its distal end to connect securely to the insufflation catheter. The size of the catheter depends on the patient's airway. An FG14 catheter with an ID of 3 mm is usually used. The Mediplast Company (Mölndal, Sweden) supplies specially designed insufflation catheters with one distal and four side holes. Gas flow through the side holes prevents air entrainment and, during surgery in the upper airway, pushes blood and tissue fragments upward. Sjöstrand (1980) summarized the major technical characteristics of HFPPV as:

1. A ventilatory frequency of 60 breaths/min and an inspiratory/expiratory ratio $\leqslant$ 1:2.

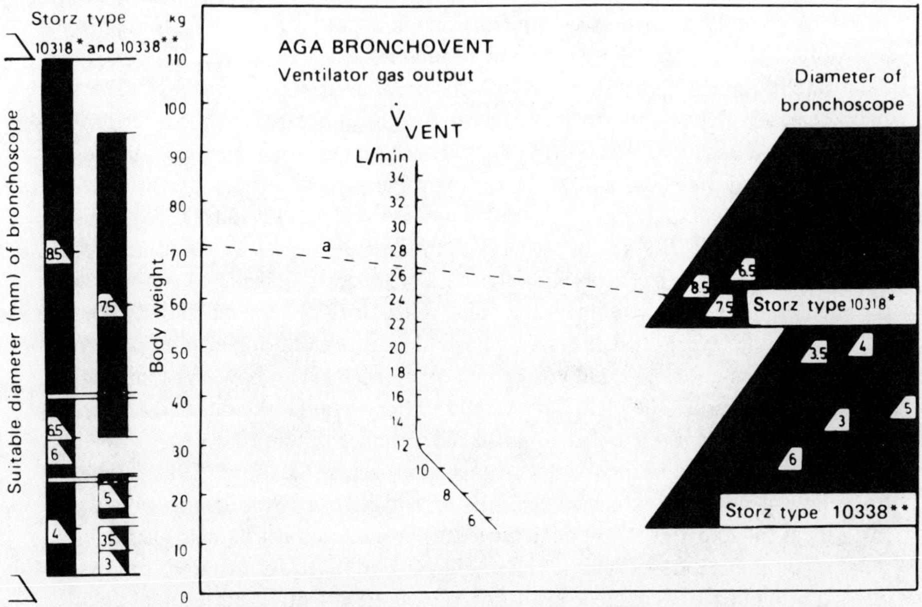

Figure 1 Ventilation nomogram for "bronchoscopic" HFPPV with the Bronchovent. *With AGA sidearm adapter (318 390 004) and side-stopper (318 300 006). **Ventilator gas supply via side-arm but with injector channel open. (Reprinted with permission from the International Anesthesia Research Society, from Borg et al., 1980.)

2. Smaller tidal volumes with lower maximal and mean airway pressure, and therefore lower transpulmonary pressures. Functional residual capacity should, however, be higher than with conventional IPPV/CPPV.
3. Positive intratracheal and negative intrapleural pressures throughout the ventilatory cycle.
4. Less circulatory interference than with conventional IPPV/CPPV.
5. Reflex suppression of spontaneous respiration (under certain conditions) at normocapnia.
6. Decelerating inspiratory flow without end-inspiratory plateau.
7. More efficient pulmonary gas distribution than in conventional IPPV/CPPV.

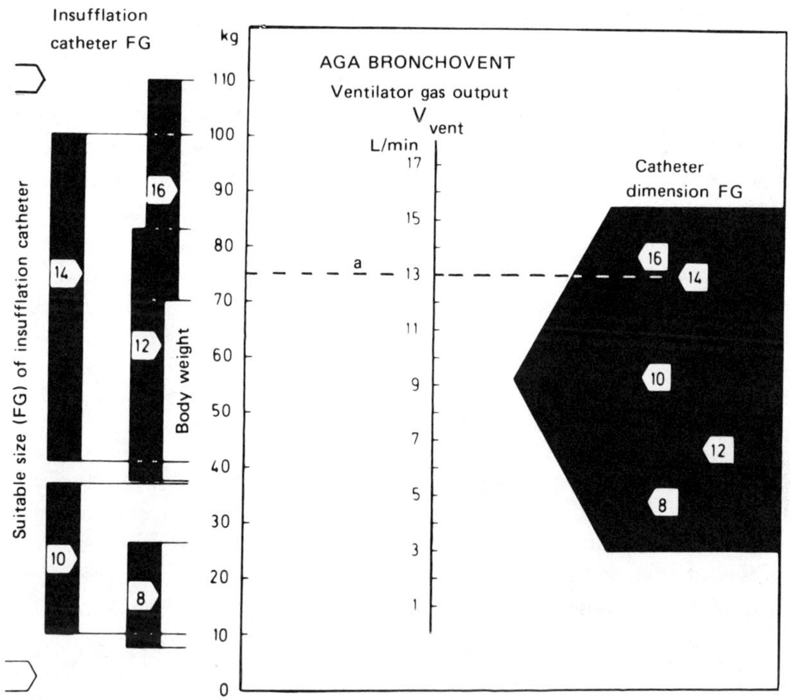

Figure 2 Ventilation nomogram for "laryngoscopic" HFPPV with the Bronchovent (courtesy of Sjöstrand, 1980).

II. Intraoperative Applications of HFPPV

A. Otolaryngology

Peroral endoscopies and surgery are among the most accepted indications for high-frequency positive-pressure ventilation (Scheck et al., 1983). During peroral surgical procedures, the small insufflation catheter allows the surgeon unencumbered access to the airway. Extensive clinical use (Borg et al., 1980; Sjöstrand, 1980) has proved the usefulness and efficacy of this ventilatory technique for procedures lasting from a few minutes to more than 2 hr.

Bronchoscopy

The Wolf and Storz rigid bronchoscopes have both been used with HFPPV (Eriksson and Sjöstrand, 1977; Borg et al., 1980). The ventilator can be connected to the fixed side-arm (Storz 10315) or into a special pneumatic valve adaptor (Wolf

8210). Exhalation takes place through the bronchoscope and in the space between the bronchoscope and the tracheal walls. During rigid bronchoscopy, ventilation can be maintained by insufflation through a catheter placed in the trachea before the bronchoscope is inserted. Gas exchange can be maintained even when the bronchoscope is advanced into one main bronchus, preventing ventilation of that lung. A flexible fiberoptic bronchoscope can be used in intubated patients if the endotracheal tube is wide enough to negotiate the bronchoscope easily, leaving sufficient space for insufflation and expiration. The flexible bronchoscope should be inserted through the pneumatic valve connector or the endotracheal tube. Without the endotracheal tube, HFPPV delivered through a channel of the flexible bronchoscope cannot ventilate patients properly because resistances are excessive.

Laryngoscopy

Laryngoscopy is usually a short procedure, even when a biopsy is performed. To deliver HFPPV, a specially designed insufflation catheter is placed in the trachea (Eriksson and Sjöstrand, 1977; Borg et al., 1980) (Fig. 3). In adults, the distal tip of the catheter should be positioned 1.5-4 cm above the carina for proper ventilation of both lungs. It is advisable to place a marker 8-10 cm above the

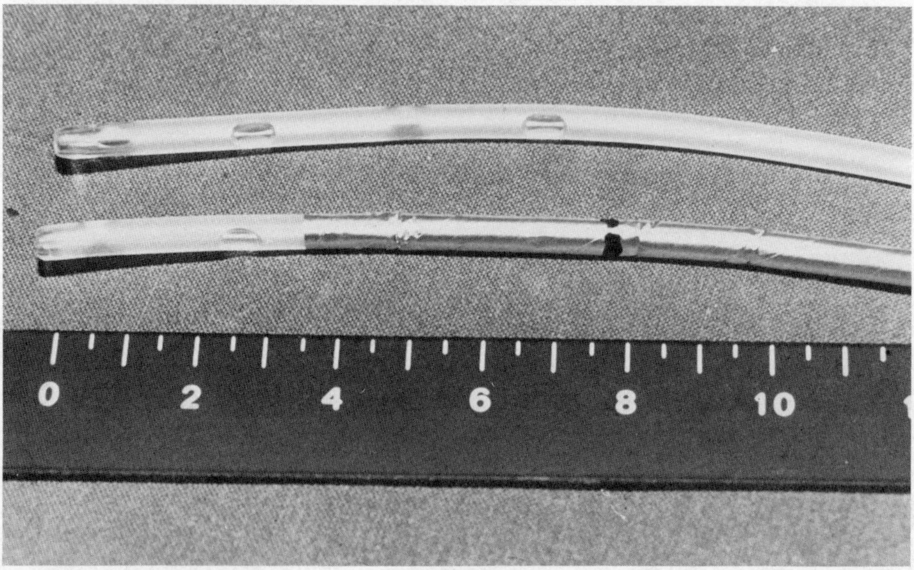

Figure 3 Insufflation catheter (Mediplast, Mölndal, Sweden) for laryngoscopic HFPPV (above) and for laser surgery in the upper airway (below).

distal tip of the catheter, to identify the point that should lie at the level of the vocal cords. Proper positioning of the insufflation catheter is very important, if the rapid gas flow exiting from the central hole of the catheter must ventilate both lungs equally. Gas flow through the side holes is much smaller, but sufficient to prevent air entrainment and inhalation of blood or tissue fragments from the glottic area. Since the internal diameter of the insufflation catheter is small, gas pressure in the catheter must be relatively high during inspiration. To prevent excessive pressures in the lungs, the ventilator is equipped with a pressure transducer, which actuates an audiovisual alarm and automatically disconnects gas flow.

This event may be triggered by coughing, chest compression, or laryngospasm and, during laryngoscopy or bronchoscopy, when the surgeon obstructs free expiration. As soon as the pressure falls below 20 cm H_2O the ventilator automatically resumes function. The nasal route is preferable for insertion of the insufflation catheter. The surgeon's approach is less obstructed and the risk of accidently extracting the catheter during instrumentation of the airway is minimal. It is advisable to ascertain, before anesthesia, whether both nostrils are patent. When possible, the left nostril is preferred because the surgeon carries out the endoscopic procedure from the right corner of the mouth. The insufflation catheter is coated with a silicone-lidocaine spray and inserted into the pharynx of the anesthetized patient. The laryngoscope is then inserted and the catheter advanced into the trachea, occasionally with the aid of a Magill forceps. The catheter is advanced until the marker is positioned between the vocal cords, and then is connected to the ventilator and taped securely to the nose. Adequacy of ventilation is verified by auscultation of the lungs. Sometimes, during difficult intubations in patients with tracheal stenosis, the tip of the catheter may twist 180° upwards in the trachea, redirecting gas flow from the bronchi to the mouth. Physical examination should always be sufficient to verify this problem.

Laryngeal Microsurgery

Microscopic surgery of the larynx is another indication for the use of HFPPV (Borg et al., 1980). Patients are intubated with the insufflation catheter previously described. It is important that the gas flow from the ventilator not induce movement of the insufflation catheter. Similarly, immobility of the vocal cords must be guaranteed, to prevent major difficulties for the surgeon. Exact positioning of the insufflation catheter in the trachea is of the utmost importance.

Laser Surgery in the Larynx

The use of laser beam for airway surgery is becoming more and more important. The major indications are papillomatosis and tumors of the larynx and the glottic area. Since both the surgeon and the anesthesiologist are sharing the very narrow entrance to the upper airway, laryngeal laser surgery poses specific problems. Adequate space must be provided for surgical manipulations, while maintaining life-supporting gas exchange. Ignition of flammable material in the airway must be prevented. HFPPV satisfies the needs of the anesthesiologist and the surgeon alike. Adequate ventilation can be maintained during prolonged anesthesia, while the narrow insufflation catheter leaves ample room for endolaryngeal laser surgery (Scheck and Mallios, 1984).

HFPPV has been successfully employed in 250 patients during carbon dioxide laser treatment in the upper airway. The technique proved safe and effective (Fig. 4).

To prevent ignition, the insufflation catheter should be covered with aluminum foil (15-μm thick), extending toward the catheter tip as far as possible, but leaving at least two side holes patent (Fig. 3). The aluminum foil must be suitably shaped to guarantee firm contact with the insufflation catheter and minimal damage to the nasal mucosa during insertion (Fig. 5). The insufflation cathe-

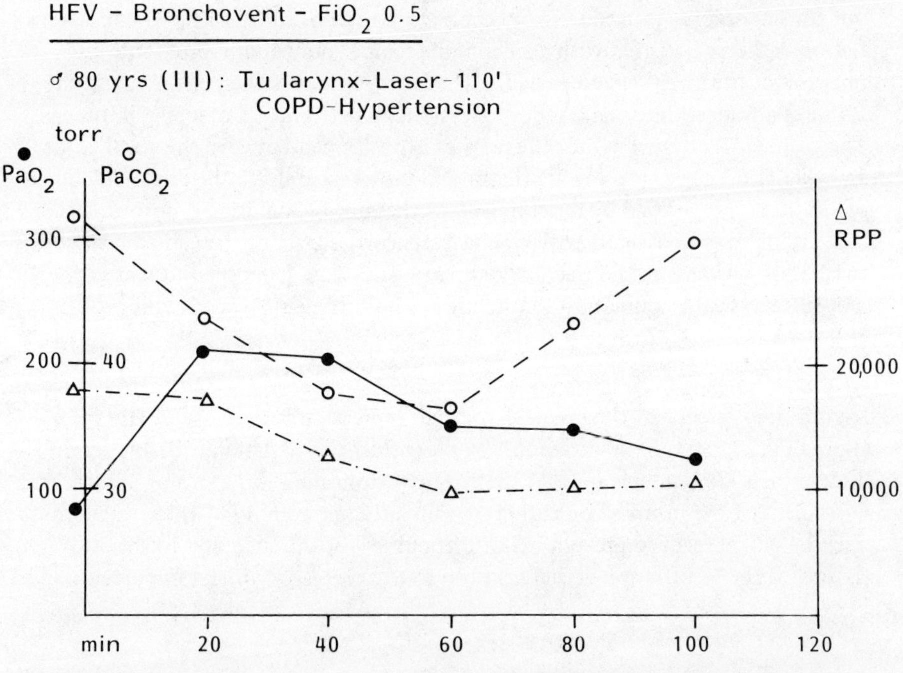

Figure 4 Arterial oxygen and carbon dioxide tension and rate pressure product (RPP) in an 80-year-old man classified ASA type III (chronic obstructive pulmonary disease, hypertension). Laser surgery of a laryngeal tumor, Bronchovent, gas flow 15 liters/min, FiO_2 0.5, insufflation catheter FG 14.

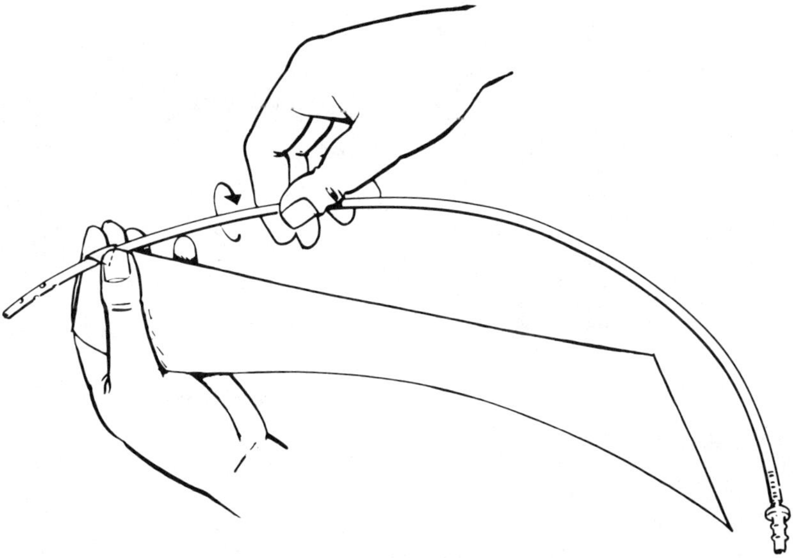

Figure 6 Preshaped aluminum foil to be fixed onto the insufflation catheter.

ter should be lubricated with a silicone spray. In a few cases of extremely bulky laryngeal tumors, which preclude insertion of the PVC catheter, a rigid metal tube, such as a metal suction catheter with an internal diameter of 2.5 mm, can be employed (Fig. 6). When this technique is used with the Bronchovent, $PaCO_2$ levels usually rise slowly, and should be carefully monitored. Occasionally, space-occupying lesions may preclude free exhalation around the catheter. In this case, a second catheter is inserted orally parallel to the insufflation catheter

The main risks of laser surgery of the upper airway are ignition of the endotracheal tube and inhalation of PVC fumes. Protection of the catheter from the laser beam is essential. The technique of wrapping the catheter with household-quality aluminum foil has proven to be satisfactory in experimental laser exposure, as well as in practice. An effective protocol of protective measures has been suggested by Schramm et al. (1981). A minor drawback of thin foil is that it may be lacerated when the catheter is introduced using the Magill forceps. Sturdier aluminum adhesive tape has sharp edges, which may seriously damage the nasal and laryngeal mucosa, if the catheter is bent. Ideally, catheters of flexible, nonflammable material should be manufactured, but they are not yet available. Spontaneous respiration and artificial ventilation with an injector cannula outside the airway without an endotracheal tube or insufflation catheter during laser surgery of the upper airway may lead to poor ventilation, pneumothorax, aspiration of resected material, and overdistention of the stomach.

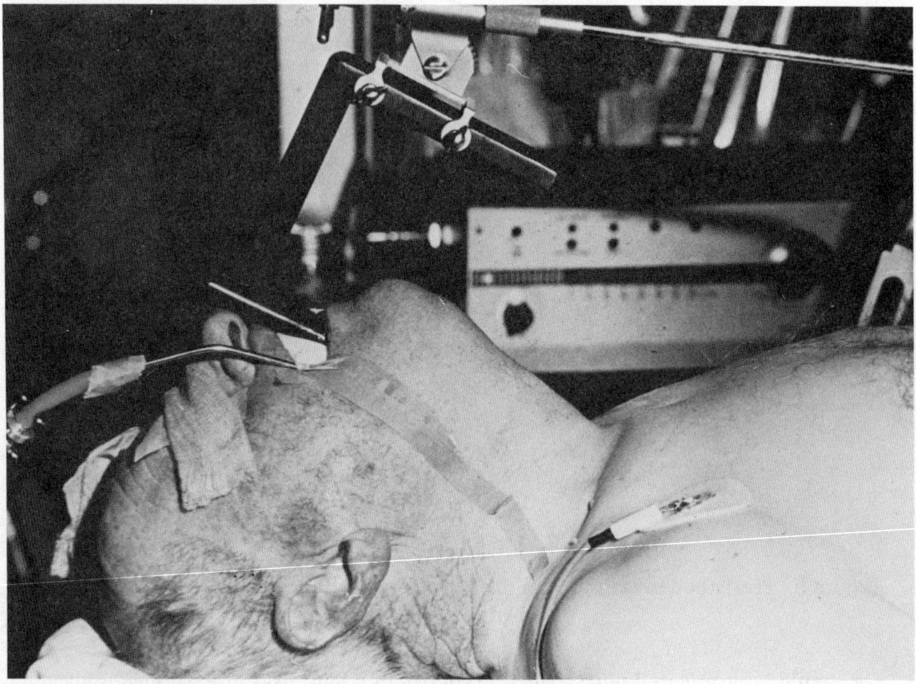

Figure 6 HFPPV with the Bronchovent and a metal suction tube.

Esophagoscopy

To perform esophagoscopy with HFPPV, the insufflation catheter may be positioned in an endotracheal tube or in the trachea, as during laryngoscopy. The technique has proved safe and satisfactory for laser treatment of diverticula in 26 patients (Scheck, 1983, unpublished data).

Tracheotomy

In patients suffocated by large malignancies in the glottic area, emergency tracheostomy is often the only life-saving treatment. Intubation with an armored tube of sufficient diameter is not always possible or may be contraindicated with friable, hemorrhagic tumors. In such cases, HFPPV can be used with a 3-mm insufflation catheter. When this approach is not possible, percutaneous transtracheal ventilation (Klain and Smith, 1977) may be performed, using a plastic or steel needle. It is difficult to apply this method of ventilation with the Bronchovent, since the resistance of the small-diameter needle raises airway pressure, automatically stopping the ventilator.

Ventilation through an existing tracheostomy is simple. The insufflation catheter is positioned with the tip just above the carina. Care must be taken not to push the catheter into a main bronchus. HFPPV has been successful during placement or replacement of laryngeal stint.

B. Thoracic and Cardiac Procedures

Thoracic Surgery

IPPV delivered by the SV-900 servoventilator (Siemens-Elema, Solna, Sweden) was compared to HFPPV delivered by the Bronchovent in patients scheduled for open chest surgery (Malina et al., 1981). Tidal volumes during HFPPV were approximately 25% smaller than estimated anatomical dead space. Ventilation synchronous movements of the lungs were evaluated as well as the development of atelectasis and the operating conditions for the surgeon. During HFPPV the exposed lung was moderately expanded and gas exchange remained adequate although there were only minor movements of the lung during insufflation. The low but constantly positive airway pressure maintained the lungs expanded even during open chest surgery. Ventilation could be confirmed even during suctioning of the airways. For sleeve pneumonectomy when the carina was also excised (Fig. 7), a high-frequency positive-pressure ventilator with personal modifications was used (El-Baz et al., 1983). An anastomosis between the trachea and the main bronchus was performed while the patient was ventilated through an insufflation

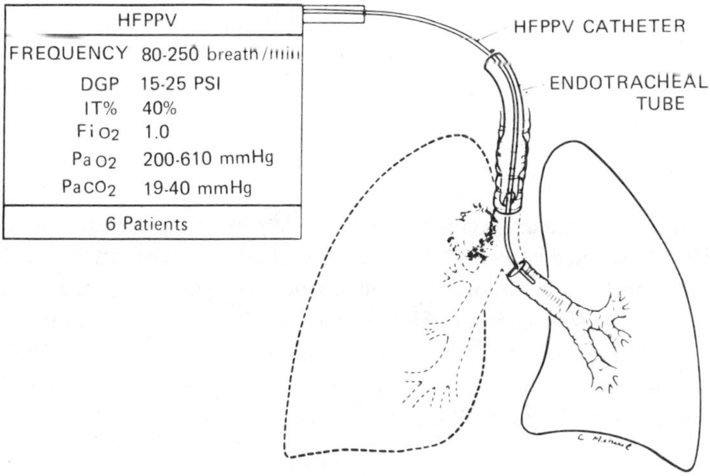

Figure 7 HFPPV for sleeve pneumonectomy (reproduced from El-Baz, 1983, by permission).

catheter positioned into an endotracheal tube. The small tidal volumes minimized movements of bronchi and other mediastinal structures.

Thoracoscopy

HFPPV was useful during thoracoscopies. The limited movement of the lungs during ventilation facilitates detailed examination of the lung surface (Scheck, 1983, unpublished data).

Tracheal Stenosis

HFPPV has been successfully used during surgery for tracheal stenosis and subsequent tracheoscopies (Eriksson et al., 1975).

Cardiac Surgery

Respirator and hemodynamic effects of HFPPV and IPPV in patients undergoing open heart surgery were compared (Swartzman et al., 1983). Patients were adequately ventilated with both types of ventilation and no differences in cardiac function were observed in the pre- or postbypass period.

C. Neurological Surgery

Experimental studies (Borg et al., 1982; Bunegin et al., 1983; Todd et al., 1981) showed substantially reduced brain movements during the use of different HFV systems when compared with IPPV. Confirmation of this finding may encourage the clinical use of HFV for microsurgical procedures in humans. Spontaneous respiration is often depressed after neurosurgical procedures. In the immediate postoperative period, HFPPV may help to provide adequate gas exchange as long as respiration is depressed. Most patients easily adapt to the ventilatory support without the requirement for sedation, which is often undesirable after neurosurgical interventions.

D. Plastic Surgery

In neonates and infants undergoing repair of a cleft lip or palate (Heyman et al., 1977), HFPPV worked very satisfactorily. Anesthesia included halothane for induction, droperidol and fentanyl for maintenance, and pancuronium bromide for muscle relaxation. Ventilation at 60 breaths/min with an insufflation time of 32% resulted in moderate hypocapnia and an arterial PO_2 above normal. Repeated measurements of blood gases were required to maintain the hyperventilation. After reversal of curarization, the infants did not fight the ventilator.

E. HFPPV for Patients in Poor Physical Condition

A clinical investigation was conducted in patients with pulmonary or cardiovascular pathological conditions or mechanical obstructions of the upper airway (Scheck and Mallios, 1984). The study considered more than 600 patients, 155 of whom were classified in the ASA physical fitness groups III and IV.

An air-oxygen mixture was used for all patients; FiO_2 varied between 0.3 and 0.7 but was 0.5 in the vast majority of cases. Various endoscopic precedures and laser surgery were performed. Gas exchange was adequate during short procedures as well as after interventions lasting more than 90 min.

F. Postoperative and Intensive Care

HFPPV and other HFV systems have been successfully used for the treatment of severe hyaline membrane disease (Bland et al., 1980) in preterm infants, adult respiratory distress syndrome (Bjerager et al., 1977; Carlon et al., 1979, 1980), respiratory failure (Wattwil et al., 1983), bronchopleural fistulae (Carlon et al., 1980), and weaning. It has also been successful in emergency situations to support patients with bleeding tumors of the upper airway or acute glottis edema.

G. Anesthesia During HFPPV

To prevent pollution of the operating room, inhalation anesthetics should not be used with open ventilatory techniques. Patients should be supported with oxygen enriched air only (FiO_2 0.3-0.5) and total intravenous anesthesia. After endoscopic procedures, the shortest possible period of unconsciousness is desirable.

The most effective anesthetic procedure combines a short-acting hypnotic agent, such as etomidate or methohexitol, a very-short-acting narcotic analgesic, alfentanil, and succinylcholine for muscle relaxation. These drugs are used for induction as well as maintenance. Discrete drug injections often fail to produce stable anesthesia, and continuous infusions are preferable. An effective technique combines 125 mg etomidate or 500 mg methohexitol with 5 mg alfentanil in a 250-ml glucose/saline solution. The infusion is started after induction of anesthesia and is administered with a volumetric infusion pump. Stable anesthesia is usually achieved with infusion rate of 200 mg/hr for the first 10 min. The respective dosages are: etomidate 25 μg/kg per min or methohexitol 100 μg/kg per min and alfentanil 1 μg/kg per min. This infusion rate is followed by a constant administration of 100 ml/hr (Mallios and Scheck, 1983).

A second infusion of a 0.1% solution of succinylcholine is used when the vocal cords must be immobilized for microlaryngeal surgery or laser treatment. For other surgical procedures not involving the vocal cords, nondepolarizing relaxants may be used.

III. Conclusions

Methods of artificial ventilation which use supraphysiological frequencies are being actively studied by researchers and clinicians to identify their proper place in medical practice.

The experience gathered by many different investigators demonstrates that high-frequency positive-pressure ventilation is an effective tool, which provides definite advantages to patients undergoing bronchoscopy, laryngoscopy, and surgery of the glottic region and upper airway.

There is no convincing clinical evidence that HFPPV is superior to IPPV during anesthesia for neurological or plastic surgery. Postoperative use might be beneficial after intracranial surgery. In critical care, bronchopleural fistulae appear the most valid indication for HFPPV or other modalities of high frequency ventilation.

Potential disadvantages of HFPPV include:

1. Wastefully high gas flows
2. Uncontrollable alveolar minute volume
3. Need for devices markedly different from those delivering IPPV
4. Poor control of humidification

Development of new mechanical ventilators, with low compressible volume and enhanced monitoring, will greatly facilitate widespread use of this new modality of ventilatory support.

References

Bjerager, K., Sjöstrand, U., and Wattwil, M. (1977). Long-term treatment of two patients with respiratory insufficiency with IPPV/PEEP and HFPPV/PEEP. *Acta Anaesth. Scand. Suppl.* **64**:55.

Bland, R. D., Kim, M. H., Light, M., and Woodson, J. L. (1980). High frequency mechanical ventilation in severe hyaline membrane disease: an alternative treatment? *Crit. Care Med.* **8**:275.

Borg, U., Eriksson, I., and Sjöstrand, U. (1980). High frequency positive pressure ventilation (HFPPV): A review based upon its use during bronchoscopy and for laryngoscopy and microlaryngeal surgery under general anaesthesia. *Anesth. Analg.* **59**:594.

Borg, U., Eriksson, I., Sjöstrand, U., and Wattwil, M. (1981). Experimental studies of continuous positive pressure ventilation (CPPV) and high frequency positive pressure ventilation (HFPPV). *Resuscitation* **9**:1.

Borg, U., Babinski, M., Bunegin, L., Sjöstrand, U. H., and Smith, R. B. (1982).

Abolished intracranial pressure fluctuations with high frequency ventilation. *Anaesthesia* **37**:407.

Briscoe, W. A., Forster, R. E., and Conroe, J. H. (1954). Alveolar ventilation at very low tidal volumes. *J. Appl. Physiol.* **7**:27.

Bunegin, L., Borg, U. R., Helsel, P., Sjöstrand, U. H., Albin, M. S., and Smith, R. B. (1982). Cerebral blood flow during HFPPV and IPPV at normal and elevated ICP. *Anesthesiology* **57**:A465.

Carlon, G. C., Ray, C., Kahn, R. C., and Howland, W. S. (1979). High frequency positive pressure ventilation for prolonged respiratory support. *Anesthesiology* **51**:S189.

Carlon, G. C., Ray, C., Klain, M., McCormack, P. M. (1980). High frequency positive pressure ventilation in a patient with broncho-pleural fistula. *Anesthesiology* **52**:160.

El-Baz, N., El-Ganzouri, A., and Ivankovich, A. (1983). High frequency positive pressure ventilation for major airway surgery. In *Perspectives in High Frequency Ventilation.* Edited by P. A. Scheck, U. H. Sjöstrand, and R. B. Smith. The Hague, Martinus Nijhoff, pp. 216-226.

Eriksson, T., and Sjöstrand, U. (1980). Effects of high frequency positive pressure ventilation (HFPPV) and general anesthesia on intrapulmonary gas distribution in patients undergoing diagnostic bronchoscopy. *Anesth. Analg.* **59**:585.

Eriksson, I., Nilsson, L. G., Nordström, S., and Sjöstrand, U. (1975). High frequency positive pressure ventilation (HFPPV) during transthoracic resection of tracheal stenosis and during preoperative bronchoscopic examination. *Acta Anaesth. Scand.* **19**:113.

Eriksson, I., and Sjöstrand, U. (1977). Experimental and clinical evaluation of high frequency positive pressure ventilation (HFPPV) and the pneumatic valve principle in bronchoscopy under general anaesthesia. *Acta Anaesth. Scand. Suppl.* **64**:83.

Eriksson, I., Jonzon, A., Sedin, G., and Sjöstrand, U. (1977). The influence of the ventilatory pattern on ventilation, circulation, and oxygen transport during continuous positive pressure ventilation. *Acta Anaesth. Scand. Suppl.* **64**:149.

Forrest, J. B., and Chambers, C. (1983). Effects of volatile anaesthetics on tracheal mucociliary transport. *Canad. Anaesth. Soc. J.* **30**, Suppl. part II: 577.

Frank, I., Noack, W., Lunkenheimer, P. P., Ising, H., Keller, H., Dickuth, H. H., Rafflenbeul, W., and Jacobsen, M. (1975). Light and electron microscopic investigations of pulmonary tissue after high frequency positive pressure ventilation (HFPPV). *Anaesthesist* **24**:171.

Heijman, K., Heijman, L., Jonzon, A., and Sjöstrand, U. (1972). High frequency positive pressure ventilation during anaesthesia and routine surgery in man. *Acta Anaesth. Scand.* **16**:176.

Heijman, L., Nilsson, L. G., and Sjöstrand, U. (1977). High frequency positive pressure ventilation (HFPPV) in neonates and infants during neurolept analgesia and routine plastic surgery and postoperative management. *Acta Anaesth. Scand. Suppl.* **64**:111.

Henderson, Y., Chillingworth, F. D., and Whitney, J. L. (1915). The respiratory dead space. *Am. J. Physiol.* **38**:1.

Jonzon, A., Sedin, G., and Sjöstrand, U. (1973). High frequency positive pressure ventilation (HFPPV) applied for small lung ventilation and compared with spontaneous respiration and continuous positive airway pressure (CPAP). *Acta Anaesth. Scand. Suppl.* **23**.

Jonzon, A., Oberg, P. A., Sedin, G., and Sjöstrand, U. (1980). High frequency low tidal volume positive pressure ventilation. *Acta Physiol. Scand.* **80**:21.

Klain, M., and Smith, R. B. (1977). High frequency percutaneous transtracheal jet ventilation. *Crit. Care Med.* **5**:280.

Malina, J. R., Nordström, S. G., Sjöstrand, U. H., and Wattwil, L. M. (1981). Clinical evaluation of high frequency positive pressure ventilation (HFPPV) in patients scheduled for open-chest surgery. *Anesth. Analg.* **60**:324.

Mallios, C., and Scheck, P. A. (1983). Total intravenous anesthesia during high frequency ventilation. In *Perspectives in High Frequency Ventilation.* Edited by P. A. Scheck, U. H. Sjöstrand, and R. B. Smith. The Hague, Mattinus Nijhoff, pp. 198-203.

Mankikar, D., Ramanathan, S., Rock, I., and Turndorf, H. (1982). Hemodynamic effects of HFPPV and IPPV during acute hemorrhage. *Anesthesiology* **57**: A466.

Öberg, P. A., and Sjöstrand, U. (1969). Studies of blood pressure regulation. Common carotid artery clamping in studies of the carotid sinus baroreceptor control of the systemic blood pressure. *Acta Physiol. Scand.* **75**:276.

Scheck, P. A., and Mallios, C. (1984). Peroral endoscopies using intravenous anesthesia and high-frequency ventilation. *Crit. Care Med.* **12**:803.

Scheck, P. A., Mallios, C., and Knegt, P. (1983). High frequency ventilation for laser surgery of the larynx. In *Perspectives in High Frequency Ventilation.* Edited by P. A. Scheck, U. H. Sjöstrand, and R. B. Smith. The Hague, Martinus Nijhoff, pp. 204-211.

Scheck, P. A., Mallios, C., Knegt, P., and Van der Schans, E. J. (1984). High frequency ventilation in laser surgery of the larynx. *Clin. Otolaryngol.* **9**: 203.

Schramm, V. L., Mattox, D. E., and Stool, S. E. (1981). Acute management of laser ignited intratracheal explosion. *Laryngoscope* **91**:1417.

Sjöstrand, U. (1980). High frequency positive pressure ventilation. A review. *Crit. Care Med.* **8**:345.

Sjöstrand, U. (1982). High frequency ventilation. *Acta Anaesth. Belg.* **34**:259.

Sjöstrand, U. H., and Eriksson, I. A. (1980). High rates and low volumes in mechanical ventilation: not just a matter of ventilatory frequency. *Anesth. Analg.* **59**:567.

Swartzman, S., Babinski, M. F., Smith R. B., Saunders, T., Trinkle, K., and Grover, F. (1983). HFPPV and IPPV in open-heart surgery. *Anesthesiology* **59**: A79.

Todd, M. M., Toutant, S. M., and Shapiro, H. M. (1981). The effects of high-frequency positive pressure ventilation on intracranial pressure and brain surface movement in cats. *Anesthesiology* **54**:496.

Wattwil, L. M., Sjöstrand, U. H., and Borg, U. R. (1983). Comparative studies of IPPV and HFPPV with PEEP in critical care patients. I: A clinical evaluation. *Crit. Care Med.* **11**:30.

5

High-Frequency Positive Pressure Ventilation

Use in Neonatal and Adult Intensive Care

ANDREW GETTINGER and D. DAVID GLASS

Dartmouth-Hitchcock Medical Center
Dartmouth Medical School
Hanover, New Hampshire

This chapter will focus on the application of high-frequency positive-pressure ventilation (HFPPV) in the management of neonatal and adult respiratory failure. Before doing this we will discuss some of the problems in defining high-frequency positive pressure ventilation, and in comparing work done in different institutions with differing methodologies and ventilators. In addition to reviewing the literature, we will describe our use of high-frequency ventilation in the intensive care units of the Dartmouth-Hitchcock Medical Center during the past 4 years. We will discuss the hemodynamic effects of high-frequency ventilation, problems with humidification, and questions about barotrauma.

What is high-frequency positive-pressure ventilation? Is it just a matter of rate, as some authors have suggested, or is it dependent on the design and performance characteristics of the specific ventilator? Can a conventional ventilator deliver high-frequency positive-pressure ventilation just by increasing the rate and decreasing the tidal volume? Recent reviews (O'Rourke and Crone, 1983; Gillespie, 1983; Gallagher et al., 1982), while acknowledging differences in the mechanisms of gas displacement, have suggested distinctions between the three types of high-frequency ventilation based on rate: HFPPV occurring at rates between 50 and 150 breaths/min; high-frequency jet ventilation (HFJV) occurring at rates from 60 up to 400-600 breaths/min; and high-frequency oscillation (HFO) occurring at rates from 400-3000 breaths/min. However, Sjostrand (1980) further characterized the pattern of HFPPV as having the following characteristics:

1. A frequency of about 60-100 breaths/min with less than 30% of the respiratory cycle spent in inspiration
2. Smaller tidal volumes (than conventional convective ventilatory techniques) leading to lower peak and mean airway pressures
3. Positive intratracheal but negative pleural pressures throughout the respiratory cycle
4. Less cardiovascular effects than conventional IPPV/CPPV
5. Decelerating inspiratory flow without an inspiratory plateau
6. Efficient pulmonary gas distribution

Sjostrand stressed that, in order to meet these goals, ventilators capable of HFPPV must include the following features: a negligible compression volume, minimal internal compliance, and no increase in functional deadspace. To these ends, Sjostrand (1983) developed a system of gas delivery based on the "pneumatic valve" principle. A mixture of conditioned gas is intermittently delivered through the side port of a specially designed connector allowing ventilation without entrainment of gas, although the system has no unidirectional valves. A further modification, "System H," featured the addition of a valve on the expiratory limb, which is closed during inspiration. This improved the efficiency of the system by reducing gas vented during inspiration. The use of a double-lumen endotracheal tube with an insufflation to expiration lumen diameter ratio of 1:10 and an expiratory valve further inproved ventilatory efficiency and allowed for the use of positive end-expiratory pressure: "System J." Other investigators (Bland et al., 1980; Abu-Dbai et al., 1983) have used conventional ventilators set to deliver reduced tidal volumes or pressures and high rates to administer HFPPV. Still other investigators (Whitwam et al., 1983) have reported clinical results with prototype ventilators using rates consistent with HFPPV but methods of gas delivery based on jet injectors (HFJV). HFJV is distinguished from HFPPV not by the rate but by the presence of entrainment, provided by a gas reservoir. It becomes a difficult to attempt to characterize clinical experiences with high-frequency ventilation when either the mechanism of gas exchange is not known or when the system combines features of both HFPPV and HFJV.

The method of high-frequency ventilation used at the Dartmouth-Hitchcock Medical Center combines elements of both HFPPV and HFJV but the precise mechanism of gas displacement has not been characterized. The ventilator, designed by John H. Emerson, consists of a rotating ball valve, controlled by a variable-speed motor. The valve "interrupts" a flow of gas to which an additional mixture of heated, humidified gas is added distal to the ball valve. The combina-

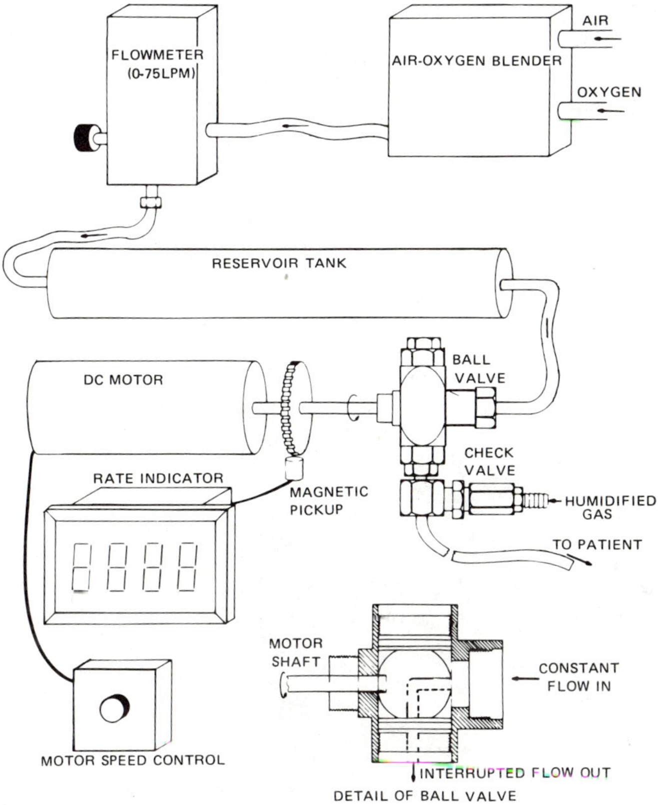

Figure 1 Schematic drawing of Emerson Airway Flow Interrupter used for HFPPV.

tion of gases is then directed via minimally compressible, low volume tubing into the proximal airway (Fig. 1). This is accomplished in one of two ways: via a #3.0 pediatric endotracheal tube introduced through a Norman elbow and into an adult endotracheal tube (Fig. 2) or more distally in the trachea via a double-lumen high-frequency endotracheal tube (National Catheter Corp.) (Fig. 3). Exhalation occurs

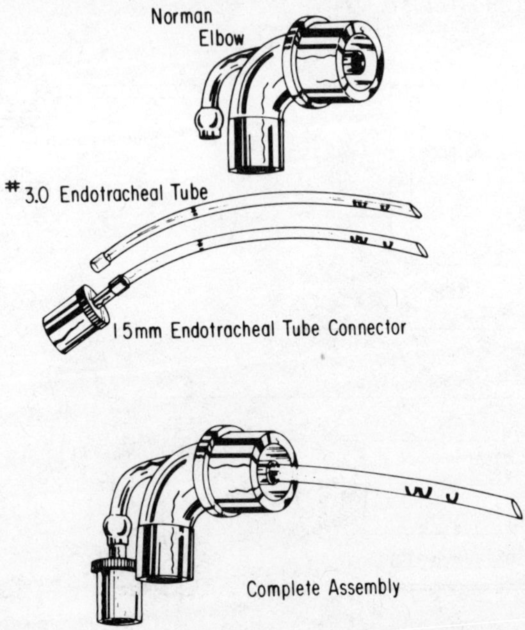

Figure 2 Modified Norman elbow used to introduce HFPPV into the proximal airway at the endotracheal tube connector.

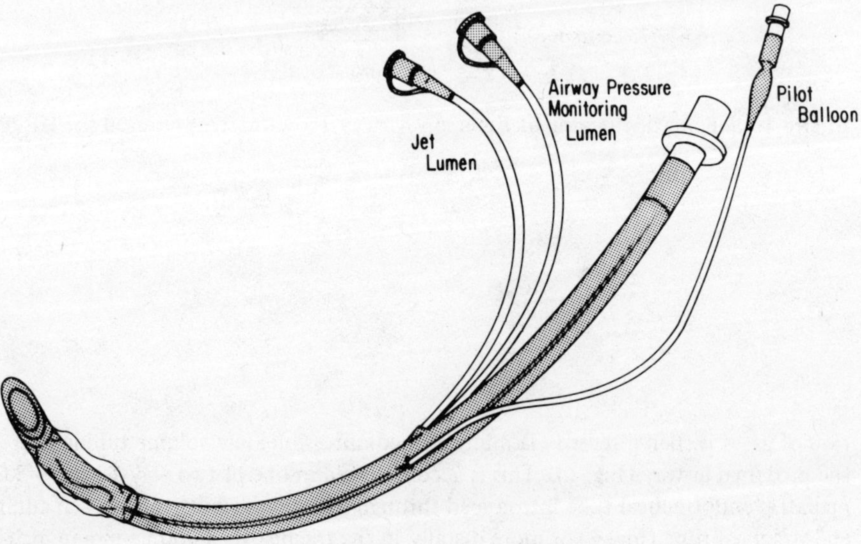

Figure 3 National Catheter Corp. Hi-Lo jet endotracheal tube.

passively by the circuit on the attached conventional Emerson volume ventilator. The addition of the conventional ventilator provides a means to add positive end-expiratory pressure (PEEP) to the system and permits the interposition of conventional intermittent mandatory ventilation together with the high-frequency ventilation. The use of the conventional ventilator also allows release of excessive airway pressure, via a pop-off valve, limiting the extent of barotrauma.

We will focus in the remainder of the chapter on our observations regarding the use of high-frequency positive-pressure ventilation in intensive care, the published experience of Dr. Sjostrand and his colleagues, and that of others in both adult and pediatric populations. Reviews of HFJV, HFO, and use of HFPPV in the operating room appear elsewhere in this text.

I. Neonatal HFPPV

Respiratory failure requiring mechanical ventilation in the premature or newborn infant can present difficult management problems. Barotrauma, including pneumothorax and/or pulmonary interstitial emphysema, is a frequent and serious complication. Bland and colleagues (1980) reported a series of 24 consecutive preterm infants with respiratory failure secondary to hyaline membrane disease who were ventilated mechanically at rates from 60 to 100 breaths/min with peak inspiratory pressures of 15-25 cm H_2O and PEEP of 4-6 cm H_2O. Support was supplemented with periods of manual ventilation at rates of 100-180 breaths/min. Eighteen of the infants were ventilated with the Bourns LS 104-105 respirator, two with a Baby Bird respirator, and the remaining with both ventilators at different times. The infants were ventilated if they were apneic or bradycardic, had a $Paco_2 > 55$ torr with a $pH < 7.25$, or a $Pao_2 < 50$ torr despite CPAP (up to 10 cm H_2O) and $Fio_2 > 0.8$. Ninety-two percent of the infants survived and there was a low incidence of major complications. The authors suggest that their approach is viable and worthy of controlled trials comparing it to conventional methods.

HFPPV has been used extensively intraoperatively, especially for procedures involving the airway. In 1977, Sjostrand and his colleagues (Heijman et al., 1977) reported the use of their open "pneumatic valve" system in 19 children ranging in weight from 2.1 to 16.8 kg. Two of these patients were ventilated with HFPPV postoperatively. Both underwent intra-abdominal procedures in the first 2 days of life. One was ventilated for 13 hr postoperatively, the other for 6 days. Upper-airway and endotracheal pressures were monitored. HFPPV rate was 60 breaths/min with an inspiratory time of 32%. Arterialized capillary blood values were evaluated to assess the adequacy of ventilation. No complications were reported. Both neonates were described as calm and without spontaneous respiratory efforts while ventilated with HFPPV. In a more recent report from the same institution

Wattwill (1982) describes the use of HFPPV in seven children less than 1 year old and 32 neonates less than 100 hr old with infant respiratory distress syndrome (IRDS). No complications were noted in the children. There were five cases of pneumothorax in the neonates. It is difficult to assess the significance of this complication due to the frequency of barotrauma in neonates ventilated for IRDS because of the nature of the disease and poor pulmonary compliance.

Several other groups (Karl et al., 1983; Frantz et al., 1983) have used another system, the Emerson airway flow interrupter, in the management of neonates with respiratory failure. We will describe their findings in this section, although the frequencies used exceed those commonly considered as HFPPV. Frantz et al., (1983) studied two different groups of infants. One group consisted of 10 infants with IRDS in the first 2 days of life who were stable on conventional ventilation (Baby Bird) but required $FiO_2 > 0.40$ and/or peak inspiratory pressures > 25 cm H_2O. They were ventilated with the Emerson flow interrupter for approximately 1 hr. Blood gas values and airway pressures were evaluated. Five additional infants with severe IRDS who developed progressive pulmonary interstitial emphysema (PIE) during conventional mechanical ventilation were switched to high-frequency ventilation. Of note, these five infants had failed to respond to the form of HFPPV with conventional ventilators employed by Bland and co-workers (1980). In Frantz's study, the flow interrupter was directed at right angles to the endotracheal tube. The expiratory limb was distal to the endotracheal tube and had a greater impedance than that of the infant's lungs. Distending airway pressure was maintained with a variable diameter orifice, placed distally in the expiratory limb. Frequencies varied from 30 to 1200 breaths/min. In the 10 patients with IRDS, comparable arterial blood gases were obtained with lower *peak* tracheal pressures and similar *mean* tracheal pressures. No adverse effects were observed except a transient metabolic acidosis (responsive to fluid therapy), in one patient. The institution of high-frequency ventilation in the group with PIE allowed two infants to be weaned from all ventilatory support within 72 hr. A third infant with bronchopulmonary dysplasia required 26 days of high-frequency ventilation before being weaned from respiratory support. During that time attempts to reinstitute conventional ventilation were unsuccessful. The remaining two patients showed initial improvement in their arterial blood gases followed by deterioration and death 2 days after the switch to high-frequency ventilation. The authors suggest that high-frequency ventilation may reduce preexisting barotrauma or prevent its development in IRDS and that controlled trials are necessary.

Karl and colleagues (1983) reported transient improvement using the Emerson flow interrupter in four seriously ill infants with hypoplastic pulmonary parenchyma and persistent fetal circulation associated with congenital diaphragmatic hernia. These patients had failed to respond to manual ventilation at rates of up to 200 breaths/min and therapy with both tolazoline and indomethacin. Respiratory alkalosis, improved oxygenation, and reduced ductal shunting were obtained with high frequency rates of 375-1800 breaths/min. Mean airway pressures were less than 15 mmHg. Karl's technique differs from that of Frantz because the flow interrupter is directed down the endotracheal tube with the exhalation at right angles to the tube. Airway pressure is controlled by varying the resistance in the expiration port. Karl concludes that high-frequency ventilation offers a means to ventilate neonates who have failed to respond to conventional ventilation but that in this group of critically ill infants the use of high-frequency ventilation was successful only for short periods of hours to days. There were no survivors.

II. Adult HFPPV

As with infants, adults have also been successfully ventilated with conventional ventilators set to frequencies consistent with HFPPV. Abu-Dbai and colleagues (1983) reported on a group of 10 patients with respiratory failure of diverse causes in whom modified conventional ventilators were used to produce HFPPV. Bennett MA-1B and MA-2 ventilators with low-compliance tubing, rates of 66-70 breaths/min, tidal volumes of 1-3 ml/kg, and peak flow rates of 100 or 125 liters/min were used. Airway pressures at the distal end of the endotracheal tube, hemodynamic variables, and both arterial and mixed venous blood gases were measured at 15-min intervals after a 2-hr equilibration period. Following the first 45-min data collection, the patient was switched to conventional ventilation (12-16 breaths/min; tidal volume 10-15 ml/kg) for 1 hr followed by a second 45-min trial of HFPPV. Oxygenation and ventilation did not change substantially. Oxygen delivery improved as a result of the increase in cardiac output. PEEP and oxygen concentrations were constant. In this varied group of patients one patient was diagnosed as being status asthmaticus, a condition which many believe is not responsive to high-frequency ventilation.

In 1977 the first long-term treatment of respiratory failure managed with HFPPV was reported. Bjerager, using an early prototype ventilator with a "pneumatic valve," was able to reduce the amount of sedative agents given to two patients. Heavy sedation had been required to prevent discoordination between ventilator and these patients using conventional ventilation. At a rate of 60 breaths/min and an inspiratory time of 32% of the cycle, one patient was ventilated for 6 days before being weaned from ventilatory support. A second patient developed adult respiratory distress syndrome (ARDS) following aortic surgery and was ventilated with HFPPV to reduce the amount of sedatives she required. Her course was further complicated by coagulopathy leading to intrapulmonary hemorrhage after 10 days of HFPPV. Before she died 19 days later, attempts to change from HFPPV to conventional ventilation failed secondary to agitation of the patient and inadequate alveolar ventilation. It is tempting to speculate whether some of the "large crusts" and later "pencil-thick organized clot" were solely a result of the patient's disease or complications from inadequate humidification reported in some high-frequency systems (Nordin et al., 1981). In any case, these two patients demonstrated the potential use of prolonged HFPPV.

Wattwill and colleagues (1983a,b) and Sjostrand (1983) reported more recently on a group of 10 patients in respiratory failure who were ventilated with HFPPV (System H) and conventional ventilation. Both clinical parameters and intrapulmonary gas distribution were measured. The comparison was made when the "acute phase of the disease had subsided." The patients had adequate oxygenation with an FiO_2 of 0.3 and 10 cm H_2O of PEEP. Cardiac index and gas exchange were not affected by HFPPV. Comparable carbon dioxide elimination was provided with lower tidal volumes and lower mean airway pressures than with conventional ventilation. Respirator-induced fluctuations in intravascular pressure monitors were eliminated with HFPPV. The need for sedatives to achieve ventilator-patient coordination was reduced from 20 to 50% with HFPPV. The uniform reduction in arterial oxygenation during suctioning was comparatively less with HFPPV than with conventional ventilation. In the companion article (Wattwill et al., 1983b), the effect on intrapulmonary gas distribution was observed using a nitrogen washout technique. HFPPV was found to deliver ventilation with the highest linear velocity. The resulting turbulence produced gas mixing in conducting airways. No instances of barotrauma were recorded in these patients. The authors suggest that HFPPV is equivalant to conventional ventilation in cardiac performance and oxygen transport, advantageous because of the reduced need for sedatives, superior in allowing suctioning of the airway to occur while ventilation continues, and potentially superior in terms of a lesser incidence of barotrauma.

HFPPV has also been used in conjunction with conventional ventilation in the treatment of unilateral lung disease (Miranda et al., 1981). A 53-year-old victim of a motor vehicle accident suffered a left-lung contusion with nine associated rib fractures. The injury caused hypoxemia and hypercarbia which were unresponsive to conventional ventilation and differential lung ventilation via a Robert-Shaw double-lumen endobronchial tube. The addition of HFPPV (Amsterdam infant ventilator set at 10 liters/min, frequency 60 breaths/min, I/E of 1:1, and PEEP of 25 cm H_2O) to the left lung while conventional ventilation continued to the right lung allowed for better overall ventilation and oxygenation. HFPPV continued for 24 hr and independent lung ventilation an additional 24 hr. The patient was weaned from mechanical ventilation and extubated 10 days later. While this report is limited to one patient, we will subsequently describe a comparable approach to the management of unilateral lung disease.

HFPPV at the Dartmouth-Hitchcock Medical Center was introduced into clinical practice in 1979 (following preliminary laboratory evaluation) as a "heroic" measure in a patient with severe refractory respiratory failure who was not responsive to conventional support with IMV and high levels of PEEP. Our technique has evolved over the intervening years as our clinical experience with HFPPV has expanded. We will discuss the evolution of our current method, indications for HFPPV, and results in 50 of our patients. This represents approximately one-third of our clinical experience for which data are presently available.

As previously mentioned, we have used the Emerson airway flow interruptor to provide HFPPV. This device has a fixed I/E ratio of 33%. Flow rates can be varied up to 70 liters/min and frequency can be varied up to 3000 breaths/min. Humidification was initially provided via a constant volumetric infusion of saline dripped into the proximal airway and nebulized by the gas flow, but was not adequate. Typically there was an initial prompt mobilization of airway secretions which then became tenacious and inspissated and became a potential cause of airway obstruction. This system humidified but did not warm the gases. Additional concern about the projectile effects of nebulized saline on tracheobronchial mucosa was expressed following postmortem histopathological study. Distinguishing between pathological changes associated with the disease and that resulting from treatment modalities is always problematic. Work on experimental animals, done by Dr. Klain and colleagues (Nordin et al., 1981) in Pittsburgh using HFJV, suggests that there is a narrow window of humidification that will preserve mucociliary transport: too little results in dry inspissated secretions, too much causes pooling in the airways and impairs gas exchange. No doubt this is also the case with HFPPV. Currently we add 5-10 liters/min of warmed, humidified gas to the bulk of the HFPPV gas as it exits from the flow interrupter (a distance of 60-90 cm away from the proximal airway). Formal continuous monitoring of humidity is not routine, but the new system has greatly reduced previous problems with humidification. Intermittent direct visualization of the trachea and major bronchi via fiberoptic endoscopy is performed when indicated both to remove secretions and to assess the adequacy of humidification.

Another issue in the development of HFPPV has been the need to incorporate safeguards into the apparatus to monitor inadvertent disconnections or development of excessive airway pressures (and to respond to them automatically). This need has led us to incorporate the HFPPV into the circuit of a conventional Emerson model 3 PV volume ventilator. The alarm used with the volume ventilator serves as a disconnect monitor when the two ventilators are used together. Also, a manually set pop-off valve will automatically release pressure when its preset limit is exceeded. In contrast to other systems, flow from the high-frequency system is not automatically stopped but pressure is limited.

The use of the conventional ventilator circuit also allows for PEEP to be incorporated into the expiratory limb with a water column. The need for PEEP in addition to HFPPV, HFJV, or HFO is highly controversial and probably dependent on the individual ventilator and how it is used. Our experience has been better in terms of oxygenation and reduced A-a gradients when PEEP (usually a low level of 5-10 cm H_2O) has been used with HFPPV.

A final advantage to having the conventional ventilator in the circuit with the flow interrupter is the ability to add conventional IMV breaths to HFPPV simultaneously. Our early experience with HFPPV was that oxygenation initially improved dramatically but then frequently deteriorated with time. Brief periods of manual ventilation were again followed by improved oxygenation. The incorporation of low rates of MINV (2-4 breaths/min) at reduced tidal volumes (to avoid excessive airway pressures) accomplishes the same end. Experimental support for this approach has been reported in two animal models of lung injury treated with HFO and conventional ventilation (Kolton et al., 1982). When a sustained inflation was combined with HFO, oxygenation improved. The authors suggest that the high peak inspiratory pressure of conventional breaths opens alveoli with elevated critical opening pressure, expanding lung volume, and permitting high-frequency ventilation to occur at a more favorable point of the pressure/volume hysteresis curve.

Until recently, the conventional IMV breath was superimposed in HFPPV, which was delivered continuously. We are currently evaluating a design modification in the Emerson flow interrupter that allows the HFPPV to be shut off automatically with the initiation of each conventional IMV breath. This may provide more flexibility in the size and inspiratory time of the conventional "sigh" IMV breath.

Our indications for HFPPV have expanded as our clinical experience has accumulated. Initially HFPPV was limited to those patients with severe ARDS in whom conventional ventilation with high levels of PEEP produced inadequate oxygenation, unacceptable hemodynamic compromise, or uncontrollable barotrauma. In an attempt to avoid oxygen toxicity, most intensive care physicians increase PEEP to achieve adequate oxygenation with FiO_2 of less than 0.5 or 0.6 (Shapiro et al., 1984). Our experience has been that HFPPV may be a better choice when PEEP levels exceed 12-15 cm H_2O. Asymmetrical pulmonary disease may respond to selective independent lung ventilation with HFPPV to the affected side and conventional ventilation to the unaffected side. Problems with ventilation (carbon dioxide elimination) that are difficult to manage with conventional ventilation may be improved with HFPPV. This is especially true where the cause is airway disruption through a bronchopleural fistula. An additional application of HFPPV may be in the patient with impaired right ventricular function. HFPPV might serve to unload the right ventricle by avoiding high peak and mean airway pressures or by mechanically limiting harmful dilation of the free wall of the right ventricle, especially in the absence of the pericardium following cardiac bypass procedures (Gettinger, 1983, unpublished data).

The initiation of HFPPV can result in periods of hemodynamic instability as well as potential periods of inadequate ventilation and/or oxygenation. To reduce this risk, during the transition we ventilate all patients with an FiO_2 of 1.0. Instability results from the precarious conditions of patients selected for HFPPV and also reflects the empirical nature of the technique. The initial high frequency settings are little more than educated guess-work. The introduction of continuous mixed venous oxygen saturation monitoring via reflectance spectrophotometry (oximetric catheter) and transcutaneous carbon dioxide monitoring has reduced the frequency of problems during the transition to HFPPV.

The records of 50 patients, representing approximately one-third of our clinical experience, with HFPPV have recently been reviewed. Patients varied in age from 3 weeks to 82 years. Most of our experience is with adult patients with diffuse pulmonary disease of varying causes. Ten of these patients were ventilated with HFPPV selectively to one lung by a double-lumen endobronchial tube (National Catheter Co.). An additional subgroup of seven patients had atelectasis not responsive to conservative measures (chest physiotherapy, bronchodilator therapy, position changes, suctioning, and bronchoscopy) that was treated with HFPPV through a conventional endotracheal tube. Duration of high-frequency ventilation varied from 2 hr to 28 days with a mean of 6.3 days. During that time no deaths were attributed to HFPPV. HFPPV flow rates varied from 15 to 60 liters/min with a mean of 26 liters/min. Increasing the flow rate generally improved carbon dioxide elimination. The frequency varied from 100 to 600 breaths/min. In our system increasing the rate up to about 250 breaths/min directly correlated with improved oxygenation but had an inverse correlation with carbon dioxide elimination (Kuwik, 1983, unpublished data). Although both slowing the rate and increasing the flow rate improved carbon dioxide elimination, flow rate had a stronger influence.

Improvement in oxygenation, as defined by a greater than 25-mmHg decrease in the A-a O_2 difference following the change to HFPPV, occurred in 38/50 patients (76%). The A-a O_2 difference improved in these patients by a mean of 137 ± 16 SEM mmHg with a range of 27–417 mmHg.

Two of the seven patients with refractory atelectasis showed radiographic improvement. Five of the seven demonstrated improved oxygenation, (which suggested improved ventilation/perfusion mismatch or recruitment of atelectactic areas that were not appreciated radiographically. Residual radiographic atelectasis resolved in two of these patients when HFPPV was applied to the atelectatic lung selectively via an endobronchial tube.

In the group of 50 patients, 10 were ventilated with selective HFPPV applied with endobronchial tubes for unilateral lung disease (including the 2 patients previously discussed). Seven of these patients did well and were successfully weaned from mechanical ventilatory support and extubated.

The application of HFPPV by selective endobronchial intubation appears to be a viable method of managing major airway disruption secondary to surgery or trauma. Questions, however, remain about the development of barotrauma in patients on HFPPV. It was impossible retrospectively to identify the cause of the barotrauma in this group of patients. That will require a prospective study with

HFPPV compared with conventional ventilation and high PEEP to provide a comparison group.

In this chapter we have discussed HFPPV, problems in its definition, and its clinical application in neonatal intensive care and adult intensive care. It is our hope that the work by many groups presented in this chapter will serve as in impetus for further study of HFPPV. Only then will we be able to define better the clinical applications and limitations of HFPPV.

References

Abu-Dbai, J., Flatau, E., Lev, A., Kohn, D., Monis-Hoss, I., and Barziley, E. (1983). The use of conventional ventilators for high frequency positive pressure ventilation. *Crit. Care Med.* **11**(5):356-358.

Bjerager, K., Sjostrand, U., and Wattwil, M. (1977). Long-term treatment of two patients with respiratory insufficiency with IPPV/PEEP and HFPPV/PEEP. *Acta Anaesth. Scand.* **64**(suppl):55-68.

Bland, R. D., Kim, M. H., Light, M. J., and Woodson, J. L. (1980). High frequency mechanical ventilation in severe hyaline membrane disease. *Crit. Care Med.* **8**(5):275-280.

El-Baz, N., Faber, L. P., and Doolas, A. (1983). Combined high-frequency ventilation for management of terminal respiratory failure: A new technique. *Anesth. Analg.* **62**:39-49.

Frantz, I., Werthammer, J., and Stark, A. R. (1983). High-frequency ventilation in premature infants with lung disease: Adequate gas exchange at low tracheal pressure. *Pediatrics* **71**:483-488.

Gallagher, T. J., Klain, M. M., and Carlon, G. C. (1982). Present status of high frequency ventilation. *Crit. Care Med.* **10**:613-617.

Gillespie, D. J. (1983). High-frequency ventilation: A new concept in mechanical ventilation. *Mayo Clin. Proc.* **58**:187-196.

Heijman, L., Nilsson, L.-G., and Sjostrand, U. (1977). High-frequency positive-pressure ventilation (HFPPV) in neonates and infants during neuroleptal analgesia and routine plastic surgery, and in postoperative management. *Acta Anaesth. Scand.* **64** (Suppl):111-121.

Karl, S. R., Ballantine, T. V. N., and Snider, M. T. (1983). High frequency ventilation in neonates with congenital diaphragmatic hernia. *International Symposium on High Frequency Ventilation.* Edited by G. C. Carlon and W. S. Howland. New York, Memorial Sloan-Kettering Cancer Center, p. 116.

Kolton, M., Cattran, C. B., Kent, G., Volqyesi, G., Froese, A. B., and Bryan, A. C. (1982). Oxygenation during high-frequency ventilation compared with conventional mechanical ventilation in two models of lung injury. *Anesth. Analg.* **61**:323-332.

Miranda, D. R., Stoutenbeck, D., and Kingma, L. (1981). Differential lung ventilation with HFPPV. *Intensive Care Med.,* **7**:139-141.

Nordin, U., Keszler, H., and Klain, M. (1981). How does high frequency jet ventilation effect the mucociliary transport? *Crit. Care Med.* **9**:146.

O'Rourke, P. P., and Crone, R. K. (1983). High-frequency ventilation: A new approach to respiratory support. *JAMA* **250**(20):2845-2847.

Shapiro, B. A., Cane, R. D., and Harrison, R. A. (1984). Positive end-expiratory pressure therapy in adults with special reference to acute lung injury: A review of the literature and suggested clinical correlations. *Crit. Care Med.* **12**(2):127-141.

Sjostrand, U. (1980). High-frequency positive-pressure ventilation (HFPPV); A review. Crit. Care Med. **8**:345-364.

Sjostrand, U. (1983). Development of high frequency positive pressure low-compression ventilation. *Int. Anesthesiol. Clin.* **21**(3):11-32.

Sjostrand, U. (1983). High frequency positive pressure ventilation (HFPPV) in ARDS. *Acta Anaesth. Scand.* **78** (suppl):26-27.

Wattwill, L. M. (1982). Evaluation of HFPPV in experimental and clinical practice. *Acta Univ. Ups* **41**:6.

Wattwil, L. M., Sjostrand, U. H., and Borg, U. R. (1983a). Comparative studies of IPPV and HFPPV with PEEP in critical care patients. I: A clinical evaluation. *Crit. Care Med.* **11**(1):30-37

Wattwill, L. M., Sjostrand, U. G., Borg, U. R., and Eriksson, I. A. (1983b). Comparative studies of IPPV and HFPPV with PEEP in critical care patients. II: Studies on intrapulmonary gas distribution. *Crit. Care Med.* **11**(1):38-43.

Whitwam, J. G., Chakrabarti, M. K., Konarzewski, W. H., and Askitopoulou, H. (1983). A new valveless all-purpose ventilator. *Br. J. Anaesth.* **55**:1017-1022.

6

High-Frequency Jet Ventilation

Technical Evaluation and Device Characterization

GRAZIANO C. CARLON, SAUL MIODOWNIK, and COLE RAY, Jr.

Memorial Sloan-Kettering Cancer Center
New York, New York

I. Mechanical Structure of High-Frequency Jet Ventilators

Beneficial clinical applications of high-frequency jet ventilation (HFJV) requre a complete understanding of the principles affecting gas delivery in this modality of mechanical ventilatory support.

Generally, respiratory rate is higher and tidal volume smaller on HFJV than on conventional ventilation. Rather than absolute values, however, the most significant differences rest with the method by which gas transport is accomplished.

Flow from a high-pressure gas source is gated by a timing device, which determines respiratory rate and inspiratory/expiratory (I/E) ratio. In earlier models, pneumatic and fluidic control circuits were employed (Klain and Smith, 1976; Calkins et al., 1982; Lyons et al., 1981), but at present most jet ventilators are electronically controlled. This approach permits the generation of precise timing signals for both rate and I/E ratio, which do not depend on gas source pressure and do not interact with each other, as is the case with pneumatic circuits (Bunegin et al., 1983). Synchronization of ventilator cycles with other electronic devices (intraaortic balloon pump, ECG, etc.) is greatly facilitated (Otto et al., 1983; Miodownik et al., 1980). A wide variety of analog and digital circuits are currently available. Advances in microprocessor-based devices will soon allow computer control of HFJV, as part of a closed-loop ventilatory support system.

To most end users, the electronic circuitry represents only an academic interest, while the pneumatic components are of more direct importance for the safe application of the technique.

Development of a common vocabulary which refers to the landmarks of a common geography should be among the first priorities of the investigator. For instance, a major advantage ascribed to HFJV is the maintenance of acceptable blood gas values at lower airway pressures. Closer observation indicates that investigators may not necessarily refer to a common concept when using this ubiquitous term. Definitions that are adequate and appropriate for conventional mechanical ventilation cannot be directly applied to HFJV. On VCV, the "Y" connector between tracheal tube and inspiratory and expiratory line represents the point of highest airway pressure. On HFJV, the jet injector is usually inserted distal to the "Y" connector, so that pressure monitored at that site would provide misleading information. Gas flowing from the injector causes a pressure drop in the immediate vicinity of the cannula, while pressure increases distally. Furthermore, pressure measurements obtained near the injector are affected by the artifacts generated by high gas velocities and turbulence. Consequently, the distal tip of the endotracheal tube is a preferable site to measure pressure, and represents a convenient and accessible location within the patient's pulmonary tree. Acquiring pressure at a consistent place more precisely reflects changes in the operational characteristics of HFJV (driving pressure, I/E ratio) as well as in lung mechanics (resistance, compliance).

Alveolar pressure is often cited as a variable which should be observed when applying HFJV, but direct access to that area of the lungs is virtually impossible. Indirect determinations, such as pleural or esophageal pressure, are very unreliable. Discrepancies between alveolar and airway pressure are probably far more significant at rates approaching the resonant frequency of lung segments (10-30 Hz), such as are obtained on high-frequency oscillation (Fletcher, 1983). At this time, the importance of alveolar pressure should most likely be discounted on HFJV.

The meaning of each term describing "airway pressure" should be reevaluated on HFJV.

1. Peak pressure: The highest pressure value in the phasic respiratory waveform
2. Mean pressure (distending pressure): The planimetric average of the waveform taken over an appropriate time interval
3. Positive end-expiratory pressure (PEEP): Airway pressure at the end of expiration, during the pause between breaths

Peak pressure is relatively easy to measure and little disagreement exists as to its meaning, but considerably greater confusion applies to mean and end-expiratory airway pressures. On HFJV, mean airway pressure indicates the constant force available for airway distention. At higher respiratory rates, distal airway segments no longer exhibit the pulsatile component of airway pressure observed at the carinal level (Fletcher, 1983; den Dunnen and Moslert, 1983; Baum et al., 1983). Mean pressure obtained during HFJV is often compared to that of VCV, but the comparison is only meaningful if a sufficient interval is allowed for averaging pressure measurements on VCV. For instances with a mechanical rate of 10 breaths/min, the interval between breaths is 6 sec. A mean pressure measurement taken over any interval shorter than this will not accurately measure the patient's mean airway pressure. Ideally, a mean measurement is taken over several cycles to average perturbations due to the patient's spontaneous respiratory activity. Consequently, mean airway pressure measurements at VCV rates must be so qualified. End-expiratory pressure is often used as a determinant of mean lung volume on VCV, but its significance on HFJV is not the same, since mean pressure on HFJV is often several cm H_2O greater than PEEP, and it is the factor determining mean lung volume (Carlon et al., 1983b).

II. Components of High-Frequency Jet Ventilators

A schematic representation of an ideal jet ventilator is shown in Figure 1. Gases under a pressure of 5-50 psi are delivered to the inspiratory line when the gating mechanism opens. Ideally, opening and closing periods should be nearly instantaneous, and the gate function should be minimally affected by driving pressure and distal pneumatic impedance. Response time of the gating mechanism becomes a significant factor at higher respiratory rates (several hundred breaths/min). Although electronic controllers generate remarkably precise time signals, the mechanical action cannot have the same degree of accuracy. Selection of an I/E ratio at respiratory frequencies which approximate the response time limits of the valve requires carful consideration. Since the valve opening and closing times are, in fact, nonzero, they must be taken into consideration if operation is attempted at high rates. Assuming $T_{open} = T_{close} = 5$ msec, it is readily apparent that effective operation cannot be achieved at rates whose period approaches $T_{open} + T_{close} = 10$ msec or 100 Hz. If the valve is given insufficient time to open and close, it will "float" and pass a steady stream of gas, and effectively be in a continuous inspiratory phase. Even at substantially lower rates than 100 Hz, the opening and closing times of the valve occupy a substantial portion of the available I/E ratio the user has selected on the front panel of the ventilator. Consequently, at rates of 10 Hz (600 beats/min) and an I/E ratio of 1:2 (33% on-time), a substantial portion of the expected gas flow is wasted while the valve is opening or closing. At these settings, the 5-msec valve time is equivalent to 5% of the available time (Fig. 2).

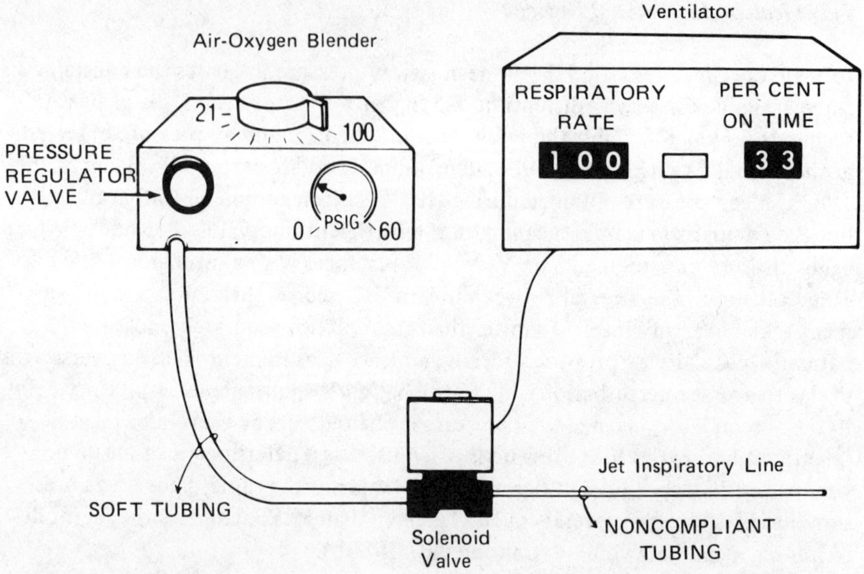

Figure 1 The ideal jet ventilator system consists of all components shown.

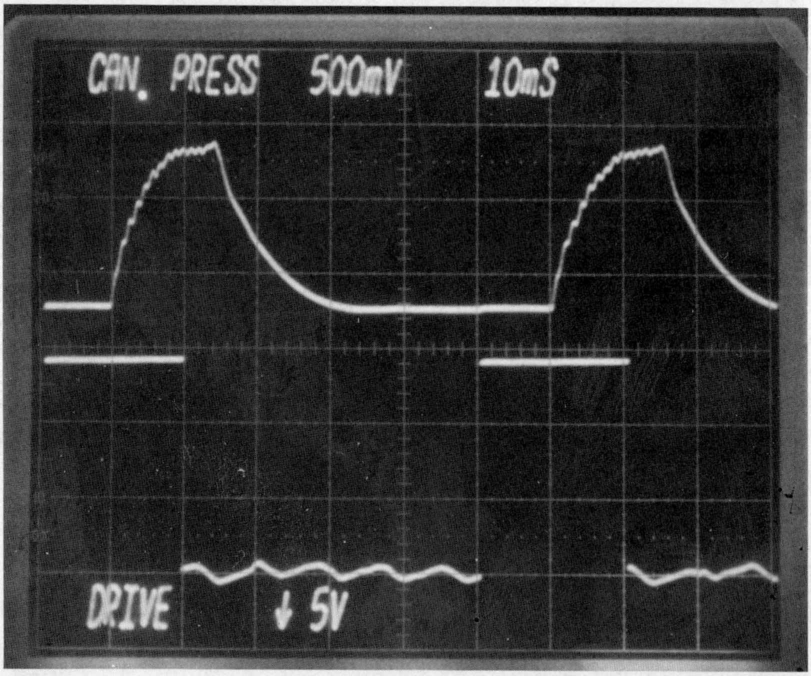

Figure 2 Cannula pressure changes (top line) are out of phase by approximately 50 msec with opening and closing of the solenoid valve (second line).

After the valve opens, gas enters the tubing forming the inspiratory line. A pressure wave moves toward the patient, ultimately causing gas flow out of the cannula. Again, time becomes a crucial factor. Volume, resistance and compliance of the connecting tubing and the diameter and length of the injector cannula will determine the time required to reach peak pressure and flow rate at the cannula, as well as the time required for flow to cease. At the driving pressures used on HFJV, significant gas can be stored as a compressible volume within connecting tubing, even when this is relatively uncompliant. The charging and discharge times of the connecting tubing and cannula determine the maximum respiratory rate and range of I/E ratios that can be used (Fig. 3). Inappropriate selection of connecting tubing may hamper understanding of the operation of HFJV.

In the HFJV system used at Memorial Sloan-Kettering Cancer Center, the connecting tubing used stores approximately 1.2 cc/psi of driving pressure. At driving pressures of 30 psi, and respiratory rates of 100/min, this yields 36 cc of additional tidal volume per breath or 3.6 liters additional minute ventilation, which may represent 10% or more of the total minute ventilation delivered to the patient, and will account for a proportional share of mean airway pressure. This

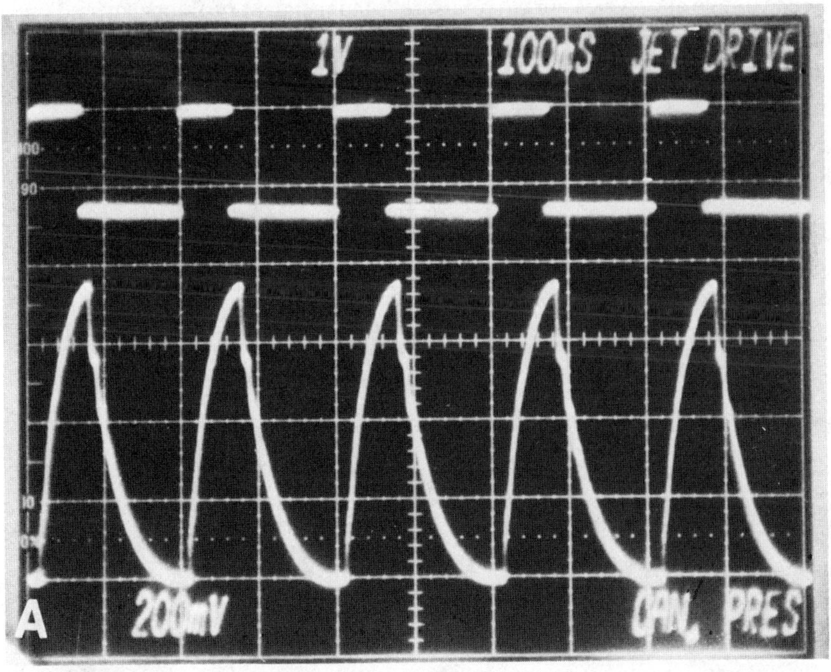

Figure 3 The exponential pressure decay in the jet inspiratory line augments the volume delivered to the patient and increases mean airway pressure.

added volume contributes little or nothing to the peak airway pressure, since this latter value decreases exponentially with time as soon as the solenoid valve closes.

A. "Inadvertent" PEEP and Other Physiological Implications

Many reports have appeared in the literature, describing an event variously defined as "inadvertent PEEP" or "auto PEEP" on HFJV (Beamer et al., 1983; Klain et al., 1980; Chakrabati and Sykes, 1980). These observations may be related to the characteristics of the tubing connecting the valve to the injector. All effects are more pronounced at higher frequencies, and to reduce effective expiratory time. Eliminating the connecting tubing and placing the valve mechanism near the injector cannula may allow the system to operate as a signal source connected to a resistor-capacitor analog of the lung. The model predicts that there should be no increase in mean pressure developed across the lung if the percentage on time (I/E ratio) is held constant, while the frequency is increased. Eliminating the injector tubing allows maintaining a constant mean airway pressure at frequencies greater than 750 breaths/min. When the interconnecting tubing is eliminated, the total compressible volume of the gas delivery system is reduced to almost zero cc. If the valve cycling times are also very short, the total delivered volume and, hence, airway pressure is independent of frequency and only dependent on input amplitude (driving pressure) and duty cycle (I/E ratio) (Fig. 4).

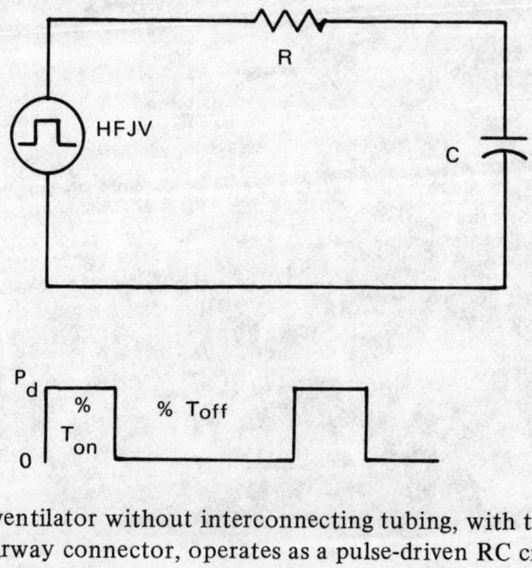

Figure 4 A jet ventilator without interconnecting tubing, with the valve placed at the patients airway connector, operates as a pulse-driven RC circuit. Mean pressure and flow are independent of pulse frequency and dependent only on amplitude (P_d: driving pressure) and duty cycle (I/E ratio).

Another component of inadvertent PEEP arises from time-dependent emptying of different lung regions (Pepe and Marini, 1982). During the inspiratory phase of a HFJV breath, pressure forces flow into the alveoli, which are equivalent to millions of resistor-capacitor elements arranged in parallel. The time required to fill or empty each element is determined by the product of its resistance and compliance. This value, defined as the time constant, defines the duration of time necessary to fill or empty 67% of the alveolar volume in response to a step change in pressure. It follows from this definition that three time constants are required to exchange 95% of the initial volume.

Several important clinical effects derive from this relationship. During mechanical ventilation, the force supporting inspiration (airway pressure) is higher than that responsible for expiration (alveolar elastic recoil). Accordingly, the expiratory time constant will be longer than the inspiratory. If frequency is excessively increased or expiratory time excessively shortened, alveoli will fill but not empty, resulting in a continuous increase in FRC. This effect may vary widely from region to region, or even from microregion to microregion, and cannot be effectively duplicated by simple one- or two-compartment mechanical test lungs. Because the magnitude of this effect in individual lung regions is impossible to predict and difficult to measure under routine clinical conditions, HFJV rates and inspiratory/expiratory ratios should be conservative so that the patient is only exposed to the amount of PEEP set by the threshold resistor valve. Studies in both animals and humans indicate that at rates below 150 and inspiratory time percentages less than or equal to 40, clinically significant gas trapping is not a problem on high-frequency jet ventilation (Carlon et al., 1983a,b; Colgan et al., 1983).

B. Injector Cannula

The inspiratory line of a jet ventilation system terminates in an injector through which gases are delivered into the patient's airway. The injector is a high-resistance throttle, which converts driving pressure into a constant flow independent of downstream pneumatic impedance. The velocity of gas exiting from the injector cannula will be inversely related to its diameter, as will its ability to entrain and move forward surrounding static gas. The injector is often inserted into the swivel adapter of the endotracheal tube.

C. Entrainment

Jet ventilators may take two divergent pathways, determined by their entrainment characteristics. When gas begins to flow from the tip of the cannula at high velocity, it pulls along ("entrains") static gases resident near the proximal end of the endotracheal tube, causing a local pressure drop. If an additional source of gas is provided, a greater gas volume will be moved down the endotracheal tube than that directly delivered through the injector cannula. HFJV with entrainment can be described as a jet pumping mechanism, which is a well-defined physical principle (Kroll, 1947; Gosline and O'Brien, 1934). When entrainment occurs, the characteristics of the additional gas source become as important as those of each other component of the system. The primary factors controlling the ratio of directly jetted-to-entrained gas are the position of the cannula with respect to the entrainment source, and the coaxial orientation of the injector within the swivel connector (Wood and Eurenius, 1982). Figures 10 through 15 show the ratios of directly jetted-to-entrained gases as functions of environmental pneumatic impedance upstream and downstream of cannula and swivel connector. Entrainment is dramatically affected by the position of the cannula within the swivel connector and its coaxial configuration within the endotracheal tube. If the cannula tip is directed at an angle toward the tube wall, a Coanda or wall attachment effect takes place, and entrainment is drastically reduced, regardless of downstream impedance. Clinical HFJV injector systems which rely on entrained volume to achieve the desired level of ventilatory support must be designed to guarantee a stable, central position of the cannula.

When entrainment is not desired or available, the entire tidal volume delivered to the patient originates from the injector tip. Higher driving pressures are necessary to achieve the same minute volume delivered by systems relying on entrainment.

D. Measurement of Physiological Variables

Characterization of high-frequency jet ventilation requires carful measurement of pressure and flow at various points in the respiratory circuit. It is desirable to determine most of the following variables:

1. Tidal volume delivered through the endotracheal tube as a function of driving pressure
2. When entrainment is used, effects of downstream pneumatic impedance on the ratio of directly jetted-to-entrained gases
3. Entrainment ratio and delivered volume as a function of cannula diameter
4. Peak and mean airway pressure (at carinal level), as a function of driving pressure, airway impedance and respiratory rate

Different HFJV systems may yield very dissimilar results under the same clinical or test conditions, since multiple factors can influence the outcome of these measurements.

Figure 5 illustrates a bench test set-up that allows one to acquire all desired data. Flow and volume are measured at points labeled "F" and pressure at points labeled "P." Accurate flow measurements are difficult to obtain in the immediate

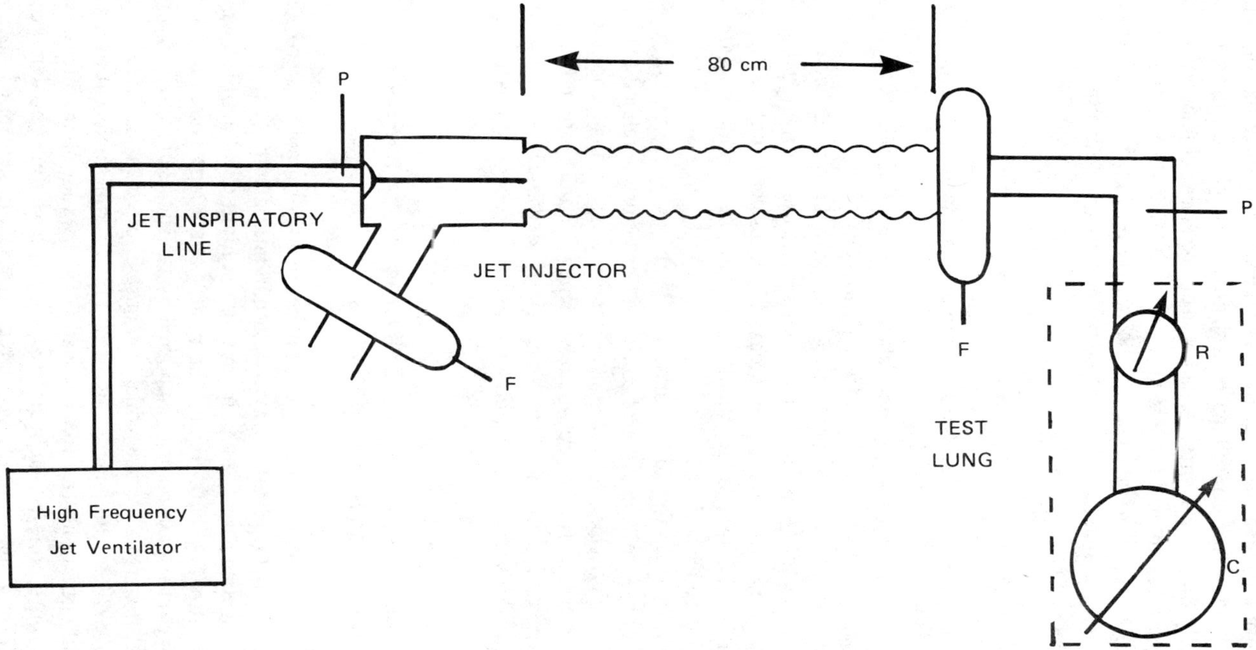

Figure 5 Diagram of a bench system which can be used to characterize high-frequency jet ventilators. Pressure is measured at points "P" and flow at points "F." An 80-cm airway hose is placed between the jet injector and the flow transducer, that then connects to the lung model.

proximity of the cannula tip, since the instantaneous velocities and pressures occurring in that region exceed the range of resistance screen pneumotachographs and ultrasound flowmeters. Consequently, a significant length of corrugated tubing (approximately 80 cm) was interposed between the swivel connector, where the jet injector was located, and the test lung where the first flow measurement was obtained. Clinical performance cannot be exactly predicted on the basis of results obtained with simple bench models, but these may provide useful indicators of directional change.

E. Safety Considerations

To be clinically practical, HFJV systems require proper characterization in two areas that do not directly affect gas delivery.

The first is the availability of proper alarms. The second relates to the proper humidification of delivered gases to the patient's airway.

At this time, HFJV is a relatively new modality that evokes concern because of its unfamiliar range of operating characteristics. The use of driving pressures of 10-50 psi and respiratory rates of hundreds of breaths per minute justify trepidation in clinical applications of HFJV, although clinical experience to date does not support undue concern.

To ease users' discomfort, useful and reliable alarms should be added to every high-frequency ventilator. Alarm configurations must be related to the specific function of each device, and sweeping generalizations are inappropriate. There is, however, one alarm feature which we believe is indispensible in all ventilators. Airway overpressure should be immediately identified, and ventilator operation automatically and immediately discontinued to prevent unacceptable risks of barotrauma.

III. Humidification of Gases Delivered by High-Frequency Jet Ventilators

More than 25 years of clinical experience with ventilatory support has provided a universal consensus that optimal airway function in intubated patients requires conditioning of inspired gases. A minimum water content of 30 mg/liter, which corresponds to saturation (100% relative humidity) at a temperature of 30.1°C, appears necessary. This statement is supported by the successful and widespread use in Europe of the artificial nose, which can raise inspired gas humidity to approximately 30 mg/liter. Brain and co-workers (1971) confirmed that over a wide range of ambient conditions, the upper airway normally adds 30 mg/liter of water to inspired gas. Furthermore, MacIntire et al. (1983) have found no demonstrable airway dysfunction in mechanically ventilated patients whose inspired gases were humidified to approximately 30 mg/liter with a heat exchanger.

On high-frequency jet ventilation, tidal volume may be entirely delivered through the jet injector or partly originate from gases entrained by the frictional drag of the high-velocity jet stream. The contribution of entrainment is highly variable, and depends on the type of HFJV application and the specific characteristics of the system used. The relative effects of temperatures and humidities of both gas sources must be taken into consideration when entrainment occurs.

The early experience of the authors (Carlon et al., 1981) and subsequent radionuclide imaging studies add to the complexity of the humidification problem. Unlike conventional ventilation, jet ventilators may cause pronounced regional effects. Certain areas, such as the carina and the medial aspects of the mainstem bronchi, are in the path of high-velocity gas streams, while the lateral aspects of those same airways are only subjected to the low-velocity flow of entrained gases. If humidification were restricted to entrained gas only, severe regional dessication of the areas exposed to the jet stream may occur, with hemorrhagic mucosal necrosis, inspissation of secretions, and, ultimately, airway occlusion.

Humidification of the jet stream may be accomplished by heated humidification of the high-pressure gas proximal to the gating mechanism or by aerosolization of water or saline into the gases distal to the injector cannula.

The first method has been utilized in at least two high-frequency jet ventilators (Bunnel et al., 1975; Sjostrand, 1980). The latter method, aerosolization, is simpler to implement, but less amenable to quantification. The solution to this problem requires accurate determination of the ratio of directly delivered-to-entrained gases, with the ventilator operating within a wide physiological and pathophysiological range of resistances, compliance, and PEEP. Once entrainment ratios have been established, the volume of directly delivered gases can be easily derived and the amount of water which should be added can be calculated. For example, if the patient is receiving 30 liters/min of total ventilation with a 1:1 entrainment ratio, the entrained gas should be conditioned by adding 44 mg/liters, with an ultimate goal of providing at least 30 mg water/liter total flow. Practically, these requirements can be met as follows.

Total required water	30 liters min × 30 mg/liter = 900 mg/min
Entrained water	15 liters/min × 44 mg/liter = 660 mg/min
Balance to be added to jet	240 mg/min

Administration of 240 mg/min × 60 min/hr requires a constant infusion of 14.4 ml/hr water, which value is in good agreement with the authors' clinical experience with the Memorial Sloan-Kettering Cancer Center/Bear Medical system's high-frequency jet ventilator. Most of approximately 400 patients who received HFJV have in fact required 15-20 ml water/hr.

However neatly the theory may fit the clinical experience, several points should be kept in mind. First, wide differences in flow patterns and entrainment ratios occur from one model of high-frequency jet ventilator to another, and between the same ventilator models when injection techniques are changed. Second, the device used to aerosolize the water should produce few large particles. Simply pumping the correct amount of water into the high-pressure gas upstream of the injector, as is often done, may result in the acceleration of large drops, or slugs, of water to high velocity. The force of impact equals one-half the mass times the square of velocity and every means should be utilized to minimize particle size, especially when the injection site is in the mid- or distal trachea near the carina. Lastly, gamma camera images of Tm^{99m} sulphur colloid aerosolized by the Memorial Sloan-Kettering Cancer Center/Bear Medical Systems humidifying injector cannula, placed at the proximal end of a standard endotracheal tube, show preferential distribution of the contrast in the central airway (Sjostrand, 1980) (Fig. 6). This indicates that continuous bathing of the central structures in the humidified high-velocity flow may be sufficient for safe support if the entrained gas humidity level is also adequate.

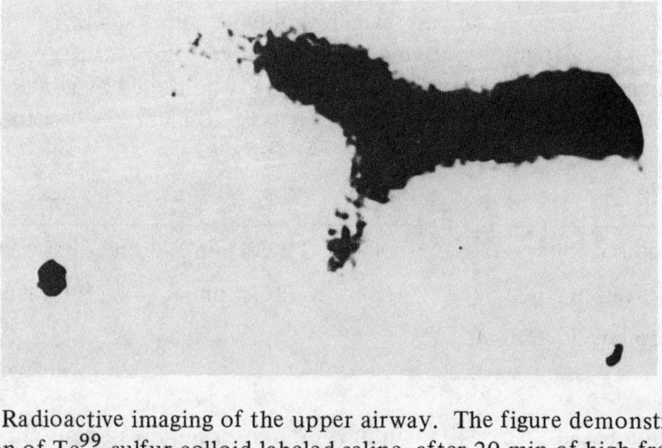

Figure 6 Radioactive imaging of the upper airway. The figure demonstrates the distribution of Tc^{99} sulfur-colloid-labeled saline, after 20 min of high-frequency jet ventilation. One mCurie of radioactive contrast was administered in 10 ml of water, at a rate of 20 ml/hr.

IV. High-Frequency Jet Ventilation of Disrupted Airways

The ability of high-frequency jet ventilation to maintain oxygenation and CO_2 clearance in the presence of large bronchopleural fistulae and other sources of pathological gas leak has been well-documented (Carlon et al., 1980). Long-term successful ventilatory support has been achieved in patients with airway defects equal in cross-sectional area to a main-stem bronchus. A satisfactory explanation of these observations can be obtained if positive pressure ventilation of the lung is considered as a pneumatic-to-electrical circuit analog.

The physical similarities between the properties of an ideal gas and the behavior of free electrons in a conductor are well enough understood to allow useful application of electrical circuit analysis techniques to both mechanical and physiological pneumatic systems. These analogies are summarized in Table 1. Throughout this section, reference will usually be made to the electrical model, although occasionally the concepts may be reiterated for the pneumatic model to allow better understanding.

Figure 7 shows the electrical circuit equivalent of a pair of lungs ventilated in parallel with a large central airway leak. Since lung ventilation is bidirectional, the appropriate electrical analog is that of an alternating current circuit, in which current is distributed to competing paths according to the inverse ratios of their total opposition to current flow (impedance).

Impedance is the function of three opposing elements: resistance (R), which is essentially frictional; capacitive reactance (X_c), which is related to capacitance (rate of charge build up per unit of voltage); and inductive reactance (X_1), an inertial factor which can be safely ignored in the pneumatic model. Resistance does not vary with frequency, while capacitative reactance does, in accordance with the expression

$$X_c = \frac{1}{2\ fc}$$

Table 1 Analogs

Pressure	(P)	=	Voltage	(E)
Flow	(V)	=	Current	(I)
Resistance	(R)	=	Resistance	(R)
Compliance	(C)	=	Capacitance	(C)

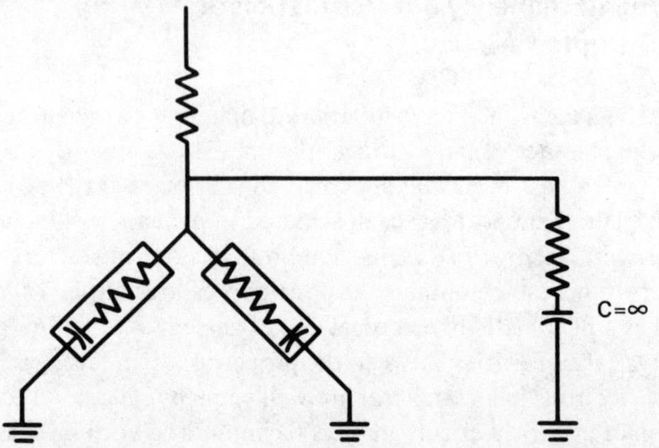

Figure 7 Circuit diagram of lung resistance and compliance elements with a parallel leak path, comparable to the one that may be caused by a bronchopleural cutaneous fistual. The leak-path compliance (C) is nearly infinite.

where f is the frequency in Hz (cycles per second) and c is the capacitance (equivalent to compliance in a pneumatic circuit).

Flow through a given circuit element is determined by the ratio of that element's Z_t, or total impedance, to the Z_t of other circuit elements. The combination of R with the time-dependent X_c is accomplished by vector addition (Fig. 8). The final value is calculated at the hypotenuse of the triangle formed by the two vector quantities: $Z_t = (X_c^2 + R^2)$. (Fig. 8A) (Javid and Breuner, 1967). This vector relationship has great significance for the frequency-dependent nature of airway leaks, as a reexamination of Figure 1 will show. A leak into the atmosphere, with its virtually infinite capacitance (compliance), results in a zero X_c for the leak path due to the virtually infinite value of c in the denominator of $X_c = 1/2$ fc. Thus the leak path essentially has only resistance, while lung flow paths have both resistive and capacitive components to their impedances. As frequency rises from 10 (0.16 Hz) to 100 beats/min (1.6 Hz), to use rates consistent with VCV and HFJV, the capacitive reactance of the lung will fall by approximately 90%. Total impedance of the lung will drop, while total impedance of the leak will remain unchanged, inducing a redistribution of flow which favors the lung component (Fig. 8B).

Airway and lung leaks often occur as slits or rents in the rather elastic tissue of the lungs. During positive-pressure ventilation, high peak airway pressure opens the hole, enlarging its cross-sectional area. This situation is analogous to substituting a voltage-controlled for a fixed resistor in the leak path, so that the higher the voltage, the lower the resistance. Under pressure, a slit in an elastic substance

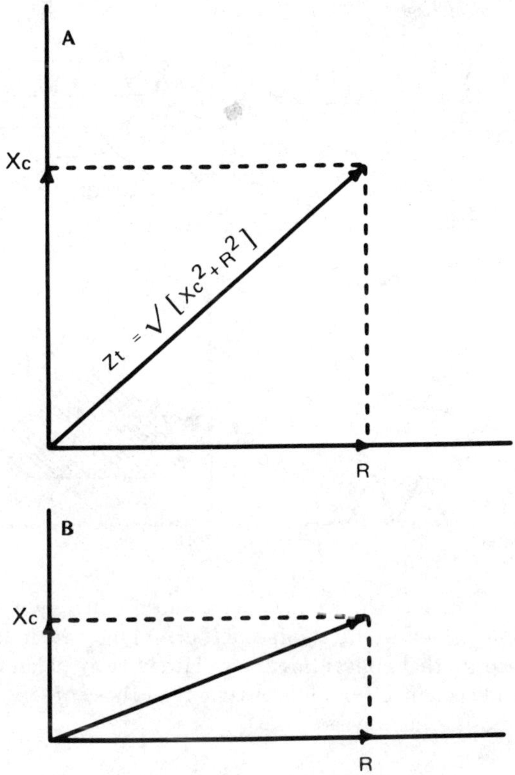

Figure 8 (A) Z_t or total impedance results from the vector addition of capacitive reactance (vertical axis) and resistance (horizontal axis). (B) At high frequencies, lung X_c is reduced and therefore Z_t falls to values approaching R, causing a proportional increase in flow to the lung.

expands into an ellipse (Fig. 9, top), whose area A = a x b, where a is the dimension of the long axis and b is the radius or one-half the diameter of the short axis. For instance, if the radius of the slit doubles, the cross-sectional area also doubles. Since flow varies with the square of the area, this modest expansion of the slit will increase by four times the flow through the leak.

In addition to the higher peak pressures generated on conventional ventilation, time is also a factor in determining leak flow (Fig. 9, bottom). The fraction of the respiratory cycle spent at higher airway pressure is much greater during conventional ventilation. Thus, both the period of time during which the area of disruption is enlarged and the pressure gradient across the defect are larger on VCV.

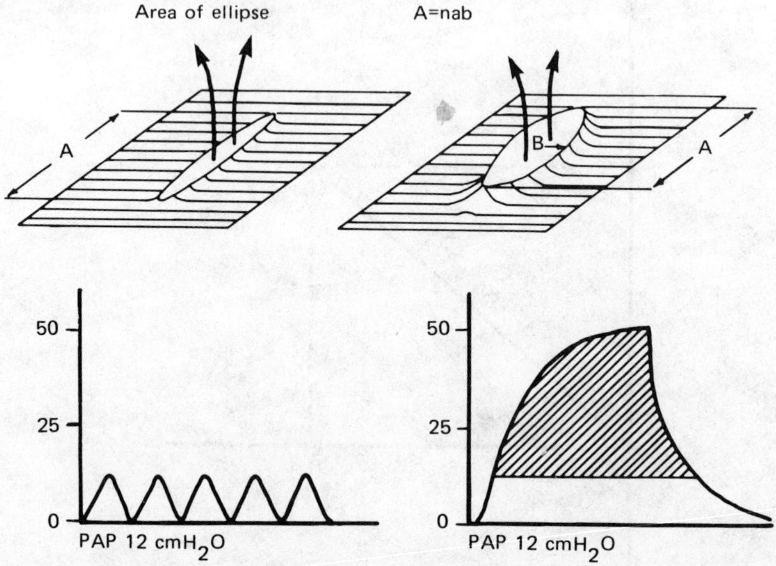

Figure 9 The upper drawings show a pressure-induced doubling in the width of an elliptical lung rent, which would result in a fourfold increase in leak flow. The lower drawings illustrate that conventional ventilator airway pressures (right graph) are higher and sustained for a longer time than those observed on HFJV (left graph). PAP, positive airway pressure.

The inevitable consequence is the loss of a much larger portion of total minute volume through the defect.

HFJV, which delivers peak pressures approximately one-half those of conventional ventilation, (den Dunnen and Mostert, 1983), will lose less gas through leak paths through two different mechanisms (Carlon et al., 1983a), one frequency-dependent, the other pressure dependent.

V. Laboratory Testing of High-Frequency Jet Ventilators

Bench evaluation of high-frequency jet ventilators should satisfy our technical and scientific curiosity for determining modalities of gas transport characteristic of each device considered, while providing practical clinical guidelines for use. Bench tests should evaluate the influence on tidal volume and proximal airway pressure of different load factors, occurring distally to the injector cannula, such as airway resistance and pulmonary compliance. The most specific characteristic of the jet ventilator—delivery of tidal volume through a narrow injector cannula and entrainment of additional gas by jet drag action—are also subjects well worth investigating.

To establish the behavior of the high-frequency jet ventilator build at Memorial Hospital under a variety of circumstances reproducing potential clinical conditions, a series of tests were performed.

A. Gas Flow and Pressure in the Absence of Load

The use of high-frequency jet ventilators has been advocated for clinical conditions in which major airways are disrupted, such as tracheoesophageal fistulae and tracheo- or bronchopleural fistulae. The theoretical aspects of gas flow and the extent of volume loss through the pathological opening have already been discussed. For each pressure gradient across the fistula, a constant flow of gases will be lost through the opening, without reaching the distal airway. On HFJV, entrainment is inversely proportional to distal airway load. This characteristic acts as an automatic correction mechanism, since the larger the fistula, the lower the distal load, and the greater the entrainment.

The experimental model selected to illustrate this characteristic used a high-frequency jet ventilator, with the injector cannula inserted into an endotracheal tube through a tightly sealed connection The endotracheal catheter had been placed into a corrugated tube approximately 80 cm in length, open at its distal end, to reproduce a wide open airway. A Hans-Rudolf pneumotachograph, located at the opening of the corrugated tube opposite to the injector cannula, measured tidal volume delivered with each jet pulse. Three needles were inserted into the corrugated tube, one immediately distal to the opening of the endotracheal tube, the other two evenly spaced along the remaining length of the corrugated tube. The needles were connected to pressure transducers calibrated for accuracy and linearity. Digital and analog pressure values were displayed on a digital storage oscilloscope; gas flow speed was derived from the time interval between peak pressures at two different measuring ports. The route of entrainment was the open limb of the swivel connector through which the injector had been inserted. The entrainment port could be sealed when desired. To test the potential consequences of modest restriction of the exhalation path, endotracheal tubes of two diameters, 7 and 10 mm, representing a difference in resistance of approximately four times, were used. Cannulas of two different sizes, 14- and 18-gauge (1.62 and 1.06 mm internal diameter, respectively) were employed as injectors. Driving pressure was progressively increased from 5 to 45 psig in increments of 5 psig. Respiratory rate was constant at 100 breaths/min. I/E ratio was always 1:2. Altogether 36 experimental conditions were studied.

The experiment (Figs. 10, 11) demonstrated that entrainment was a very significant component of the total tidal volume delivered, and its importance was

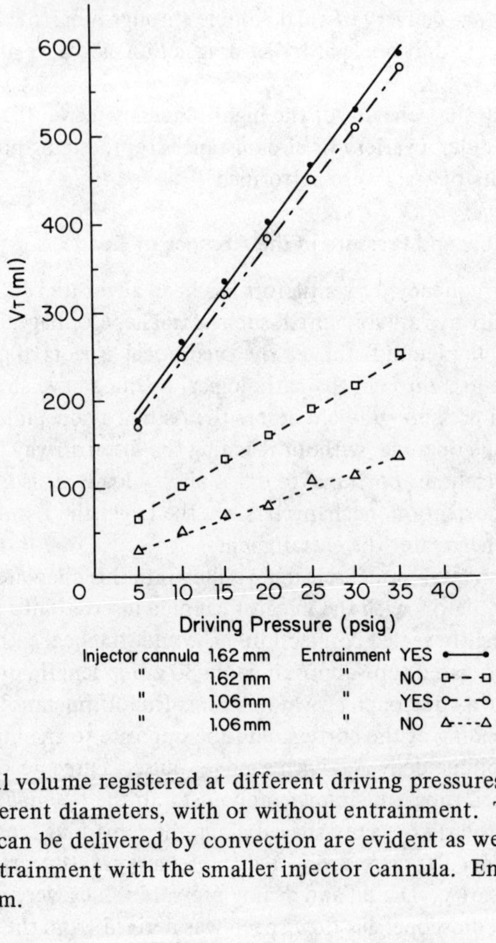

Figure 10 Tidal volume registered at different driving pressures, with injector cannulas of different diameters, with or without entrainment. The very large volumes which can be delivered by convection are evident as well as the greater proportional entrainment with the smaller injector cannula. Endotracheal tube diameter is 7 mm.

substantially greater with the smaller injector cannula. Without entrainment, tidal volume delivered through the larger injector cannula was approximately twice that of the smaller cannula in all experimental conditions. When entrainment was added, tidal volume delivered from the two cannulas was identical. Entrainment is determined by the product of gas pressure and velocity, which are two variables inversely proportional to each other. The lower gas pressure occurring at the tip of the smaller cannula was offset by the greater gas speed. Total gas flow, directly delivered and entrained, was approximately 10% higher with the larger tube (10 mm). This finding, of little clinical significance, is probably related to greater gas turbulence in the proximity of the injector nozzle, when tube diameter is smaller.

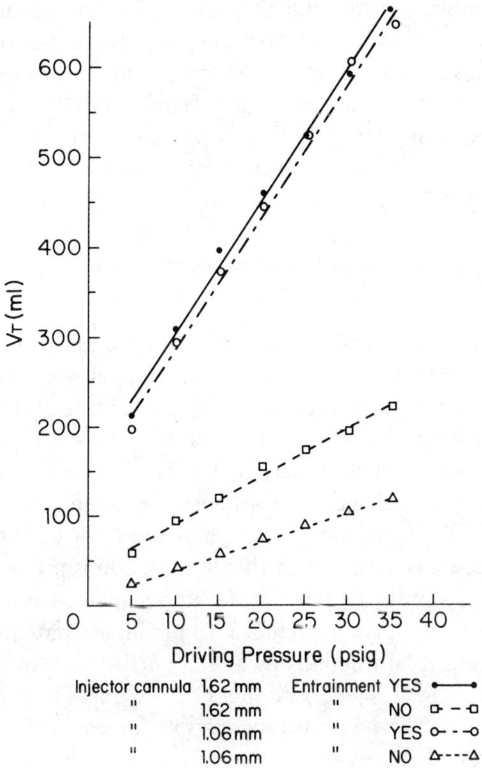

Figure 11 Same as Figure 10 except that the endotracheal tube had a 10-mm diameter. All volumes increased by approximately 10%, indicating that resistance can be affected by the size of the endotracheal tube even at relatively large diameters.

Pressure tracings obtained during the experiment revealed extremely transient pressure spikes, lasting a few milliseconds only, substantially less than the time during which the solenoid valve remained open, which was 200 msec. The amplitude of the pressure spike did not change at different points in the airway. The gas flow velocity profile indicated that the faster component moved at a speed approximating the speed of sound. This observation confirms findings of other authors, also reported in this book and lends support to the theory of gas exchange in multiple stages. Most of the gas flow was delivered at a much lower pressure, barely higher than baseline, confirming experimentally the clinical advantages of high-frequency jet ventilation in the presence of major airway disruption.

The number of patients with severe airway disruption who cannot be supported with conventional ventilation is very small. The interest in developing alternative modalities of mechanical support cannot be supported only by the possibility of treating this disease entity. By far the most common reason for admission to intensive care units is acute respiratory failure, usually characterized by hypoxemia and occasionally by hypercapnia. Potential applications of high-frequency jet ventilation in the support of patients with abnormal lungs are clearly of major interest to physiologists and clinicians.

B. Volume and Pressure with Varying Compliance and Resistance

In pathological conditions two mechanical properties of lung function, compliance and resistance, are usually abnormal. An experiment was designed to evaluate the influence of varying resistance and compliance on tidal volume, entrainment, and pressure recorded in a simple lung model. The experimental structure previously described was used, with the distal end of the corrugated tube attached to a test lung, which allows changes of resistance and compliance. Tidal volume was measured by placing a pneumotachograph between the corrugated tube and the test lung. Pressure was measured at the three locations previously described; resistance was 5 and 20 cm H_2O/liter per sec; compliance 20 and 50 ml/cm H_2O. The entrainment port was open or occluded, to permit separate measurement of the two components of tidal volume, one directly delivered through the jet injector and the entrained gases. Injector cannulas of two diameters (1.06 and 1.62 mm) were used. Driving pressure was progressively increased from 5 to 45 psig, in increments of 5 psig, as in the previous experiment. Only the 10-mm diameter endotracheal tube was used during these experiments. Respiratory rate and I/E ratio were maintained constant. The total number of experimental conditions was 144 (Figs. 12-15).

Experimental results indicate that distal airway resistance is the factor most influencing both tidal volume delivered through the injector cannula and, to a far greater extent, entrained volume. Even application of a small resistance resulted in a drastic decrease of entrainment from the values observed with the open load model. Further increases in resistance, to levels comparable to those observed in some forms of pulmonary disease, virtually eliminated entrainment. Changes in compliance within a rather wide range had a much smaller effect on gas delivery, which was constant at different compliances, if resistance was consistant, airway pressure was proportional to tidal volume, which was, in turn, entirely determined by flow rate, since inspiratory time was constant (Fig. 16, 17).

The results of this investigation have significant clinical implications, since they demonstrate that entrainment may not constitute a significant component of the total tidal volume delivered on high-frequency ventilation, when airway resistances are increased even slightly, as is frequently the case in patients with

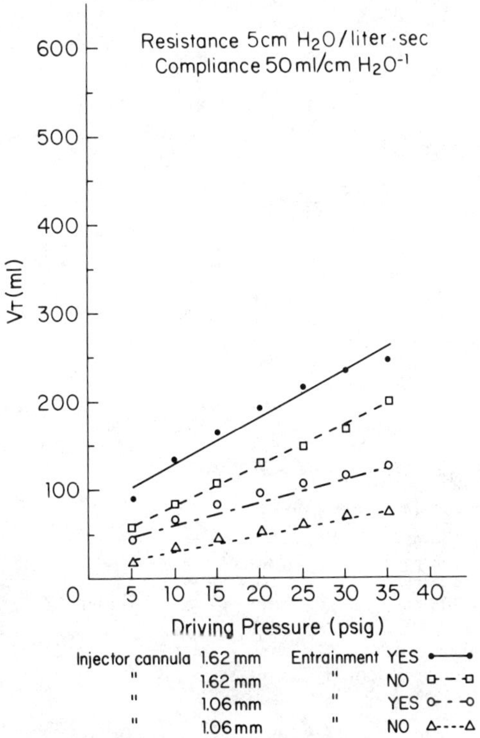

Figure 12 Tidal volume registered at increasing driving pressure in the presence of a distal airway load. Injector cannula is of two different diameters. Entrainment is alternately present or absent. The very sharp reduction of tidal volume delivered, as compared to the noload condition (Figs. 14, 15), is apparent. Entrainment is far more affected by higher load than volume directly delivered through the injector cannula.

acute respiratory failure. Furthermore, the application of high-frequency jet ventilation in diseases characterized by a marked increase in airway resistance might not be appropriate. The study design did not allow differentiation between airway resistances caused by proximal obstruction, such as tracheal or bronchial tumors, and those caused by bronchospasm in smaller airways, as in asthmatic patients. Nonetheless, the available information is sufficient to warrant caution in the administration of high-frequency jet ventilation in patients with increased airway resistance.

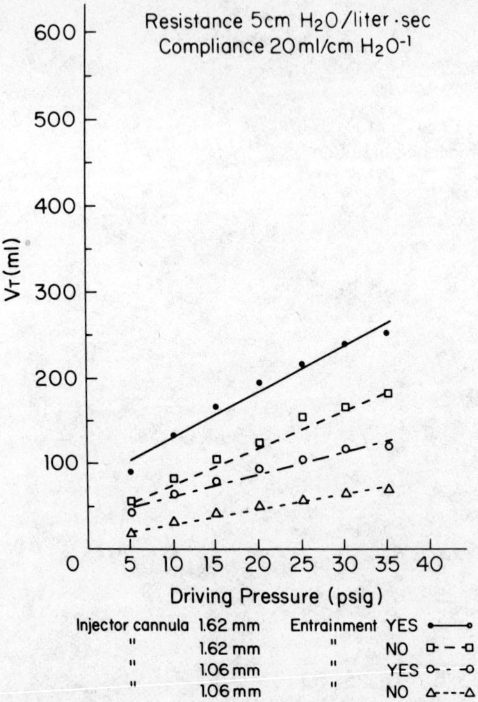

Figure 13

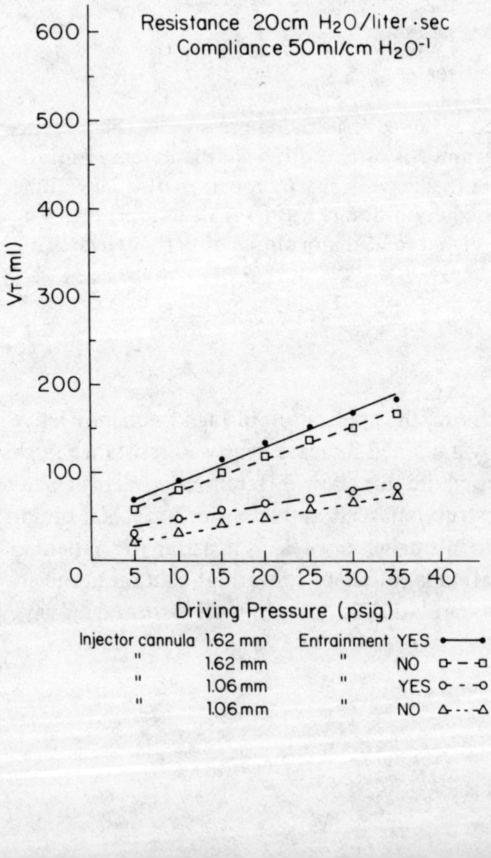

Figure 14

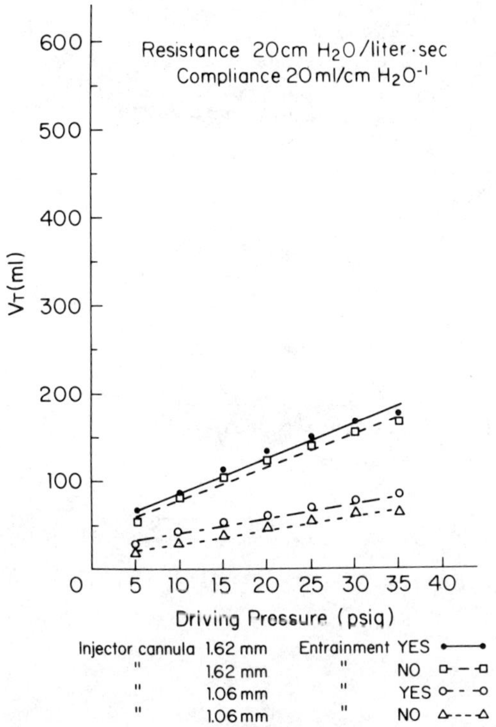

Figure 15

Figures 13-15 Same conditions as in Figure 12 except that resistance is increased and/or compliance decreased. The tidal volume directly delivered through the injector cannula is not affected by the added load, while entrainment virtually disappears at higher resistance. Compliance changes are of lesser significance.

C. PEEP and Demand Valves

Under most circumstances, application of positive end-expiratory pressure (PEEP) is necessary in patients with acute respiratory failure who require mechanical ventilation. To maintain a constant PEEP level throughout all phases of the respiratory cycle, and to prevent excessive gas consumption, gas flow is usually provided by a demand valve, only during the inspiratory phase. The inertia and response times of currently available valves have been designed for spontaneous breathing, not for the far faster rates of HFJV. Changes in airway pressure or flow rates necessary to open the demand valve are also quite different, according to the type of device used, and can occasionally be very high. For all these reasons,

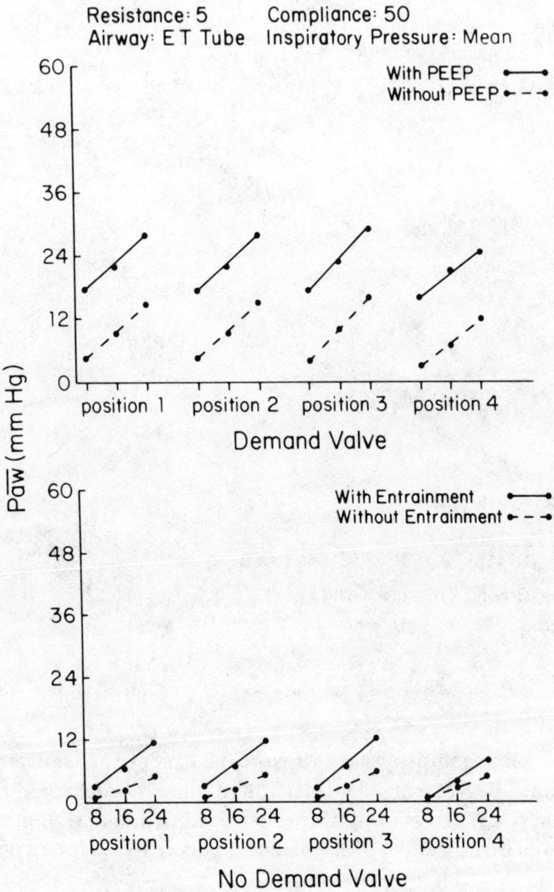

Figure 16 Mean inspiratory pressure measured while driving pressure was progressively increased from 8 to 24 psig. Pressures were measured immediately distal to the opening of the endotracheal tube (position 1), between the distal opening of the endotracheal tube and the test lung model used to generate variable resistance and compliance (position 2), immediately before the insertion of the corrugated tube into the test lung (position 3), and distally to the test lung itself (position 4). For some measurements, an open entrainment port was used; for others entrainment was obtained from a demand valve with or without 10 cm of PEEP applied. In all experimental conditions, the mean inspiratory pressure was proportional to tidal volume and flow rate.

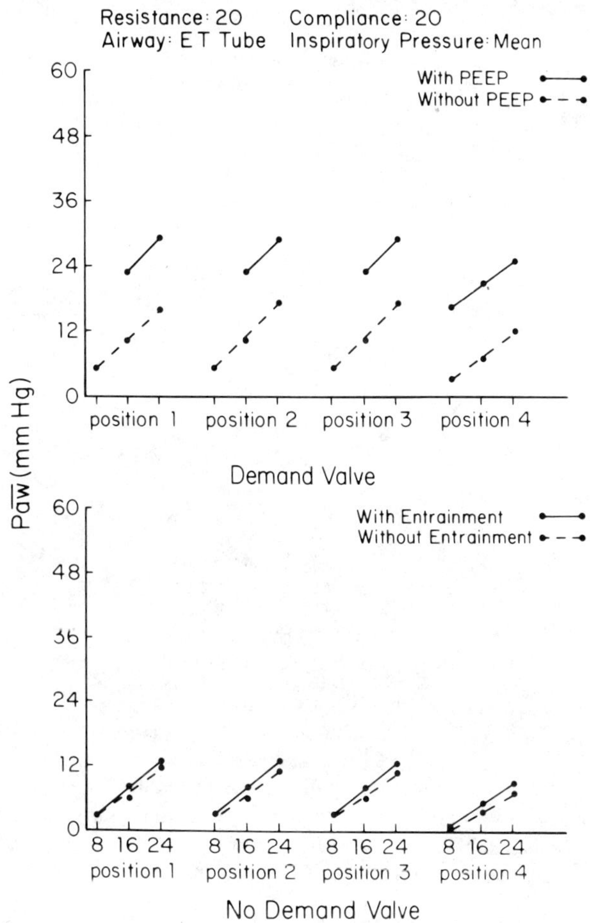

Figure 17 Same as Figure 16 except that resistance has been increased and/or compliance decreased. Mean inspiratory pressure is primarily affected by tidal volume.

it may not be prudent to assume that entrainment through a demand valve is identical to open entrainment.

The test model previously described was used to evaluate the effects of PEEP and demand valves on gas flow and airway pressure. The experimental conditions were similar to those described in the two previous experiments, but entrainment was provided by a Bear Medical demand valve. Two different levels of PEEP were used: 0 and 10 cm H_2O. Injector cannulas were of two diameters

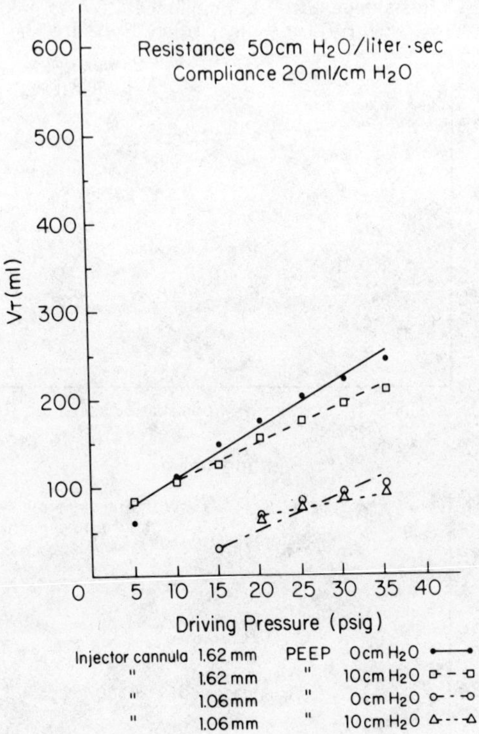

Figure 18 Tidal volume measured while driving pressure was progressively increased. Entrainment was obtained from a demand valve in all experimental conditions. Tidal volume was not affected by PEEP and was slightly lower than that measured with the open entrainment technique (Fig. 16).

(1.06 and 1.62 mm). Driving pressure was progressively increased from 5 to 45 psi. Respiratory rate and I/E ratio were kept constant. In each experimental condition, tidal volume and airway pressure were measured as previously described. Altogether 36 different combinations were investigated (Figs. 18-21).

The results of the experiment indicated that the addition of PEEP slightly reduced gas flow through the larger injector cannula, and significantly reduced entrainment. With the smaller injector cannula, directly delivered volume was even further reduced, and entrainment completely abolished. At higher resistances, total gas flow was so low as to prevent reliable measurement. These results should be expected, since PEEP essentially adds a resistance to gas flow to the lower airway. At 0 PEEP, tidal volume is lower and peak inspiratory pressure substantially higher when a demand valve is used, compared to open entrainment (Figs. 22, 23). Examination of the pressure wave form is notable for its biphasic aspect. An initial slow pressure rise is followed by a delayed sharp increase, which affects peak rather than mean inspiratory pressure values (Figs. 24, 25). This observation must be attributed to a delay in the response of the demand valve. In the early phase of inspiration, flow rate is only composed of the jet flow; later on, when the demand valve opens, a positive-pressure breath is delivered after the solenoid valve has already closed. These considerations may significantly affect gas delivery on HFJV and interpretation of clinical results.

In conclusion, experimental verification of specific characteristics of high-frequency jet ventilators, which may affect clinical efficacy, was performed in a

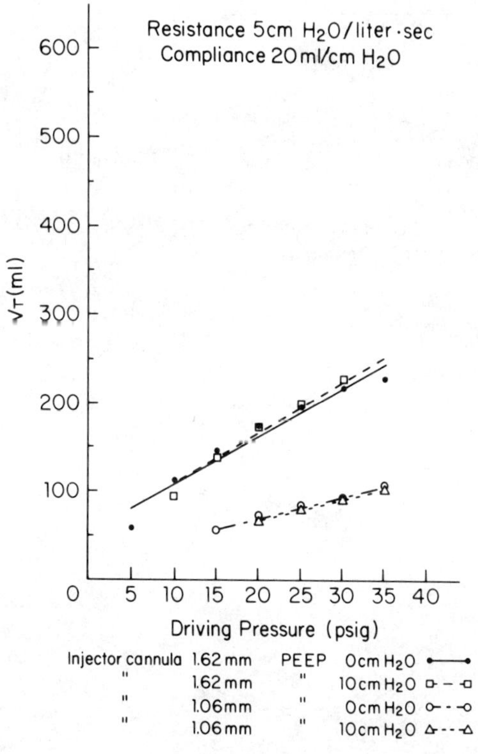

Figure 19 Same experimental conditions as Figure 18 except that resistance is increased and/or compliance decreased. At higher resistance the demand valve function was impaired, so that tidal volume decreased, falling below measurable levels in some circumstances.

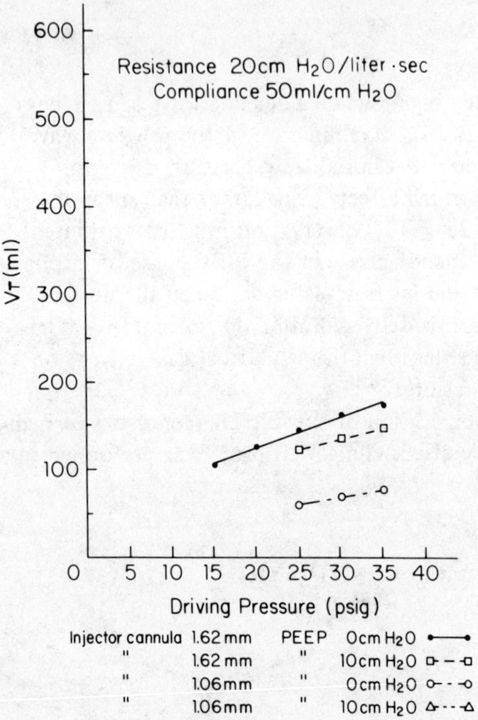

Figure 20

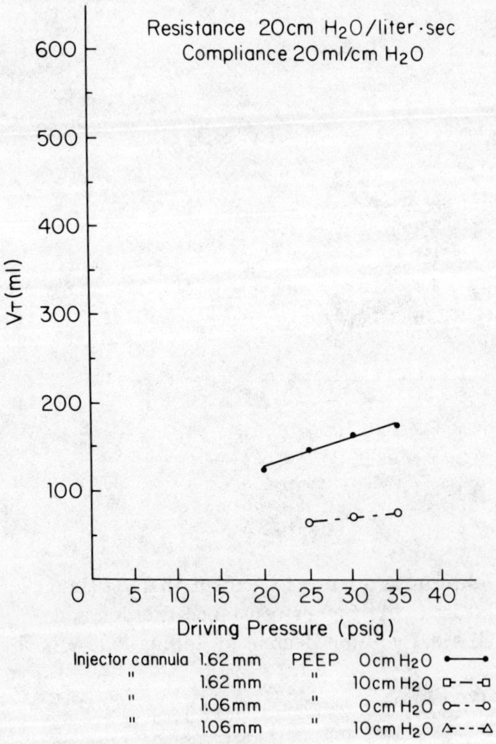

Figure 21

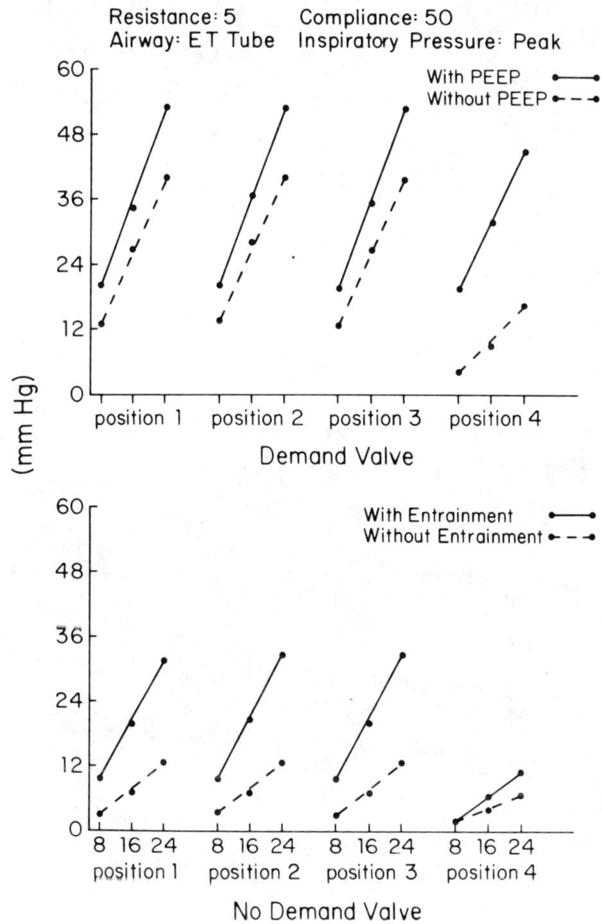

Figure 22 Peak inspiratory pressure measured while driving pressure was progressively increased from 8 to 24 psig. Measuring ports were placed as previously described (Fig. 16). Peak inspiratory pressure was substantially higher when the demand valve was used, compared to the same experimental conditions with open entrainment, although tidal volume was lower.

Figures 20 and 21 Same experimental conditions as Figure 18 except that resistance is increased and/or compliance decreased. At higher resistance the demand valve function was impaired, so that tidal volume decreased, falling below measurable levels in some circumstances.

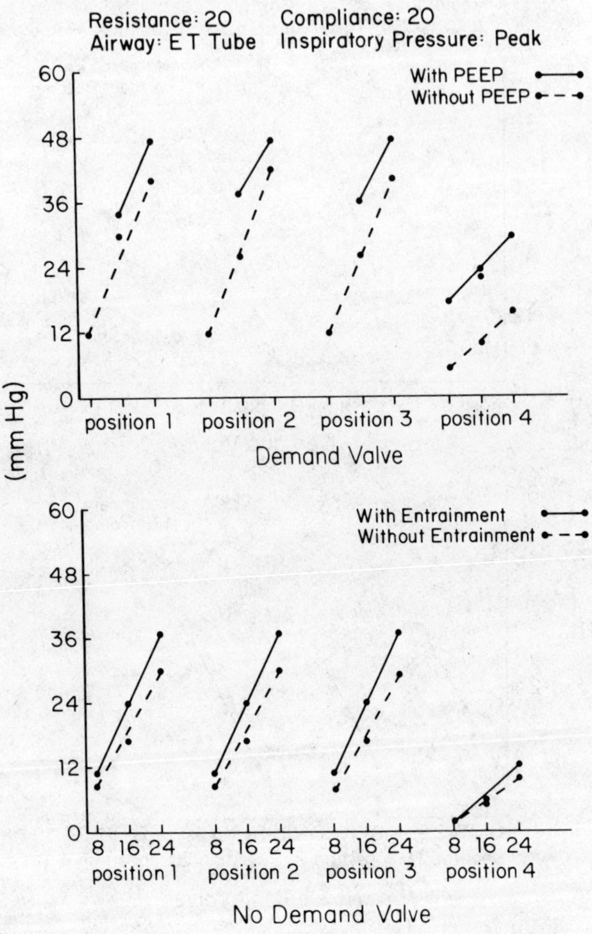

Figure 23 Same as Figure 22 except that resistance has been increased and/or compliance decreased.

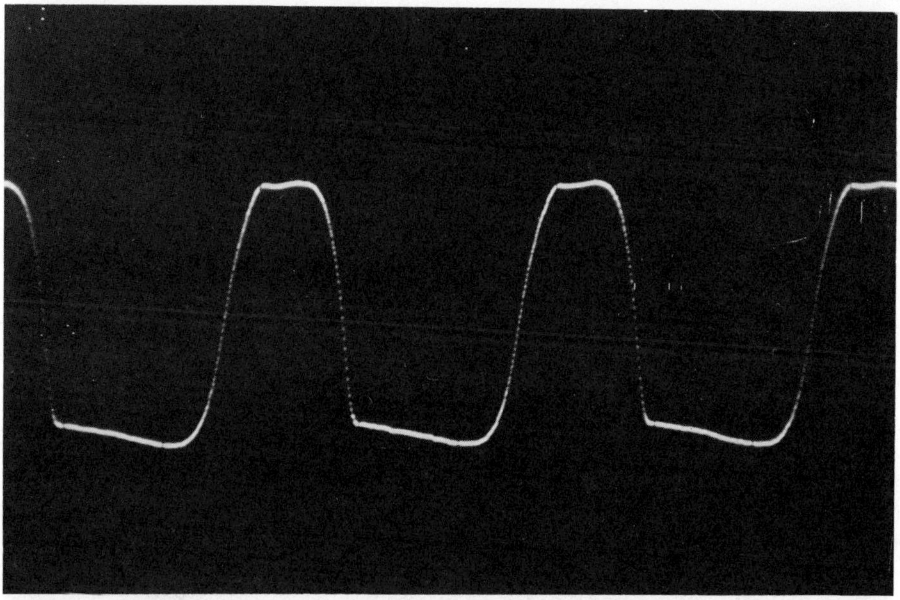

Figure 24 Pressure waveform recorded from position 3 of the corrugated tube connecting endotracheal tube and test lung. The experimental conditions were: driving pressure 30 psig, cannula diameter 1.62 mm, resistance 5 cm/liter per min, compliance 50 mg/cm H_2O, tidal volume 170 ml. There is a sharp increase of airway pressure, followed by a steady plateau while the demand valve is open, and then a sharp decrease upon closure of the valve.

simple test lung model. The experiments confirmed the usefulness of the device in the presence of airway disruption. In patients with diseased lungs, when distal airway load is present, entrainment is less significant and the majority of the tidal volume is directly delivered through the injector cannula. Addition of PEEP does not affect tidal volume, but when entrainment is provided through a demand valve, the response time of the device may substantially influence tidal volume and airway pressure.

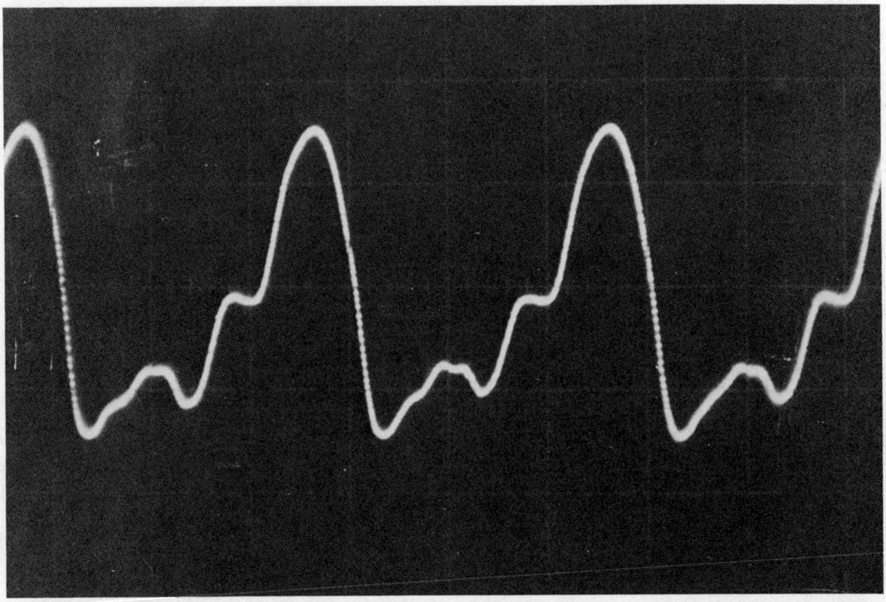

Figure 25 Same experimental conditions as Figure 24 except that entrainment was obtained through a demand valve. Initial pressure rise is slower; later a substantial pressure spike occurs at the closure of the solenoid valve which can be attributed to the delayed closure of the demand valve. The pressure spike is responsible for the sharply higher peak inspiratory pressure observed with this experimental condition, compared to open entrainment, even though tidal volume was comparable.

References

Baum, M., Benzer, H., Goldschmid, W., and Mutz, N. (1983). Pressure flow pattern and gas transport using various types of high frequency ventilation. In *Perspectives in High Frequency Ventilation.* Edited by P. A. Scheck, U. H. Sjostrand, and R. B. Smith. The Hague, Martinus Nijhoff, pp. 51-58.

Beamer, W. C., Prough, D. S., Royster, R. L., et al: (1983). High frequency jet ventilation produces Auto-PEEP. In Proceedings: International Symposium on High Frequency Ventilation. Memorial Sloan-Kettering Cancer Center, pp. 63-66.

Brain, J. D., Proctor, D., and Reid, L. M. (1977). *Respiratory Defense Mechanisms.* New York, Marcel Dekker.

Bunegin, L., Borg, U., and Sjostrand, U. H. (1983). Letters to the Editors. *Anesth. Analg.* **62**:122-123.

Bunnel, J. B., Karlson, K. H., and Shannon, D. C. (1978). High frequency positive pressure ventilation in dogs and rabbits. *Am. Rev. Respir. Dis.* **117**(2) (abstr.).

Calkins, J. M., Waterson, C. K., Hammeroff, S. R., and Kanel, J. S. (1982). A simple flueric high frequency jet ventilator. *Anesth. Analg.* **61**:138-141.

Carlon, G. C., Ray, C. Jr., Klain, M., and McCormick, P. M. (1980). High frequency positive pressure ventilation in the management of a patient with bronchopleural fistula. *Anesthesiology* **52**:160.

Carlon, G. C., Miodownik, S., Ray, C. Jr., and Kahn, R. C. (1981). Technical aspects and clinical implications of high frequency jet ventilation with a solenoid valve. *Crit. Care Med.* **91**(1):47-50.

Carlon, G. C., Howland, W. S., Ray, C. Jr., Midownik, S., Griffin, J. P., and Groeger, J. S. (1983). High-frequency jet ventilation: A prospective randomized evaluation. *Chest* **84**:551-559.

Carlon, G. C., Ray, C., Griffin, J., Midownik, S., and Groeger, J. S. (1983b). Tidal volume and airway pressure on high frequency jet ventilation. *Crit. Care Med.* **11**:83-86.

Chakrabarti, M. K., and Sykes, M. K. (1980). Cardiorespiratory effects of high frequency intermittent positive pressure ventilation in the dog. *Br. J. Anaesth.* 475-481.

Colgan, F. J., TenEyck, L. G., and Sawa, T. (1983). Ventilation requirements during high frequency ventilation. Crit. Care Med. **11**(3):173-176.

den Dunnen, W. L., and Mostert, T. (1983). Pneumatic controlled circulation. In *Perspectives in High Frequency Ventilation.* Edited by P. A. Scheck, U. H. Sjostrand, and R. B. Smith. The Hague, Martinus Nijhoff, pp. 122-131.

Fletcher, P. R. (1983). Alveolar pressure during high frequency ventilation. In *Perspectives in High Frequency Ventilation.* Edited by P. A. Scheck, U. H. Sjostrand, and R. B. Smith. The Hague, Martinus Nijhoff, pp. 92-97.

Gosline, J. E., and O'Brien, M. P. (1934). *The Water Jet Pump.* Berkeley, University of California Press.

Javid, M., and Brenner, E. (1967). *Analysis of Electrical Circuits,* 2nd ed. New York, McGraw-Hill.

Klain, M., and Smith, R. B. (1976). Fluidic technology. *Anaesthesia* **31**:750-757.

Klain, M., Smith, R. B., and Babinski, M. (1980). Limits of high frequency percutaneous transtracheal jet ventilation using a fluidic logic controlled ventilator. *Can. Anaesth. Soc. J.* **27**:351-356.

Kroll, A. E. (1947). The design of jet pumps. *Chem. Engin. Progr.*, p. 21-24.

Lyons, D., Stenzler, A., Steinberg, H., et al: (1981). The airway mechanics of jet ventilation. *Otolaryngol. Head Neck Surg.* **89**:364-369.

MacIntyre, N. R., Anderson, H. R., Silver, R. M., et al: (1983). Pulmonary function in mechanically ventilated patients during 24 hour use of a hygroscopic condenser humidifier. *Chest* **84**:560.

Miodownik, S., Ray, C., and Carlon, G. C. (1980). The digitally programmable cardiac synchronized jet ventilator: An effective research tool. AAMI 15th Annual Meeting 1980, Proceedings, p. 183.

Otto, C. W., Quan, S. F., Conahan, T. J. III, Calkins, J. M., Waterson, C. K., and Hameroff, S. R. (1983). Hemodynamic effects of high frequency jet ventilation. *Anesth. Analg.* **62**:298-304.

Pepe, P. E., and Marini, J. J. (1982). Occult positive end-expiratory pressure in mechanically ventilated patients with airflow obstruction: the auto-PEEP effect. *Am. Rev. Respir. Dis.* **126**:166-170.

Sjostrand, U. (1980). High frequency positive pressure ventilation (HFPPV); A review. *Crit. Care Med.* **8**(3):345.

Wood, P., and Eurenius, S. (1982). Dynamics of Venturi jet ventilation through the operating laryngoscope. *Ann. Otol. Rhinol. Laryngol.* **91**.

7

High-Frequency Jet Ventilation
Experimental Evaluation

JERRY MILAN CALKINS

University of North Carolina School of Medicine
Chapel Hill, North Carolina

High-frequency jet ventilation (HFJV) is but one mode of high-frequency venti lation (HFV) that has been used successfully to provide respiratory support. Like other methods of HFV, HFJV can achieve effective alveolar ventilation and oxygenation at rates ranging from 60 to 900/min using low airway pressures and tidal volumes less than or equivalent to anatomical dead space volume (Quan et al., 1983a,b; Gillespie, 1983).

Unfortunately, as research efforts with various HFJV techniques have progressed, meaningful comparison of results between investigations has been difficult because of the variety of mechanical systems used, a lack of standardization of controlled and measured variables for performance evaluation, and no consistency with either animal models or clinical situations. Hence, each HFJV technique has been investigated as a single entity with unique devices, experimental animal protocols, and clinical situations. Thus, in order to understand the results and appreciate inconsistencies between experimental studies, it is essential that an appreciation for various techniques and applications of HFJV be obtained.

This chapter summarizes experimental data from animal protocols obtained with diverse HFJV techniques. The discussion will be limited to a brief description of commonly used experimental apparatus and measurement techniques, the effects of design and control variables upon gas transport and exchange, physiological interactions, and potential clinical applications.

I. Experimental Apparatus and Measurement Techniques

In general, HFJV utilizes a pulsed gas stream from a high-pressure source delivered into the airway via a small catheter placed either directly into the trachea or inside an endotracheal tube. Precise pulsation of the jet is accomplished by automatic control via either fluidic or electromechanical control systems (Quan et al., 1983a,b). Fluidics is the technology of using fluids (in this situation, gases) to sense, power, or control. It is composed primarily of two major areas: pneumatics (fluidics with moving parts) and fluerics (fluidics without moving parts) (Technical Manual, 1972; Mushin et al., 1980). In 1977, Klain and Smith introduced a high-frequency jet ventilator utilizing pneumatic techniques. In this ventilator, bistable flueric amplifiers were used to control mechanical time-delay relays to regulate the inspiratory and expiratory cycle of the jet through a mechanical interfacing spool valve. In 1982, the concept of a simple flueric high-frequency jet ventilator was introduced (Calkins et al., 1982a). In this device, a single flueric component (bistable amplifier oscillator) located in the power gas stream was employed to control jet pulsations (Fig. 1). The inspiratory and expiratory cycle of the jet was regulated by the pressure imbalance which occurs cyclically between each exhaust port and its control circuit comprised of a capacitor (bottle) and variable resistor (needle valve). In the configuration shown in Figure 1, the

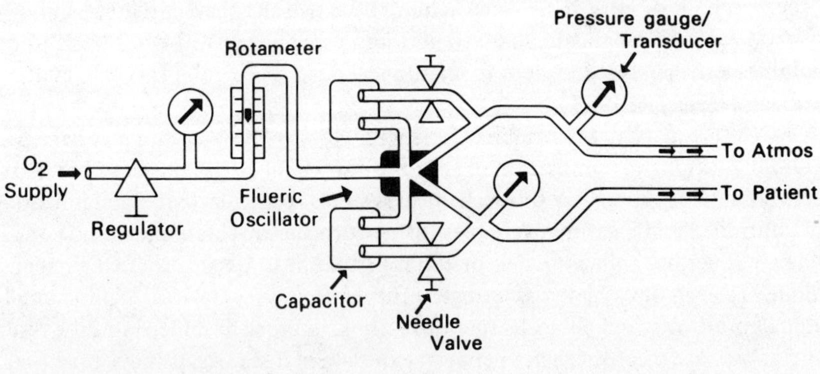

Figure 1 Schematic diagram of a flueric HFJV system. Essential components consist of flueric oscillator with two feedback control circuits consisting of capacitor (bottle) and resistor (needle valve) attached in series between each exhaust and control port. Figure from Calkins et al. (1982a). Reprinted with permission from the International Anesthesia Research Society.

exhaust stream (port) can either be vented directly into the atmosphere or used with the original patient stream for endobronchial high-frequency alternating lung ventilation (HFALV) (Hameroff et al., 1981).

Probably the simplest and most widely used devices for HFJV utilize electromechanical control systems (Carlon et al., 1981b; Calkins et al., 1982b). These units usually consist of a solenoid valve attached to an electronic controller. Programmed electrical impulses from the controller energize the coil of the valve thus opening and closing it at a selected frequency (rate) and pulse duration (valve on). An additional feature of this type of control system is the ease by which the ECG, with or without programmed delays, can be used to provide an initiating control signal (Carlon et al., 1981c; Otto et al., 1983b).

The small-diameter jet catheter can be introduced into the airway in a number of ways. It can be placed directly into the trachea via the oral or nasal pharynx with or without an endotracheal tube (Fig. 2). The most common method is to place the jet nozzle at either the proximal (Carlon et al., 1981b) or distal (Calkins et al., 1982b) tip of an endotracheal tube. When the distal location is

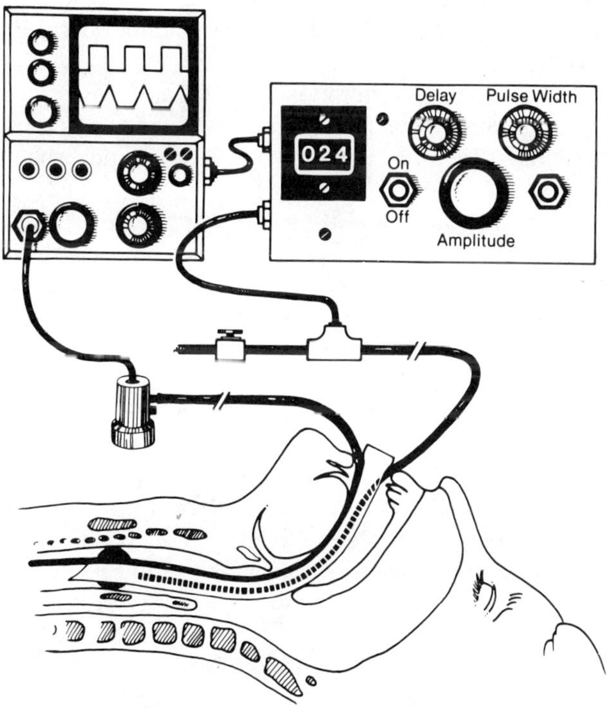

Figure 2 Introduction of jet into trachea. Jet catheter is usually placed directly into the trachea via either oral or nasal pharynx with or without an endotracheal tube.

preferred, the jet can be introduced through a catheter placed either inside the endotracheal tube or via another lumen extruded within the wall of the endotracheal or bronchial tube (Hameroff et al., 1981; Calkins et al., 1982b, 1983b). The percutaneous transtracheal route requires insertion of a catheter through the cricothyroid membrane and is effective in selected situations (Klain and Smith, 1977; Smith et al., 1980).

Selection of control variables for HFJV has been the subject of numerous discussions among investigators. Several researchers maintain that variables controlled during conventional mechanical ventilation (CMV) (respiratory rate, airway pressure, tidal volume) are also appropriate for HFJV (Workshop, 1982). However, interpretation of data must consider features peculiar to HFJV. For example, measurement of tidal volumes and different flow rates (jet, entrainment, minute ventilation) is not easy because of the inherent characteristics of jet dynamics. Volume measurement is even more difficult when HFJV is administered through uncuffed, loosely fitting endotracheal tubes or via small catheters free-floating in the trachea.

Estimates of flow rates and volumes have been made by several methods. With one technique, exhaled and entrained volumes and flow rates are measured with various types of flowmeters (Carlon et al., 1983c; Colgan et al., 1983), and total tidal volumes calculated. With this method, exhaled volumes and flow rates, and therefore calculated tidal volumes, will represent the combined values of jet and entrained sources. They may not represent the actual tidal volumes delivered to the alveoli.

Because of known transient overshoots with rapid exponential decay superimposed on a rectangular flow wave, a pitot tube flowmeter interfaced with a MINC minicomputer system for controlled collection and analysis of the data was used to determine jet flows and volumes (Watt et al., 1983). This type of measurement system has a high-frequency response and immunity to time-dependent interference by pressure variation.

In HFJV, airway pressures (peak, mean, PEEP) are considered important variables that should be measured. Investigators differ sharply on the type of airway pressure to be determined, the ideal sampling location, and the most suitable technique to provide an adequate time response (Workshop, 1982). For example, some studies report mean airway pressure values measured at the exhalation port (Carlon et al., 1981b), while others use distal peak and PEEP values (Calkins et al., 1982b; Carlon et al., 1983c). Measurements can also vary significantly as a function of the breathing circuits used.

Because of the difficulty in measuring airway pressure, many investigators prefer to use values for ventilator-driving pressures. This method does not provide complete information since these values are dependent upon the characteristics of the ventilator, delivery system, and patient (Klain, 1983).

To evaluate pressure measurement techniques, a study monitoring pressures

Table 1 Pressures Measured at Various Locations in Airway

	Distance from jet (cm)					
	Above					Below
	30	20	10	5	0	5
Peak (cm H_2O)	3.4	5.4	6.7	7.2	8.0	7.8
Mean (cm H_2O)	1.2	2.3	2.9	3.6	3.9	4.9
Trough (cm H_2O)	-1.0	-1.5	-1.8	-1.9	-1.8	+1.6

Values shown are means for six animals.

at various airway locations defined in reference to the site of introduction of the jet catheter into the airway was undertaken (Quan et al., 1982; Waterson et al., 1984). Beginning at the proximal opening of the endotracheal tube (30 cm above the jet) and moving the pressure sampling catheter distally toward the jet nozzle located at the distal tip of the endotracheal tube, peak pressures rose when approaching the jet and remained constant 5 cm distally to it (Table 1). Mean pressures also rose through the entire length of the tube. Trough pressures went from a negative value, proximal to the jet nozzle, to a positive value distal to it. These results imply that airway pressures must be measured at locations free from jet interference and referenced to the location of the measurement with respect to the jet nozzle.

The effectiveness of HFJV techniques upon ventilation and oxygenation is easily accomplished with measurements of arterial blood gas tension (ABG). However, continuous noninvasive techniques such as transcutaneous oxygen and carbon dioxide, oximetry, end-tidal CO_2 analysis, and mass spectrometry (Rolly and Versichelen, 1983) have been used. Mihm et al. (1982) have demonstrated excellent correlation of Pa_{CO_2} and end-tidal CO_2 measured during HFJV after a single large breath.

II. Experimental Work With Design and Control Variables

Prior to any discussion of HFJV design and control variables, a few simple, specific physical principles involved in the operation of any high-frequency jet ventilator must be understood. The first is the conservation of mass, which simply states that the rate of mass flowing into a system (patient) must equal the rate of mass flowing from the system (patient). If the rates are not equal, the difference must be accounted for by accumulation (pressurization) or removal (metabolism). High-frequency jet ventilators must provide gas flow into and out of a patient, with minimal accumulation and at a sufficient rate to meet metabolic demands.

In HFJV, a pulse of inspiratory gas is introduced into the airway. The magnitude of the gas pulse is determined by duration (percentage inspiratory time), waveshape (rectangular greatest), and pressures (driving, airway). In addition to these variables for a single pulse, total flow and tidal volume will also depend upon frequency. Hence, frequency inspiratory time and airway pressure are interdependent (Carlon et al., 1981b; 1983c; Calkins et al., 1982b; Klain, 1983).

Once the amount of mass delivered by an active process during the inspiratory pulse has been introduced, it must be removed. This can be accomplished passively using the elastic recoil of the lung and chest wall or actively with the application of a low negative pressure (suction) which produces a reverse flow. Passive exhalation is most commonly used by HFJV.

In either passive or active exhalation, the time allowed must be long enough to permit sufficient removal of gas. Regardless of the inspiratory technique, the gas pulse is rapidly introduced into the airways since driving pressure is significantly higher than the airway pressure. This large pressure difference produces the driving force which directly affects the flow rate, and a large gas volume is delivered in a short period of time. To remove the inspired gas volume during exhalation in the same amount of time as inspiration, either the same pressure difference between the airway and ventilator must exist between the airway and the atmosphere or the exhaust flow resistance must be much smaller. If the pressure difference is low and expiratory resistance cannot be suffuciently decreased, a longer exhalation time is required.

In addition to differences in inhalation and exhalation techniques, each HFJV system must present minimal resistance to exhalation. Any type of obstruction or exhaust resistance will drastically decrease exhalation flow. As the conservation of mass predicts, an accumulation will occur, and pressure will increase inside the respiratory system. When appropriately controlled, this characteristic generates a beneficial PEEP effect. Similarly, if the inlet flow to the airway from the jet is slightly higher than the outlet flow from the airway to the atmosphere, inadvertent PEEP can be obtained.

There is no consensus of opinion regarding the design principles and control variables required for applying HFJV in a safe and effective manner (Workshop, 1982). The results of a few studies which have investigated the influence of HFJV design principles and control parameters on arterial blood gas tensions have appeared in the literature (Carlon et al., 1981b; Calkins et al., 1982b, 1983b; Klain, 1983). The majority of those experimental protocols were conducted on healthy, paralyzed, anesthetized dogs.

A. Design Variables

For the purposes of this discussion, design variables will be defined as characteristics of the ventilator and jet delivery circuit not under continuous operational control. The design variables studied include the location for introducing the jet into the airway expressed as a distance from the carina, the ratio of jet lumen area to exhaust lumen area, and jet pressure wave shapes.

Location of Jet in Airway

With a flueric ventilator operating at a source pressure of 20 psi, 144/min frequency, a 50% inspiratory time (I/E = 1:1), and total flow of 18.5 liters/min, the jet was most effective in carbon dioxide removal when its distal opening (nozzle) was near the carina (Hameroff et al., 1981). Placement of the nozzle at the distal end of an endobronchial tube resulted in a lower $PaCO_2$ than at the proximal opening (40 ± 3 vs. 66 ± 5 torr). Catheter tip distance from the carina correlated linearly with $PaCO_2$. The position of the catheter tip did not significantly alter arterial oxygen tension (Hameroff et al., 1981).

Although the jet nozzle can be placed proximally in the airway (an alternative which may offer practical and safety advantages), the loss in efficiency must be overcome with higher driving pressures and gas consumption (Hameroff et al., 1981). Similar results for jet location and CO_2 elimination were obtained by Baum et al. (1983) with their double-lumen jet located 2 cm above the carina. It should be noted, however, that entrainment is more efficient with the jet centered in the proximal endotracheal tube. This increased efficiency in entrainment could, in some instances, lead to higher volumes and airway pressures, hence better gas exchange, than is achievable by distal placement of the nozzle at the same driving pressures.

Pulse Wave Shape

Using an electromechanical system operating at a constant driving pressure, the effect of jet pressure wave shapes upon ABG tensions was investigated in healthy dogs (Calkins et al., 1982b). A noncompliant capacitor (bottle) placed between the outlet of the solenoid and the nozzle of the jet, produced a damped sinusoidal (sawtooth) wave shape. The effect of each wave shape on ABG tensions was determined as a function of pulse duration (percentage inspiratory time) and frequency.

In general at a constant driving pressure, airway pressures increased with longer inspiratory time and higher frequency. Significant differences between wave shapes reveal higher peak, lower PEEP, and greater airway pressure differences (Δ Paw = peak - PEEP) with rectangular wave shapes (Table 2).

At a constant driving pressure, $PaCO_2$ values tended to be lower as the percentage inspiratory time and frequency increased with rectangular wave shapes, but the differences were not significant. The highest mean $PaCO_2$ values (63.7 torr) for rectangular waves occurred with the shortest percentage inspiratory (% I time) time and lowest frequency (10%, 120/min). For sawtooth waves, the

Table 2 Significant Differences Between Rectangular and Sawtooth Wave Shapes

Variables	Rectangular[a]	Sawtooth[a]
Peak airway pressure (cm H_2O)		
10% I time, 150/min	5.3 ± 0.5	3.9 ± 0.3
PEEP (cm H_2O)		
20% I time, 120/min	1.7 ± 0.3	2.1 ± 0.4
25% I time, 150/min	2.1 ± 0.4	2.7 ± 0.3
Airway pressure difference (cm H_2O)		
10% I time, 120/min	3.8 ± 0.7	2.1 ± 0.4
25% I time, 150/min	4.8 ± 0.2	3.4 ± 0.4
PaO_2 (torr)		
40% I time, 180/min	481 ± 45	437 ± 48
$PaCO_2$ (torr)		
20% I time, 120/min	47.3 ± 8.2	79.1 ± 19.0
25% I time, 120/min	30.1 ± 3.1	55.9 ± 8.9
30% I time, 150/min	33.1 ± 3.7	67.8 ± 11.3
30% I time, 180/min	43.2 ± 5.7	84.0 ± 19.3

[a]Mean ± SEM, p. $\leqslant$ 0.05.

highest $PaCO_2$ (97.3 torr) was observed with a 15% I time and a rate of 180/min. Rectangular wave shapes consistently produced a lower $PaCO_2$ than the sawtooth for the same % I time and frequency settings (Table 2). At an FiO_2 of 1.0, changing % I time, frequency, and wave shapes resulted in a minimal effect on PaO_2 (Table 2).

Rectangular pressure waveforms proved more efficient for CO_2 removal than the sawtooth shape (Calkins et al., 1982b). This suggests that an initial transient high flow may be important in obtaining an effective inspiratory volume. Although flows through the jet cannula were not measured in this study, higher driving pressures were necessary to achieve the same peak airway pressure and expiratory minute volumes with the damped wave form.

Ratio of Jet Lumen to Exhaust Lumen Areas

The ratio of the inspiratory lumen area to expiratory lumen area appears to be another determinant of CO_2 elimination. Babinski et al. (1981) investigated tracheal tubes with lumen area ratios of 1:1, 1:4, and 1:10 in healthy dogs at an I/E ratio of 1:2 and frequencies ranging from 100 to 600/min and adjusted driving pressures. They found no differences in ventilation and oxygenation between these three tubes at frequencies $<$ 300/min. However, lower intratracheal pressures existed with larger exhalation lumen areas. Similar results for ratios were observed in other studies in healthy and oleic-acid-treated dogs where ratios ranged from 1:6 to 1:11 (Calkins et al., 1983b; Carlon et al., 1983c).

B. Control Variables

Control variables are those which can be manipulated by the operator while the device is in use. Frequency, % I time (pulse duration), driving pressure (jet supply pressure), airway pressures (peak, mean, PEEP), airway pressure difference (Δ Paw = peak - PEEP), estimated tidal volumes, and minute ventilation are among those commonly investigated (Calkins et al., 1982b, 1983b; Carlon et al., 1983c; Klain, 1983; Quan et al., 1982; Waterson et al., 1984). The variables selected for these studies were chosen on the basis of the investigators' experience and the practical clinical usefulness for the safe and successful application of HFJV. Because of the interactions between variables, care must be exercised in interpreting results.

Frequency

Investigations were conducted on the effects of frequency, at a constant driving pressure, on airway pressures (peak, PEEP), expiratory flow rates, and ABG tensions (Calkins et al., 1982b; Carlon et al., 1983c; Klain, 1983). In general, the results indicated that at a given driving pressure and I/E ratio, increasing frequency increases airway pressures, exhaled volumetric flow rates (tidal volumes), and $PaCO_2$. Another study investigated the effect of frequency upon ABG tensions at a constant 30% inspiratory time and peak airway pressure (Calkins et al., 1983b). Mean $PaCO_2$ increases linearly with increasing frequency (Fig. 3). However, at constant peak airway pressure and % I time, there was no difference in $AaDO_2$ between a frequency of 100 and 300/min. During HFJV, as well as on CMV, oxygenation depends predominantly on mean airway pressure. Increasing frequency usually increases mean airway pressure, and therefore PaO_2. At higher frequencies (>450/min) there was a tendency for $AaDO_2$ to increase. The reason for this behavior was not apparent from these data (Calkins et al., 1983b).

Percentage Inspiratory Time (Pulse Duration)

Percentage inspiratory time (% I time) is the portion of total pulse cycle during which gases flow to the patient. At a constant driving pressure and frequency, increasing % I time increases expiratory flow and airway pressures, while $PaCO_2$ decreases (Calkins et al., 1982b). As shown in Figure 4, increasing % I time at a

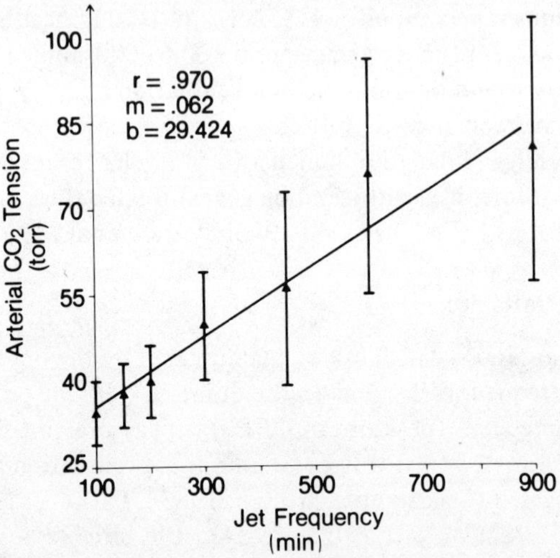

Figure 3 Frequency vs. $PaCO_2$ at constant peak airway pressure and 30% I time, CO_2 tension increases linearly with increasing frequency. Figure adapted from Calkins et al. (1983b).

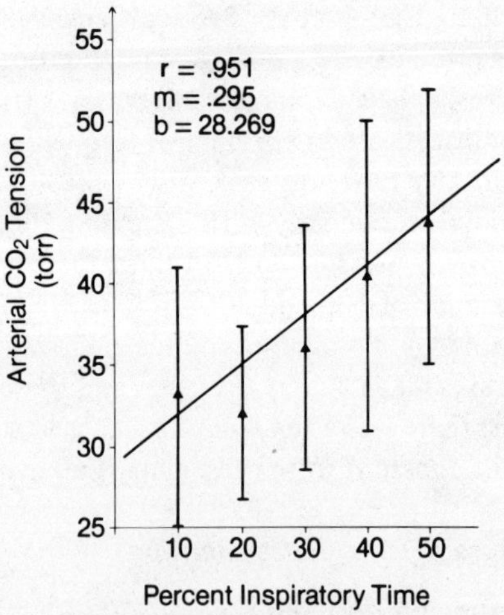

Figure 4 Percentage inspiratory time vs. $PaCO_2$. At a constant peak airway pressure and frequency (150/min), CO_2 tension increases linearly with increasing % I time. Figure adapted from Calkins et al. (1983b).

constant frequency and peak airway pressure increases $PaCO_2$ linearly. Under these conditions, increasing % I time has no apparent effect upon $AaDO_2$ (Calkins et al., 1983b).

These results suggest the need for longer exhalation phase (a passive process) at higher frequencies. This is not surprising considering the flow-volume relationship that must be established between inspiratory and expiratory volumes with greatly different driving pressures, resistances, and flow rates. Since a certain volume (mass) of gas must be delivered into the airway during inspiration, there is a limit to the degree of reduction of inspiratory time. If % I time is reduced, drive pressure must be increased to deliver the same inspired volume. Due to limits in the response time of equipment, supersonic or choke flow characteristics, and gas supply pressures, % I time cannot be lowered limitlessly. For example, at 150/min and a constant peak pressure, normocarbia is obtained at a 30% I time. However, at the same frequency and peak airway pressure both 10% and 50% I time will produce hypercarbia (Calkins et al., 1983b).

Airway Pressure

The single strongest determinant of the adequacy of ventilation is airway pressure. Numerous experimental protocols have been conducted to determine its effects upon expiratory volumes, ABG tensions, and other variables (Calkins et al., 1982b, 1983b; Carlon et al., 1983c; Klain, 1983; Waterson et al., 1984).

Increasing jet driving pressure produces increases in peak, mean, and PEEP airway pressures (Calkins et al., 1982b; Klain, 1983). Increasing peak airway pressure at constant frequency and % I time decreases $PaCO_2$ linearly (Calkins et al., 1983b). The independent effects of PEEP, mean, and airway pressure difference (Δ Paw = peak – PEEP) on ABG tensions have also been investigated (Calkins et al., 1983b; Carlon et al., 1983c; Klain, 1983; Waterson et al., 1984). Increasing PEEP and Δ Paw (Fig. 5) decreased $PaCO_2$. Mean airway pressure had no significant effect on $PaCO_2$. The single most important determinant was Δ Paw (Calkins et al., 1983b; Waterson et al., 1984). Peak airway pressures required to ob tain normocarbia were lower than those necessary on CMV. However, mean airway pressures may not be different with HFJV and CMV since in both situations they are also dependent on rates and I/E ratios.

Lendinez et al. (1983) investigated the effect of mean airway pressure, measured distal to the carina, upon ventilation (VD/VT, $PaCO_2$) using an electromechanical HFJV system with the jet introduced at the proximal end of the endotracheal tube in healthy dogs. In this investigation, either tidal volume (driving pressure) and I/E ratio or tidal volume and mean airway pressure were held constant while frequency varied. At a constant tidal volume and I/E ratio, increasing frequency resulted in higher mean airway pressure, VD/VT, and $PaCO_2$. At constant tidal volume and mean airway pressure, decreasing I/E from 1:1 (50%

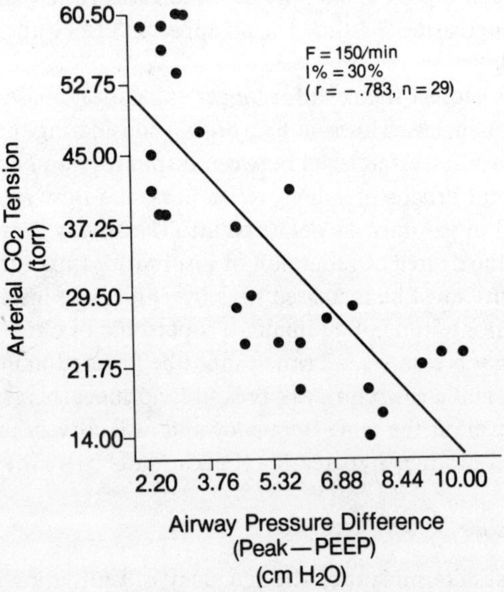

Figure 5 Airway pressure difference vs. $PaCO_2$. At a constant 30% I time and 150/min frequency, CO_2 tensions tend to decrease with an increasing airway pressure difference. Figure adapted from Calkins et al. (1983b).

I time) to 1:6 (14% I time), while increasing frequency from 100 to 200/min, produced no changes in VD/VT, but lowered $PaCO_2$. Oxygenation primarily depended on mean airway pressure. Data analysis indicated that mean airway pressure can explain only 70% of the changes in oxygenation and that the airway pressure difference (peak - PEEP) has an additional influence (Klain, 1983).

Driving Pressure

The most commonly used control variable is driving pressure adjusted to change minute ventilation (Klain, 1983). Unfortunately, it does not provide adequate information to compare different techniques. The same driving pressure may deliver completely different gas flows if different catheters or inspiratory times are used. When we discuss driving pressure, absolute values cannot be used. In most situations, however, increasing driving pressure enhances gas flow rate. The result is higher airway pressure (peak, mean, PEEP) with lower $PaCO_2$ and higher PaO_2 (Klain, 1983).

Minute Ventilation

Klain (1983) and Colgan et al. (1983) demonstrated that minute volume and alveolar ventilation are dependent upon the driving pressure, jet catheter size, and inspiratory time. Increasing each of these variables will increase delivered minute volume. At constant driving pressure, increasing frequency will not change minute volume, only divide it into smaller tidal volumes (Klain, 1983). A higher minute volume is needed to achieve the same $PaCO_2$ at higher frequencies. At constant frequency, a higher driving pressure and therefore minute volume and airway pressures (mean, peak) result in lower $PaCO_2$.

III. Experimental Evaluation of Physiological Consequences of High-Frequency Jet Ventilation

A. Respiratory System

Some authors suggest that gas exchange during HFV must rely on enhanced molecular diffusion to explain the magnitude of gas transport observed in the available time. Tantalum powder was used to coat the bronchioles and make them radio-opaque. Cinebronchography was used to evaluate dynamic changes in airway caliber produced in dogs by HFJV; these changes were then compared with those observed during IPPV and spontaneous ventilation (Quan et al., 1984a). The results indicated that on HFJV the larger airway (>3 mm) experienced proportionally greater changes in diameter. These findings were most pronounced at HFJV frequency of 450/min which induced visible movements of the large airways with only minimal motion of the small airways. The results of this study suggest that gas movement in the smaller airways does not occur by bulk flow (Quan et al., 1984a).

Despite the increasing acceptance of high-frequency jet ventilation, only recently have investigations been conducted to determine the effects of HFJV on the respiratory system. At certain pulse durations (% I time) and frequencies, HFJV-related phasic variations in heart rate, arterial blood pressure, and chest expansion have been observed (Calkins et al., 1982b). Typical wave shape patterns of this interaction are shown in Figure 6. HFJV-induced fluctuations in amplitude of chest expansion generally occurred with a rectangular jet pulse wave shape. Analysis of tracings of phasic fluctuations showed a typical "beat frequency envelope" (mathematically, the differences of two sine waves).

Maximal chest expansion occurred when peak airway pressure coincided with ventricular diastole. Maxima and minima in chest expansion occurred periodically as beat frequencies at a rate equal to the difference between heart rate and HFJV rate. Phasic changes in arterial blood pressure commonly occurred with sawtooth pulse wave shapes at a PEEP >3 cm H_2O. These phasic blood

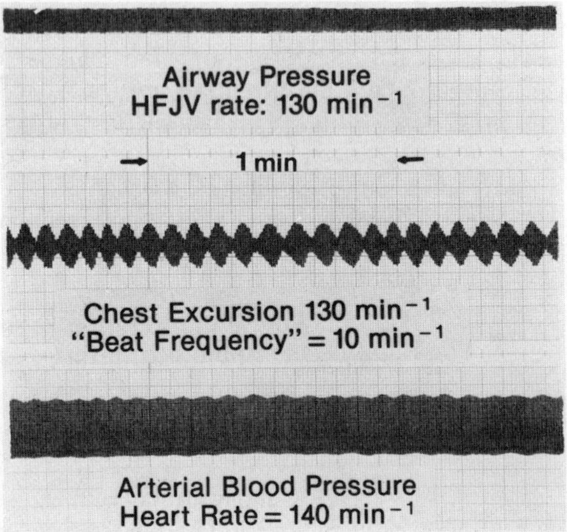

Figure 6 Phasic variations in chest expansion and arterial blood pressure. Chest excursion curve (center) demonstrates a beat frequency envelope (mathematically, the difference of two sine waves). Frequency of this wave shape is approximately heart rate minus jet frequency (140 – 130 = 10/min). Blood pressure curve (bottom) demonstrates phasic variation (not beat frequency). Figure from Calkins et al. (1982b). Reprinted with the permission from the International Anesthesiology Research Society.

pressure fluctuations were periodic but did not occur at predictable or identifiable beat frequencies.

Tallman et al. (1983) demonstrated similar phasic changes with pulmonary artery pressure. Depending upon the timing of lung inflation with HFJV and the phase of the cardiac cycle, this interaction can have marked effects on pulmonary vascular impedance, and hence pulmonary blood flow and pressure.

Recent studies have investigated potentially harmful effects of HFJV on the lungs or tracheal mucosa. Rock et al. (1976) found no tracheal mucosal damage after 2 hr of HFJV in dogs. Likewise, Smith et al. (1981) reported no damage to either the airway or lung parenchyma in a dog after 24 hr of HFJV. Keszler et al. (1982) compared the effects on lung parenchyma of HFJV and conventional IPPV administered for 24 hr by specifically searching for atelectasis and barotrauma in healthy dogs. With mean airway pressure of 4 cm H_2O, neither atelectasis nor barotrauma occurred in any of the animals receiving HFJV. However, with both ventilatory techniques, microscopic hyperaeration with some degree of polymorphonuclear cell infiltration was observed. Some adverse effects may be secondary to preconditioning of the ventilatory gases and to techniques used to introduce the catheter into the airway. As with conventional mechanical ventilation, inadequate humidification of gases delivered by HFJV impairs mucociliary transport, while adequate humidification preserves it (Klain et al., 1982). Transtracheal jet ventilation has been associated with increased incidence of tracheal mucosal damage, subcutaneous emphysema, pneumomediastinum, and pneumopericardium (Smith et al., 1975).

B. Cardiovascular System

The potential adverse cardiovascular effects of conventional positive pressure ventilation are well-known to physicians. They are related to increased airway pressure which decreases venous return to the right heart and leads to a fall in cardiac output. The magnitude of the hemodynamic effect is directly related to the amount of positive pressure applied to the airway. Since HFJV can provide adequate alveolar ventilation at much lower peak and perhaps mean airway pressures, HFJV should have less adverse effects on the cardiovascular system than conventional mechanical ventilation. However, investigators have reported improved, unchanged, and impaired hemodynamic function with HFJV under a variety of experimental conditions (Table 3) (Otto et al., 1983a). Using HFJV in patients, Dedhia (1981) found no change in cardiac output; while Carlon et al. (1981a) found either no change or an increase in cardiac output compared to conventional ventilation. Schuster et al. (1981) observed higher mean arterial pressures, but no change in either stroke or cardiac index. In their experiment, peak airway pressure was lower on HFJV than on conventional ventilation, but mean airway pressure was higher. Szele and Shavari (1981) found no differences in cardiac output, mean arterial pressure, or heart rate in intravascularly depleted dogs, although mean airway pressure was lower on HFJV than on CMV.

Some data suggest that synchronization of ventilation with heart rate during HFJV might provide circulatory assistance and increase cardiac output (Carlon et al., 1981c). In comparison to asynchronous HFJV and CMV, Carlon et al. noted a decrease in cardiac output when HFJV was synchronized with the heart rate to deliver the peak inspiratory pressure coincident with mid-diastole. However, synchronization of peak airway pressure with aortic valve opening produced no change or increase in cardiac output.

In contrast, utilizing HFJV in healthy dogs, Otto et al. (1983b) observed no difference in cardiac output compared to IPPV. However, if 15 cm of H_2O PEEP was added, there was less depression in the cardiac output during HFJV. When the high-frequency pulse was synchronized with the heart rate, no beneficial effects on cardiac output were demonstrated.

In these investigations, cardiac function was based upon both invasively

Table 3 Hemodynamic Effects of HFJV

Author	Subjects	P_{aw} with HFJV	Hemodynamic effect of HFJV[a]
Dedhia, 1981	Patients	?	=
Carlon et al., 1981a	Patients	?	= or ++
Schuster et al., 1981	Patients	Higher	=
Szele and Keenan, 1981	Dogs	Lower	=
Carlon et al., 1981c	Dogs	Higher	--
Otto et al., 1982b	Dogs	Lower	++
Calkins et al., 1984a	Patients	Lower	=

[a]++ improved; = unchanged; -- impaired
P_{aw}, mean airway pressure
Adapted from Otto et al. (1983b).

measured (pressures, cardiac output) and calculated variables (resistances, volumes, indices). Since these parameters assess myocardial status indirectly, they may not be sensitive enough to detect myocardial dysfunction. To assess left ventricular function better during HFJV and IPPV, esophageal echocardiography was utilized (Calkins and Waterson, 1984). Moynihan et al. (1981) have shown that analysis of left ventricular function by 2D echocardiography is best done using changes in area. An esophageal 3.5-mHz phased-array probe was used to assess left ventricular function in anesthetized patients undergoing low abdominal surgery on HFJV and OPPV. No significant difference between ventilatory modes on left ventricular function was observed (Table 4).

The results of these various hemodynamic investigations suggest that HFJV may be useful in clinical situations in which IPPV produces an unacceptable depression in cardiac output. Unfortunately, comparisons of the cardiovascular effects of HFJV and IPPV have not been performed in situations of parenchymal disease.

C. Renal System

On IPPV, glomerular filtration rate (GFR), urine volume, and urine sodium excretion decrease. These changes have been attributed to decreased cardiac output and a secondary increase in sympathetic tone, stimulating the renin-angiotensin system, increasing antidiuretic hormone (ADH) secretion, and reducing free water clearance (Marquez et al., 1981). More recently, alterations in renal vein pressures and renal pulsatile flow patterns, induced by IPPV, have been implicated

Table 4 Esophageal Echocardiographic Areas of Left Ventricle During IPPV and HFV

	IPPV[a] (n=34)	HFV[a] (n=30)
Areas		
Diastolic area (cm^2)	12.1 ± 0.06	12.0 ± 0.7
Systolic area (cm^2)	5.5 ± 0.4	4.9 ± 0.4
% Area reproduction	55.3 ± 1.7	58.0 ± 1.9
Airway pressure range Peak/PEEP		
High (cm H_2O/cm H_2O)	27/2	15/10
Low (cm H_2O/cm H_2O)	12/2	9/7

[a]Mean ± SEM

(Marquez et al., 1981). Results from limited studies indicate that high-frequency positive-pressure ventilation (HFPPV) does not produce a similar renal effect (Jonzon et al., 1971). The absence of ADH hypersecretion may be related to lower intrathoracic pressures. When HFPPV is utilized in experimental animals, free water clearance results in normally dilute urine and the water load excreted without delay. Marquez et al. (1981) compared renal function in swine on HFJV (100/min, I/E 0.3) with 10 cm H_2O PEEP and on spontaneous ventilation with 10 cm H_2O CPAP. Their preliminary results indicate that neither airway pressure pattern altered GFR or venous renin. However, urine volume was decreased with both ventilatory modes, but urine sodium excretion was decreased only during HFJV with PEEP.

D. Nervous System

IPPV produces changes in intrathoracic pressure during the respiratory cycle which produce large fluctuations in intracranial pressure (ICP). These fluctuations are clearly reduced on HFPPV, and the physical movement of the brain is likewise less pronounced (Todd et al., 1981). However, mean intracranial pressure does not decrease with HFPPV. In addition, HFPPV has little effect on cerebral hemodynamics (Toutant et al., 1983). Babinski et al. (1981a) demonstrated that ICP fluctuations were less in normocarbic dogs on HFJV at 100-150 min than at lower frequencies. This was also demonstrated in dogs with intracranial hypertension. Absolute values of ICP in these groups of animals were not affected by HFJV, and brain movement was reduced. In another study no significant cerebral lesions were observed by gross and histological examination, in 12 mongrel dogs supported on HFJV for 4 hr (Calkins and Waterson, 1984).

IV. Possible Clinical Applications

HFJV has been successfully utilized in a number of acute care situations (Quan et al., 1983a,b). Applications include emergency airway management during cardiopulmonary resuscitation, anesthesia, and surgical procedures, and ventilatory support of critically ill children and adults.

No form of HFJV has demonstrated a clear, significant advantage over conventional methods of respiratory support in any clinical application. For some uses, the efficacy of HFJV has been demonstrated and cost, risks, and benefits reasonably established. Because basic operational mechanisms are not understood, and clinical experience is limited, HFJV is still in the investigational stages. This discussion will be limited to investigations in animals, which address applications for which HFJV may have greater efficacy, at lower cost and risk/benefit ratio than conventional ventilation.

A. Emergency Airway Management

Klain (1983) and Smith et al. (1981) have described the successful use of percutaneous transtracheal HFJV in dogs. Their results indicated that, with this technique, it is possible to maintain gas exchange at frequencies to 200/min. Numerous investigators have substantiated these results in a variety of experimental and clinical situations (Quan et al., 1983a,b).

HFJV has been compared to IPPV during recovery of asphyxic, hypotensive animals and during CPR in animals with cardiac fibrillation (Klain et al., 1981). Both ventilatory techniques proved equally successful in maintaining oxygenation and ventilation. In nonintubated dogs, the effects of frequency and I/E ratio on aspiration during CPR were examined (Klain et al., 1983). Without chest compression, no aspiration occurred as long as expiration was less than 66% of the cycle and frequency greater than 60/min (Klain et al., 1981). With chest compression, aspiration was prevented as long as expiration was less than 50% of the respiratory cycle and frequency greater than 100/min. In a third series using the same technique, an upper-airway obstruction was created using radioopaque material and the efficacy of transtracheal HFJV in removing the obstruction was evaluated by radiocinematography (Klain et al., 1981). Material above the jet nozzle was expelled into the mouth, while material below the nozzle was propelled deeper into the lungs. Szele and Keenan (1981) demonstrated that percutaneous transtracheal HFJV at 150/min, 30% I time, with a mean airway pressure of 4 torr may prevent aspiration if the orophraynx is initially free of foreign material. If particulate matter is present, the direction of the needle becomes important. Another series of experiments investigated the potential of HFJV for cardiac assist with copulsation or counterpulsation (Klain et al., 1981). These results were discussed in a previous section. In general, HFJV did not cause hemodynamic compromise and, at 120 breaths/min, counterpulsation was achieved. In the last series of CPR protocols, the use of transtracheal HFJV for administration of cardioactive drugs was investigated. Under direct bronchoscopy, Cardio-Green (indocyanine) dye was injected and observed while rapidly dispersing to the most distal airway. Response to atropine (0.8 mg) and epinephrine (0.4 mg) administered through this route had a time of onset comparable to intravenous injection. With 0.8 mg epinephrine, a biphasic response with prolonged duration was noted. The second peak was reached after 4 min with activity lasting for 20 min (Klain et al., 1981).

B. Potential Applications in the Operating Room

HFJV has been used in numerous types of surgical procedures requiring general anesthesia, including ENT, orthopedic, and general (Quan et al., 1983c; Marquez et al., 1982). It has been used extensively for ventilation during rigid bronchoscopy, laryngoscopy, and microscopic laryngeal surgery with the laser.

Potential clinical applications also exist for neurosurgical procedures. As previously discussed, the significant decrease in cerebral motion and less pronounced ICP fluctuations without cerebral hemodynamic changes may offer advantages to the neurosurgeon. Another potential advantage of HFJV is the rapidity with which air embolisms are cleared from the pulmonary vasculature. Hoff et al. (1982a) compared the effects of IPPV and high-frequency oscillatory ventilation (HFOV) (1200/min) on the rapid intravenous infusion of 6.6 ml/kg of an air/xenon mixture into healthy mongrel dogs. In animals that did not develop an air lock, HFOV resulted in a more rapid clearance of the embolized gases from the right ventricle and lungs as compared to IPPV. When an air lock developed, cardiovascular collapse occurred with death of the animal, regardless of the mode of ventilation. These results need confirmation for HFJV.

The potential of HFJV for ventilatory support during thoracic surgical procedures and airway disruptions has also been investigated. Hoff et al. (1982b) compared percutaneous transtracheal HFJV with IPPV in healthy dogs before and after thoracotomy. Their results indicated that adequate gas exchange with low mean airway pressures was consistently obtained at frequencies of 100 and 300/min. There were no significant differences with IPPV except that the lowest PaO_2 and $PaCO_2$ were observed at 100/min. In addition, the surgical field for median sternotomy thoracotomy procedures was more quiescent during HFJV. Carlon et al. (1983b) demonstrated that HFJV provided effective ventilation with airway disruption of increasing magnitude to 0.5 cm × 2.0 cm.

The use of another technique, high-frequency alternating lung ventilation (HFALV), has been suggested for thoracic surgery (Hameroff et al., 1981). With this technique, bronchial catheters are placed in each main stem bronchus and high-frequency jet ventilation delivered alternately (180° out of phase) to each.

The inspiratory phase of one lung coincides with the expiratory phase of the other. With HFALV, a lower $PaCO_2$ and (A-a) DO_2 was obtained than with HFJV.

C. Experimental Use in Critical Care

Applications in the critical care area include adult respiratory distress syndrome, and bronchopleural fistulae (Carlon et al., 1982). HFJV has also shown promise as a life-support technique for neonates with severe respiratory distress when conventional regimens have failed (Pokora et al., 1983).

HFJV appears significantly superior to IPPV for the treatment of bronchopleural fistulae in experimental models and clinical applications. Barringer et al. (1982) compared HFJV and IPPV in the management of bronchopleural fistulae in dogs. Results from their study suggest that HFJV is beneficial in two eays. First, since peak and mean airway pressures were lower, quantitative gas flow through the fistula was reduced as much as 47% compared to IPPV. Second, the lung with the fistula could be expanded more easily with HFJV than IPPV, thus facilitating apposition of the lung to the chest wall at lower transpulmonary pressure and accelerating recovery.

Only a limited number of studies have been conducted in experimental animals with pathological lesions. They have been primarily directed to saline-lavaged rabbits to simulate infant respiratory distress syndrome (IRDS) and to dogs in respiratory failure produced by oleic acid.

In the saline-lavaged rabbit model of IRDS, high-frequency oscillation (HFO, 15-Hz) has been compared to CMV by Hamilton et al. (1983). Their observations suggest that HFO provides better oxygenation and prevents formation of hyaline membranes. Pneumothoraces occurred less frequently with HFO than CMV. In contrast, HFJV does not appear to prevent hyaline membrane formation in the same rabbit model of IRDS (Calkins et al., 1983a; Quan et al., 1984b). Furthermore, HFJV did not appear to alter the incidence of pneumothorax. However, arterial oxygenation was better with HFJV.

Working in dogs with an HCL/oleic acid model of respiratory failure, Carlon et al. (1983a) conducted two studies. In the first, CMV at a minute ventilation rate of 300 ml/min per kg and PEEP of 0 or 15 cm H_2O was compared to HFJV at 600 ml/min per kg at 100 and 150/min. In the second, CO_2 clearance and other physiological variables were compared at different minute ventilation for CMV and HFJV and different % I time for HFJV. Results indicated that HFJV could be effectively used in this model at a smaller tidal volume and reduced peak airway pressure. The best physiological results were obtained on HFJV at a rate of 100/min and tidal volume of 9 ml/kg.

V. Summary

In HFJV, small pulses of gas flowing from a high-pressure source are delivered into the airway via an accurately controlled jet. Operation of the jet is usually controlled by a fluidic or electromechanical control system. HFJV is effective at ventilatory frequencies ranging from 100 to 900/min and is associated with relatively low peak pressures and tidal volumes.

Data from studies investigating design variables indicate that the optimal jet for gas transport has a rectangular pressure/flow pulse wave shape, is more efficient when introduced into the airway close to the carina, and has a jet lumen to exhaust lumen area ratio ranging from 1:11 to 1:6. Frequency, % I time (I/E ratio), airway pressures (peak, mean, PEEP), airway pressure difference (Δ PAW = peak – PEEP), minute volume, and driving pressure have been evaluated as control variables to establish operational guidelines.

Although the exact mechanisms of HFJV are not clearly understood, alveolar ventilation is well-maintained. One major difference between IPPV and HFJV at equivalent ventilatory levels is that peak intratracheal pressure is lower. A lower intratracheal pressure should correspond to a lower intrathoracic pressure. Hence, HFJV should decrease the incidence of barotrauma and interfere less with venous return to the heart and cardiac function than CMV. Some data suggest that synchronization of ventilation with heart rate during HFJV might improve cardiac output. These results suggest that HFJV may be useful in situations in which IPPV produces an unacceptable depression in hemodynamics.

Experimental evaluation of HFJV for potential clinical situations includes airway management and CPR, anesthesia for selected surgical procedures, and respiratory failure in children and adults. Experimental evidence clearly supports use of transtracheal HFJV in situations requiring immediate control of a difficult airway. In the operating room, HFJV may offer distinct advantages for neurosurgical and thoracic procedures. Its benefits in situations in which surgeons and anesthesiologists are competing for airway, such as laryngoscopy and bronchoscopy, are generally accepted. Applications in critical care are expanding to include treatment of bronchopleural fistulae, IRDS, and ARDS.

References

Babinski, M. F., Albin, M., and Smith, R. B. (1981). Effects of high frequency ventilation in ICP. *Crit. Care Med.* **9**:159.

Babinski, M. F., Bunegin, L., Smith, R. B., and Hoff, B. H. (1981). Application of double lumen tracheal tubes for high frequency ventilation. *Anesthesiology* (Suppl.) **55**:A370.

Barringer, M., Meredith, J., Prough, D., Gibson, R., and Blinkhorn, R. (1982). Effectiveness of high frequency jet ventilation in management of an experimental bronchopleural fistula. *Am. Surg.* **48**:610.

Baum, M., Benzer, H., Goldschmied, W., and Mutz, N. (1983). Pressure flow pattern and gas transport using various types of high frequency ventilation. In *Perspectives in High Frequency Ventilation.* Edited by P. A. Scheck, U. A. Sjostrand, and R. B. Smith. Boston, Martinus Nijoff, p. 51.

Calkins, J. M., and Waterson, C. K. (1984). Clinical factors influencing the selection of high frequency jet ventilators. *Crit. Care Med.* **12**:806.

Calkins, J. M., Waterson, C. K., Hameroff, S. R., Harris, T. R., and Jones, J. R. (1982a). A single flueric high frequency jet ventilator. *Anesth. Analg.* (Cleve) **61**:138.

Calkins, J. M., Waterson, C. K., Hameroff, S. R., and Kanel, J. S. (1982b). Jet pulse characteristics for high frequency jet ventilation in dogs. *Anesth. Analg.* **61**:293.

Calkins, J. M., Militzer, H. W., Quan, S. F., Sobonya, R. E., Waterson, C. K., Otto, C. W., Conhanan, T. J. III, and Rothrock, L. S. (1983). High frequency jet vs conventional ventilation in saline lavaged rabbits. *Anesthesiology* (Suppl.) **59**:A107.

Calkins, J. M., Waterson, C. K., Quan, S. F., Militzer, H. W., Conahan, T. J. III, Otto, C. W., and Hameroff, S. R. (1983b). Effects of high frequency jet ventilation design and operational variables upon arterial blood gas tensions. In *Perspectives in High Frequency Ventilation.* Edited by P. A. Scheck, U. A. Sjostrand, and R. B. Smith. Boston, Martinus Nijoff, p. 71.

Carlon, G. C., Kahn, R. C., Howland, R. S., Ray, C., and Turnbull, A. D. (1981a). Clinical experience with high frequency jet ventilation. *Crit. Care Med.* **9**:1.

Carlon, G. C., Miodownik, S., Ray, C., and Kahn, R. C. (1981b). Technical aspects and clinical implications of high frequency jet ventilation with a solenoid valve. *Crit. Care Med.* **9**:47.

Carlon, G. C., Pierri, M. K., Ray, C., and Kreton, V. (1981c). Hemodynamic and respiratory variables with high frequency jet ventilation (HFJV) synchronized with heart rate. *Crit. Care Med.* **9**:163.

Carlon, G. C., Ray, C., Pierri, M. K., Groeger, J., and Howland, W. S. (1982). High frequency ventilation: Theoretical considerations and clinical observations. *Chest* **81**:350.

Carlon, G. C., Cole, R., Miodownik, S., Howland, W. S., Guy, Y., and Groeger, J. S. (1983). Physiologic implications of high frequency jet ventilation techniques. *Crit. Care Med.* **11**:508.

Carlon, G. C., Griffin, J., Ray, C., Groeger, J. S., and Patrick, K. (1983). High frequency jet ventilation in experimental airway disruption. *Crit. Care Med.* **11**:353.

Carlon, G. C., Ray, C., Griffin, J., Midownik, S., and Groeger, J. S. (1983).

Tidal volume and airway pressure on high frequency jet ventilation. *Crit. Care Med.* **11**:83.

Colgan, F. J., Teneyck, L. G., and Sawa, T. (1983). Ventilation requirements during high frequency ventilation. *Crit. Care Med.* **11**:173.

Dedhia, M. V. (1981). Hemodynamic effect of high frequency ventilation in open heart surgery patients. *Crit. Care Med.* **9**:158.

Gillespie, D. J. (1983). High frequency ventilation: A new concept in mechanical ventilation. *Mayo Clin. Proc.* **58**:187.

Hameroff, S. R., Calkins, J. M., Waterson, C. K., and Kanel, J. S. (1981). High frequency alternating lung ventilation. *Anesthesiology* **54**:237.

Hamilton, P. P., Onayemi, A., Smyth, J. A., Gillon, J. E., Cutz, E., Froese, A. B., and Bryon, A. C. Comparison of conventional and high frequency ventilation: oxygenation and lung pathology. *J. Appl. Physiol.* **55**:131.

Hoff, B. H., Benedetto, A. R., Nusynowitz, L., Wilson, E. A., Smith, R. B., and Pentoja, G. (1982). Rapid infusion air embolism: Effects of IPPV and high frequency ventilation (HFV). *Anesthesiology* **57**:A85.

Hoff, B. H., Smith, R. B., and Bunegin, L. (1982). High frequency ventilation in dogs with open chests. *Crit. Care Med.* **10**:517.

Jonzon, A., Oberg, P. A., Sedin, G., and Sjostrand, U. (1971). High frequency positive pressure ventilation by endotracheal insufflation. *Acta Anaesth. Scand.* (Suppl.) **43**:1.

Keszler, M., Klein, R., McClellan, L., Nelson, D., and Platt, M. (1982). Effects of conventional and high frequency jet ventilation on lung parenchyma. *Crit. Care Med.* **10**:514.

Klain, M. (1983). Gas exchange in high frequency ventilation: An experimental study. In *Perspectives in High Frequency Ventilation.* Edited by P. A. Scheck, U. A. Sjostrand, and R. B. Smith. Boston, Martinus Nijoff, p. 158.

Klain, M., and Smith, R. B. (1977) High frequency percutaneous transtracheal jet ventilation. *Crit. Care Med.* **5**:280.

Klain, M., Keszler, H., and Brader, E. (1981). High frequency jet ventilation in CPR. *Crit. Care Med.* **9**:421.

Klain, M., Keszler, H., and Stool, S. (1983). Transtracheal high frequency jet ventilation prevents aspiration. *Crit. Care Med.* **11**:170.

Klain, M., Nordin, U., and Keszler, H. (1982). Microciliary transport with and without humidification in high frequency ventilation. *Anesthesiology* **57**: A86.

Lendinez, M. J., Cambromero, J. A., Lopez, J., Galvan, B., Garcia, A., Denia, R., and Aguado, A. (1983). Airway pressure as a determining factor for ventilation and hemodynamic efficiency during high frequency jet ventilation. In *Perspectives in High Frequency Ventilation.* Edited by P. A. Scheck, U. A. Sjostrand, and R. B. Smith. Boston, Martinus Nijoff, p. 81.

Marquez, J., Klain, M., and Romano, B. (1981). Renal and cardiovascular effects between CPAP and HFJV with PEEP. *Anesthesiology* **55**:A68.

Marquez, J., Fine, J., Klain, M., Bennett, R., and Freeman, J. (1982). Clinical applications of high frequency jet ventilation in the operating room. *Anesthesiology* **57**:A464.

Mihm, F. G., Feeley, T. W.,and Rodarte, A. (1982). Monitoring high frequency jet ventilation by end-tidal carbon dioxide concentrations. *Anesthesiology* (Suppl.) **57**:A87.

Moynihan, P. F., Parisi, A. F., and Feldman, C. L. Quantitative detection of regional left ventricular contraction abnormalities by two dimension echocardiography. *Circulation* **63**:752.

Mushin, W. W., Rendell-Baker, L., Thompson, P. W., and Mapleson, W. W. (1980). Historical background to automatic ventilation. In *Automatic Ventilation of the Lungs.* 3rd edition. London, Blackwell Scientific Publications, p. 223.

Otto, C. W., Calkins, J. M., Quan, S. F., Conahan, T. J. III, Waterson, C. K., and Hameroff, S. R. (1983a). Cardiovascular consequences of high frequency ventilation. In *Perspectives in High Frequency Ventilation.* Edited by P. A. Scheck, U. A. Sjostrand, and R. B. Smith. Boston, Martinus Nijoff, p. 115.

Otto, C. W., Quan, S. F., Conahan, T. J. III, Calkins, J. M., Waterson, C. K., and Hameroff, S. R. (1983b). Hemodynamic effects of high frequency jet ventilation. *Anesth. Analg.* **62**:298.

Pokora, T., Bing, D., Mammel, M., and Boros, S. (1983). Neonatal high frequency jet ventilation. *Pediatrics* **72**:27.

Quan, S. F., Waterson, C. K., Calkins, J. M., Conahan, T. J. III, Otto, C. W., and Hameroff, S. R. (1982). Airway pressure monitoring in high frequency ventilation. *Crit. Care Med.* **10**:233.

Quan, S. F., Otto, C. W., Calkins, J. M., Hameroff, S. R., Conahan, T. J. III, and Waterson, C. K. (1983). A promising new method of ventilation. *Heart Lung* **12**:152.

Quan, S. F., Calkins, J. M., Waterson, C. K., and Otto, C. W. (1983). High frequency ventilation—current concepts. *Arizona Med.* **40**:319.

Quan, S. F., Militzer, H. W., Calkins, J. M., and Waterson, C. K. (1983). High frequency ventilation in the operating room. *AORN J.* **38**:991.

Quan, S. F., Calkins, J. M., Waterson, C. K., Conahan, T. J. III, Hameroff, S. R., and Otto, C. W. (1984). Airway movement in dogs during high frequency jet ventilation. *Crit. Care Med.* **12**(5):452-456.

Quan, S. F., Militzer, H. M., Calkins, J. M., Sobonya, R. E., Waterson, C. K., Otto, C. W., and Conahan, T. J. III. (1984). A comparison of high frequency jet ventilation with conventional mechanical ventilation in saline lavaged rabbits. *Crit. Care Med.* **12**:759.

Rock, J. J., Pfaeffle, H., Smith, R. B., Medolow, H., and Klain, M. (1976). High pressure jet insufflation used to prevent aspiration and its effect on the tracheal mucosal wall. *Crit. Care Med.* **4**:135.

Rolly, G., and Versichelen, L. (1983). Gas analysis by mass spectrometry during high frequency ventilation. In *Perspectives in High Frequency Ventilation.* Edited by P. A. Scheck, U. A. Sjostrand, and R. B. Smith. Boston, Mattinus Nijoff, p. 164.

Schuster, D. P., Snyder, J. V., Klain, M., and Grenvik, A. (1981). The use of high frequency jet ventilation during respiratory failure. *Crit. Care Med.* **9**: 162.

Smith, R. B., Schaer, W. B., and Pfaeffle, H. (1975). Percutaneous transtracheal ventilation for anaesthesia and resuscitation. A review and report of complications. *Can. Anaesth. Soc. J.* **22**:607.

Smith, R. B., Klain, M., and Babinski, M. (1980). Limits of high frequency percutaneous transtracheal jet ventilation using a fluidic logic controlled ventilator. *Can. Anaesth. Soc. J.* **27**:351.

Smith, R. B., Cutaia, F., Hoff, B. H., Babinski, M., and Geliveau, J. (1981). Long term transtracheal high frequency ventilation in dogs. *Crit. Care Med.* **9**: 311.

Szele, G., and Keenan, R. L. (1981). Does percutaneous transtracheal high frequency ventilation prevent aspiration? A word of caution. *Crit. Care Med.* **9**:163.

Szele, G., and Shavari, M. B. G. (1981). Comparison of cardiovascular effects of high frequency ventilation and intermittent positive pressure ventilation in hemorrhagic shock. *Crit. Care Med.* **9**:161.

Tallman, R. D., Peterson, S. F., and McDonald, J. S. (1983). Pulmonary blood flow during high frequency jet ventilation. *Anesthesiology* (Suppl.) **59**: A144.

Technical Manual (1972). What you should know about fluidics. National Fluid Power Association, Thiensville, WI.

Todd, M. M., Toutant, S. M., and Shapiro, H. M. (1981). The effects of high frequency positive pressure ventilation on ICP and brain surface movement in cats. *Anesthesiology* **54**:496.

Toutant, S. M., Todd, M. M., and Drummond, J. C. (1983). Cerebral blood flow during high frequency ventilation in cats. *Crit. Care Med.* **11**:712.

Waterson, C. K., Militzer, H. W., Quan, S. F., and Calkins, J. M. (1984). Airway pressure as a measure of gas exchange during high frequency jet ventilation. *Crit. Care Med.* **12**:742.

Watt, R. C., Waterson, C. K., and Calkins, J. M. (1983). Computer analysis of flow transient effects in high frequency jet ventilation. *Proc. AAMI* **18**:131.

Workshop on High Frequency Ventilation, December (1982). New Orleans. U.S. Department of Health and Human Services, Public Health Service, National Institutes of Health.

8

Clinical Applications of High-Frequency Jet Ventilation

Part A Clinical Use in the Operating Room

MIROSLAV KLAIN

University of Pittsburgh
School of Medicine
Pittsburgh, Pennsylvania

I. Introduction

Even though most attention has been paid in the last several years to the possible use of high-frequency ventilation (HFV) in respiratory failure, intraoperative application of HFV is its most common use. For example, more than 1000 patients were ventilated at the University of Pittsburgh Health Center Hospitals with high-frequency jet ventilation (HFJV) in the last 5 years, 65% of them intraoperatively. Only 25% were ventilated in intensive care units and 10% in the emergency room and postoperative recovery room (Klain et al., 1983).

High-frequency jet ventilation (HFJV) has proven itself as a worthwhile addition to our methods of airway management. It should be considered in situations where its specific advantages can offer benefit to the patient or to the overall treatment plan. These advantages are gas exchange at lower airway pressures (Klain and Smith, 1977), the possibility of ventilating even with uncuffed tubes or with a leak in the airways (Klain et al., 1982a), the ability to use small insufflation catheters and not to compete with the surgeon in ENT surgery (Babinski et al., 1980), less movement in the operative field of the chest wall (Marquez et al., 1982), good tolerance by the patient (Klain et al., 1982b), and, finally, emergency use of transtracheal ventilation in upper airway trauma or cardiopulmonary resuscitation (Klain et al., 1981).

II. Indications

Indications for intraoperative use of HFJV are summarized in Table 1.

A. Ventilation with an Insufflation Catheter

Endoscopies

Laryngoscopies and bronchoscopies are the primary indications for HFJV (Babinski et al., 1980). Laryngoscopy requires a small endotracheal tube to facilitate viewing. A small tube of 5-5.5 mm ID usually allows some view of the larynx, but the posterior commissure is obscured from the surgeon's view. Therefore, HFJV through an insufflation catheter represents a method of choice. A 14 F size is sufficient for adults and 10 F for children. Small catheters not only eliminate competition with the surgeon for the airway but also assure minimal discomfort during emergence from anesthesia and postoperatively. Even a small uncuffed insufflation catheter protects the airway from aspiration as long as frequency is at least 60 breaths/min.

For rigid bronchoscopy, an uncuffed 14 F catheter is also the easiest to use. Introduced nasotracheally under direct vision, this catheter provides satisfactory respiratory support even during insertion of the bronchoscope or if its tip is positioned distally in the main stem bronchus during bronchoscopy. The bronchoscope itself allows expiratory flow. Adequacy of ventilation is judged by observing chest movements. It is also possible to ventilate through the side arm of the bronchoscope or with an attachment on its distal end, but in this case only one side of the lungs is ventilated when the bronchoscope is positioned in the periphery.

Table 1 Intraoperative Indications for HFJV

Laryngoscopies and bronchoscopies
Microlaryngeal procedures
Airway leaks and airway surgery
When quieter operative field is needed
Independent lung ventilation
Emergency airway management

Microlaryngeal Procedures and Laser Surgery

Anesthesia for examination, manipulation, or operation within the larynx is characterized by the need to share the same space with the surgeon and to protect the airway. A standard endotracheal tube obstructs the surgeon's view. Any method that does not use an endotracheal tube in a spontaneously breathing patient does not allow control of secretions nor protect against aspiration.

Low-frequency jet used proximally through the lumen of the laryngoscope provides sufficient artificial ventilation, but does not protect the airway. A modified endotracheal tube such as the Pollard tube (Pollard, 1968), the Carden tube (Carden and Vest, 1974), or a transtracheal catheter (Spoerel et al., 1971) has been used successfully with jet ventilation and delivers sufficient ventilatory support.

Administering the jet at higher frequency will produce less intrapulmonary pressure and less potential for barotrauma, especially in expiratory obstruction. Frequencies higher than 100 breaths/min also protect the airway if the catheter tip is introduced in the midtrachea and provided with side openings. Entrainment of outside air is prevented and satisfactory prevention of aspiration occurs.

To avoid a whip effect of the catheter tip seen with a long free line catheter with one terminal opening, the catheter should have side openings to stabilize it or, similarly to the Benjamin jet tube (Benjamin and Gronow, 1979) it should have soft plastic petals at the distal end, designed to maintain it in middle position in the trachea. In such a way trauma to the tracheal wall, mucosal tear, or traumatic laceration may be avoided and even distribution of gas insured. The adult Benjamin tube is 4.0 mm in external diameter with a black mark 8 cm from its distal tip. The pediatric tube is 2.8 mm in external diameter with a similar mark 5 cm from its distal tip. The marks indicate the level of vocal cords for ease of positioning. Both tubes are 35 cm long. The jet opening at the distal end is approximately 1.7 mm ID, equivalent to a 14 gauge needle.

After preoxygenation, anesthesia is induced with a short-acting barbiturate, then Anectine (succinylcholine chloride) is given for relaxation and intubation. The tube is inserted nasotracheally and positioned in the trachea with the tip 10 cm above the carina.

For laser surgery two approaches can be taken. One is to use an endotracheal tube that also secures exhalation. It should be a metallic tube, or silastic with reflective metallic cover or wrapped with thin metallic tape or moist gauze to prevent combustion (Schiede et al., 1983). The second approach is not to use a tube at all but only an injector or transtracheal catheter for HFJV. The echalation occurs through natural airways. In any case, the patient has to be immobilized because no movement can be permitted during laser surgery.

The expiratory flow must be assured at all times. Therefore, extreme caution is indicated in the presence of a significant laryngeal obstruction. Ventilation of both lungs is checked by auscultation, and the tube is fixed to the face by tape. Anesthesia is maintained with repeated doses of fentanyl or other short-acting narcotic and succinylcholine drip is used for muscle relaxation.

Adequacy of ventilation is assessed from the movement of the chest. It is important that the endoscopist not lean on the chest and that the laryngoscope holder rests on a table, not on the patient's chest.

When the procedure is finished, the laryngoscope is withdrawn, and HFJV is continued, with a gradual decrease in the driving pressure. When the patient starts to breathe, HFJV is superimposed over spontaneous breathing. The patient usually does not cough, especially if 50 mg of xylocaine is administered IV at the end of the procedure. Ventilation is continued with gradually decreasing minute volume until the patient is ready for extubation. Before you remove the insufflation catheter, stop the ventilator completely. The patient usually does not have problems with breathing spontaneously with catheter in place, and can even talk with a hoarse voice. The catheter is then removed if the patient is breathing satisfactorily. Otherwise, controlled ventilation via the catheter can be reinstituted.

Airway Surgery and Airway Leaks

The key to successful management of anesthesia and ventilatory support during airway surgery is in the proper sharing the airway and proper monitoring. Even a tonsillectomy, which is usually a brief procedure in young healthy patients, is never a minor operation. It can have acute complications such as bleeding and airway obstruction. It is important to wait for return of protective laryngeal reflexes before extubation and to observe the patient for laryngospasm after extubation.

Reoperation for continuous posttonsilectomy bleeding is especially dangerous. To manage a bloody pharynx and possible vomiting during induction, rapid sequence with cricoid pressure is usually used. Securing the airway by high-frequency jet ventilation administered by cricothyroid membrane puncture is as effective (Miller et al., 1982).

For tracheal resection or sleeve resection it is possible to position the insufflation catheter through the operative field and ventilate satisfactorily without impairing the surgical field of anastomosis (El-Bar et al., 1983).

Short Surgical Procedures

Experimental and clinical experience in recent years shows that use of insufflation catheter could also be extended to other indications. The small uncuffed catheter does not obstruct the operative field and significantly decreases the discomfort of the patient during weaning and postoperatively.

For example, Miller et al. (1982) in a series of 50 patients inserted a 14 F insufflation catheter nasotracheally under direct vision and introduced it below the vocal cords so that the tip stayed about 10 cm above the carina. The patients were kept anesthetized by nitrous oxide/oxygen/narcotic anesthesia and paralyzed with succinylcholine. They were ventilated with a VS 600 ventilator (IDC, Pittsburgh) at a frequency of 100 cpm and an I/E ratio of 1:2.

The indications included short oral surgical procedures, ENT procedures such as reduction of nasal fractures, tonsillectomies, and outpatient surgery. Sufficient gas exchange and protection of the airways was achieved in all patients. The blood gas values from the first six patients are shown in Table 2.

After the procedure, respiratory support was slowly decreased. The patient was allowed to start spontaneous breathing and gradually take over ventilation completely. Patients felt minimal discomfort and no coughing occurred as they resumed their own breathing. This was considered a significant advantage, especially in outpatients. The method also decreased patients' postoperative discomfort.

Oral and facial surgery for trauma is easiest done with nasal intubation. But induction of anesthesia with blood and secretions in the upper airway poses a hazard. Again, transtracheal application of HFJV establishes the airway and provides sufficient time for inducing the anesthesia, letting the patient be examined, and eventually introducing a standard endotracheal tube if needed.

Postoperatively, these patients benefit from ventilatory support by HFJV as well. They can be extubated awake and with intact protective laryngeal reflexes.

B. Ventilation with an Endotracheal Tube

Quieter Operative Field

Small tidal volumes result in smaller peak airway pressures and less movement in the operative field. That can simplify surgical dissection in hepatic resection or any operative procedure below the diaphragm (Marquez et al., 1982). HFJV was therefore used in many patients for laparotomy. Less fluctuation in the surgical field also is beneficial in craniotomies and thoracotomies. Because the nondependent lung is semiexpanded and not under high pressure, the surgical dissection is facilitated and the gas exchange is superior to that achieved by one-lung ventilation (Moulaert et al., 1983).

To allow the use of PEEP, 45% of the patients in our institution were ventilated via a cuffed endotracheal tube. In half of them a "Hi-Low" jet tube (NCC, Argyle, NY) was used which has the jet channel incorporated in the wall of the tube (Fig. 1). In the other half a regular endotracheal tube was used with the jet catheter inserted through a T-connector on the proximal end of the tube (Fig. 2). In 50% of the patients an uncuffed 14 F catheter was introduced nasotracheally under direct vision and in 5% of the patients a transtracheal cannula was used.

Ventilation was established by using either the VS600 or the newer MK800

Table 2 HFJV in Routine Oral Surgery

Patient	Procedure	psi	FiO_2	Arterial pH	PaO_2	$PaCO_2$
1	Removal of impacted teeth	40	1.0	7.478	615.1	28.9
2	Removal of impacted teeth	40	1.0	7.401	495.2	32.0
3	Removal of impacted teeth	40	1.0	7.426	463.2	26.2
4	Removal of impacted and carious teeth	40	1.0	7.558	395.6	21.0
5	Mandibular odontectomy and alveolectomy	35	1.0	7.419	289.5	31.2
6	Maxillary and mandibular odontectomy and alveolectomy	40	0.5	7.467	281.6	27.1

Frequency = 100/min., I/E ratio 1:2 with nasal O_2 catheter.
Note: Arterial blood gases were drawn from the radial artery 5 min after induction of anesthesia.
Source: Miller et al. (1982).

(IDC Pittsburgh) high-frequency jet ventilator. Ventilation was controlled by adjusting driving pressure, respiratory rate, and I/E ratio, with adjustments made as warranted by arterial blood gas results. On the average, 26-30 psi of driving pressure is needed to achieve normocarbia in an adult at a frequency of 100 cpm (Table 3). Anesthetic gas delivery to the jet ventilator was through the Bird N_2O-O_2 blender, or the Veriflow air/O_2 blender. Scavenging of waste anesthetic gases was performed by attachment of the jet tube to the circle system while humidification was achieved by instillation of normal saline via the humidification port of the jet ventilator. Anesthesia was maintained by narcotics, hypnotics, and muscle relaxants.

Clinical monitoring during HFJV was carried out in routine manner. Because heart sounds are difficult to auscultate during HFJV the pulse was monitored either digitally, by plethysmography or intra-arterially.

In all patients satisfactory ventilation and anesthesia were maintained during HFJV.

C. Independent Lung Ventilation

If there is a need to ventilate each lung independently, HFJV can be used for differential lung ventilation, for example during surgery on a bronchopleural fistula

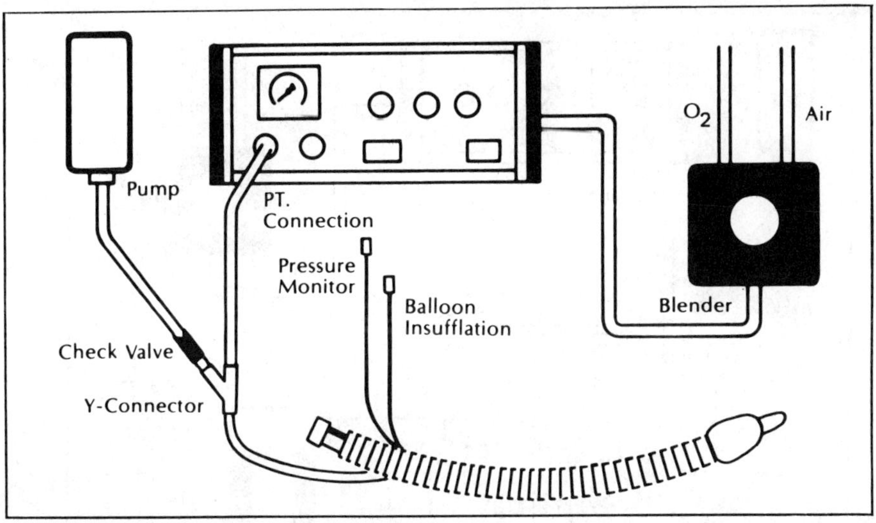

Figure 1 HFJV system with "Hi-Lo" jet tube which has the jet channel build in the wall.

(Benjaminsson et al., 1981). A Carlen's double-lumen tube or a Robertshaw tube is inserted. Each lung can be connected to a separate ventilator and driving parameters independently adjusted. If HFJV ventilator is indicated, as in bronchopleural fistula, it does not need to be synchronized with the other one. For one-lung anesthesia, the lower pressures generated do not produce a shift of blood flow to the nonventilated lung by high intrathoracic pressure and therefore the shunt is decreased (Moulaert et al., 1983). For example, one-lung HFJV was successfully used for contralateral lavage in alveolar proteinosis by Marquez (unpublished data).

D. Transtracheal Emergency Ventilation

Trauma, foreign body, tumor, or infection can compromise the airway. Such compromise is manifest by signs of stridor, tachypnea, tachycardia, and hypertension. Inspiratory stridor at rest indicates a severely compromised airway with a diameter less than 4 mm. Before general anesthesia is induced, the airway should be secured. Instead of classic awake intubation this can be achieved by transtracheal ventilation in an awake patient (Klain et al., 1981). Anesthesia can be then started with an already secured airway.

Transtracheal jet ventilation should be the method of choice for emergency airway management and respiratory support in hospital settings (Fig. 3). It was successfully used to secure the airway and prevent aspiration in cases of oral and facial trauma or upper airway trauma. In that situation a cricothyroid catheter allows ventilatory support before anesthesia is started. It is alos possible to displace a foreign body impacted at the level of the cords. In suitable cases of diffi-

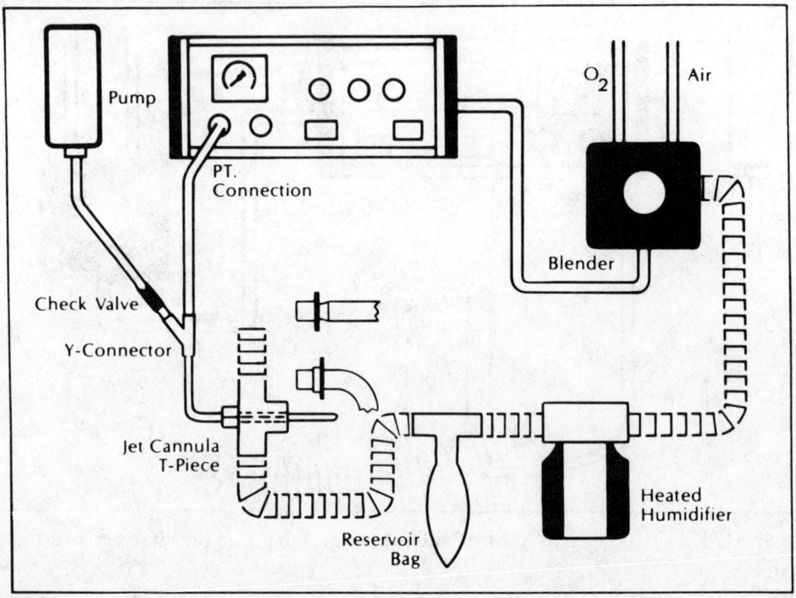

Figure 2 System for attachment of HFJV with a T-connector to any endotracheal or tracheostomy tube. Humidity is administered by a pump directly in the jet and a heated humidifier is used for entrained gas.

cult intubation this method permits one to avoid awake intubation (Marquez et al., 1982).

Laryngospasm is complete glottic closure due to continued spasm of the false cords. Removing the stimulus and administering rapid-acting muscle relaxants may be the necessary steps. Continuous positive pressure is usually recommended to break the spasm. Transtracheal high-frequency jet ventilation with cut-off alarm of the ventilator set to 50 torr can do that in most cases as well. Even for tracheostomy, high-frequency jet ventilation with 100% oxygen remarkedly relieves anxiety.

A 14-gauge needle placed transtracheally and connected to a bag system for manual ventilation cannot provide sufficient ventilatory support. In spontaneously breathing patients it can certainly be used to administer oxygen but ventilatory support cannot be used to administer transtracheally without a jet ventilator.

III. Inhalation Agent Admixture and Scavenging

Presently available vaporizers are not designed for high-pressure delivery systems. Therefore, admixture of volatile potent anesthetic agents has not been success-

Table 3 Usual Driving Pressure for HFV at Frequency 100, Inspiratory time 30%

	Procedure				
	Dental	Orthopedic	Abdominal	Thorocotomy	Craniotomy
Sample size	93	83	583	112	161
Psi					
Mean ± standard deviation	29.9 ± 7.0	27.8 ± 7.7	26.5 ± 7.8	25.9 ± 6.9	25.5 ± 7.5
$PaCO_2$					
Mean ± standard deviation	33.9 ± 4.6	34.2 ± 6.5	33.8 ± 6.3	34.5 ± 5.2	31.7 ± 6.8

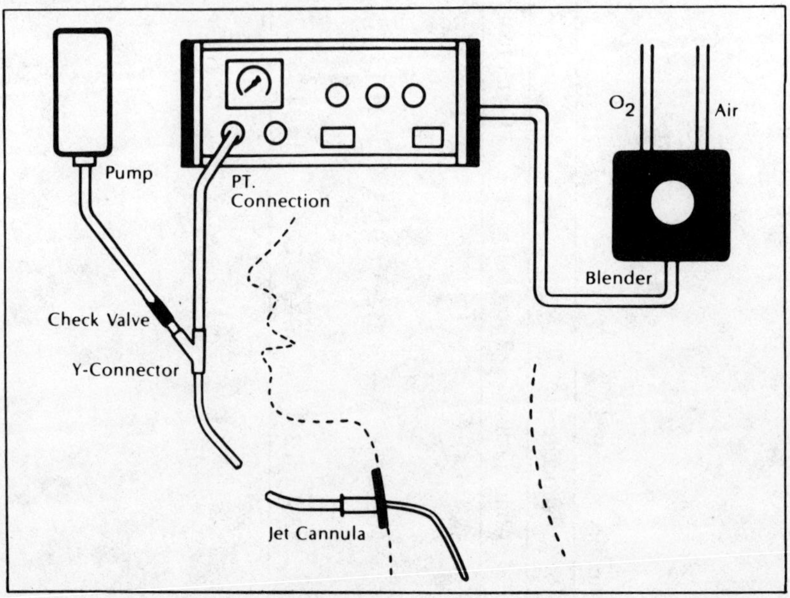

Figure 3 Transtracheal jet ventilation.

fully carried out yet and intravenous anesthesia must be used. Admixture of nitrous oxide is possible with a blender. To secure scavenging of gases, a cuffed endotracheal tube is used, which is connected to the anesthesia circle system with the relieve valve fully open for scavenging.

IV. Weaning and Postoperative Use

The indications for HFJV postoperatively are similar to those for its intraoperative use (Table 4). Prevention of barotrauma after lung surgery is one indication.

Other indications are respiratory support during tracheobronchial suctioning or fiberoptic bronchoscopy (Guntupalli et al., 1981) or during exchange of endotracheal tubes. In all these cases no other method can match the advantages of HFJV.

The second application depends on the tolerance of HFJV by the patient. The patient gradually resumes spontaneous breathing without struggling, therefore the method is suitable for assisted ventilation or weaning.

Weaning of patients from short-term respiratory support, usually after anesthetic procedures, is often accompanied by a dilemma: Patients start to

Table 4 Postoperative Indications for HFV

Barotrauma or risk of barotrauma (i.e., after surgery on airways)
For assisted ventilation
Weaning
During tracheal suctioning and bronchoscopy
For endotube exchange

breathe on their own, but their respiratory effort is not sufficient to support adequate gas exchange fully. The transition from controlled ventilation to assisted ventilation and spontaneous breathing might be long if additional sedatives are administered to calm the patient who is "fighting" the ventilator. High-frequency jet ventilation under these circumstances offers a significant advantage because it can be superimposed on spontaneous breathing and tuned to the needs of the patient without the need for additional sedation (Klain et al., 1982b).

In patients admitted to the recovery room or to the intensive care unit after surgical procedures, respiratory support is begun with HFJV at frequencies of 100-150/min and I/E ratio of 1:2. The support is decreased at 30-min intervals by decreasing the driving pressure stepwise from 40 to 10 psi in 50psi decrements, thereby decreasing the delivered minute ventilation.

All the patients were able progressively to increase their spontaneous breathing. The progress of spontaneous breathing was monitored by capnographic tracings using a mass spectrometer (Perkin-Elmer RMS III). The superimposed oscillations are clearly demonstrated on the tracing in Figure 4. As weaning progresses, the spontaneous breathing curve becomes more and more prominent and the end-tidal CO_2 reaches normal values. At this point, the patient can be extubated

V. Advantages

Gas exchange during HFJV was found to be adequate. In more than 200 arterial blood gas samples, arterial P_{O_2}, P_{CO_2}, and pH levels were satisfactory (Table 5).

Because HFJV made ventilation possible using a small uncuffed tube, procedures involving the upper airway were made less cumbersome and easier to manage. It also lowered the incidence of postoperative sore throat in patients undergoing plastic and orthopedic surgery. The lack of diaphragmatic and mediastinal movement during HFJV made this technique particularly useful in upper abdominal procedures such as cholecystectomies, gastrectomies, and hepatic

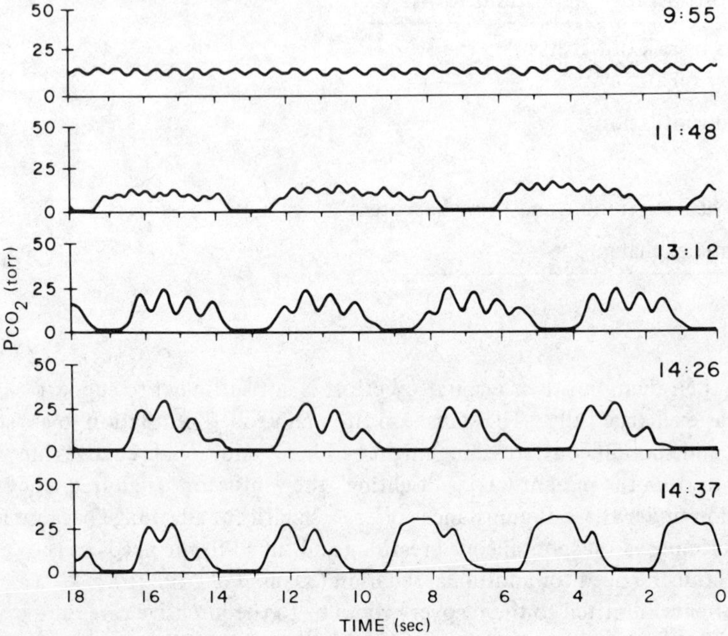

Figure 4 Capnographic tracings of a patient weaned from respiratory support by HFJV (from *Perspectives in High-Frequency Ventilation,* The Hague, Martinus Nijhoff, 1983).

transplants as well as CABG, valvular replacements, and "redo" open heart procedures.

During HFJV a lack of cardiovascular impairment was noted, particularly in those patients undergoing CABG. Cardiac index, stroke index, heart rate, and arterial blood pressure were slightly better than control values during IPPV.

During HFJV no pulmonary complications involving aspiration of foreign materials occurred when an uncuffed endotracheal tube was used (Klain et al., 1982b). Weaning from HFJV to spontaneous breathing was easily accomplished and well-tolerated in this series of patients.

Clinical use of HFJV in the operating room offers advantages in terms of airway management, hemodynamic stability, operative surgical conditions, and possibly a lower incidence of postoperative sore throat. We believe that HFJV offers a unique alternative and in some ways an improvement over the currently available methods of anesthetic techniques and ventilatory management of surgical patients.

Table 5 Gas Exchange

	PO_2/FiO_2	PCO_2	pH
Oral surgery (n=100)	455	32	7.44
Laryngoscopy/bronchoscopy (n=11)	359	42	7.34
Thoracic/cardiac (n=14)	298	40	7.37
Abdominal surgery (n=52)	290	33	7.43
Plastic/orthopedic (n=36)	370	32	7.45

Source: Marquez et al. (1982).

VI. Disadvantages

Disadvantages of HFJV are listed in Table 6. Unfamiliarity with the method or equipment must be overcome. The use of uncuffed tubes is also not universally accepted in adults. The inability to administer potent anesthetic agents is also considered a disadvantage by some.

Table 6 Disadvantages of HFV

Relatively high gas consumption
Different adjustments than conventional ventilation
Monitoring of ventilation more difficult
Insufficient alarms in some ventilators
With uncuffed tubes: Possibility of aspiration if ventilation interrupted
If used for anesthesia
With insufflation catheter, no scavenging if N_2O used
No volatile anesthetics possible at present

Clinical Applications of High-Frequency Jet Ventilation

Part B High-Frequency Jet Ventilation and Pulmonary Mechanics

PETER M. SUTER

Hôpital Cantonal Universitaire
Geneva, Switzerland

I. Introduction

High-frequency jet ventilation (HFJV) can cause significant changes in pulmonary mechanics. On the other hand, the underlying mechanical properties of the respiratory system influence the effects of HFJV on alveolar ventilation and gas exchange. Important factors that must be considered include

Ventilatory frequency

Tidal volume and minute ventilation produced by HFJV; the volume of the jet and the gas entrained

Time constants (i.e., compliance and resistance) of the ventilated lung regions

The changes caused by HFJV in the following variables have been studied:

Intrapulmonary and alveolar pressure (Benhamou et al., 1984; Cartwright et al., 1984; Rouby et al., 1983)

Lung volume; functional residual capacity (FRC) and mean lung inflation during HFJV (Benhamou et al., 1984; Cartwright et al., 1984; Rouby et al., 1983; Saari et al., 1984)

Deadspace volume (Whitwam, 1984)

Compliance (Rouby et al., 1983; Weinman et al., 1984)

Distribution of intrapulmonary ventilation (Brusasco et al., 1984; Schmid et al., 1981; Slutsky et al., 1980; Solway et al., 1984; Wattwil et al., 1983)

All these factors are relevant for the gas exchange function of the lung and can influence oxygen uptake and carbon dioxide elimination (Carlon et al., 1980, 1983; Froese and Bryan, 1981). The following sections review briefly some aspects of pulmonary mechanics as they apply to HFJV.

Intrapulmonary and Alveolar Pressures

Because tidal volumes are small during HFJV compared to conventional ventilation, it has been assumed that intrapulmonary and alveolar pressures are lower with HFJV in humans. Recent investigations, however, show that this is not always the case (Saari et al., 1984). HFJV increases mean airway and alveolar pressure progressively with increasing frequency (Saari et al., 1984) and driving pressure (Benhamou et al., 1984). The changes in mean airway pressure correlate in a number of studies (Benhamou et al., 1984; Rouby et al., 1983) with the resulting alterations in arterial oxygenation (Fig. 5), and the static "recoil" pressure parallels an increased resting lung volume (Saari et al., 1984). Airway pressure does not reflect alveolar pressure in all circumstances, but there can be a good correlation (Benhamou et al., 1984; Rouby et al., 1983) between these two variables (Fig. 6).

For clinical practice these results imply that HFJV causes an adequate arterial oxygenation depending on the mean intrapulmonary pressure produced. Up to now, there has been no evidence that HFJV provides a better pulmonary gas exchange than conventional mechanical ventilation for oxygen at similar or lower mean intrapulmonary or alveolar pressures. Meanwhile, this gas exchange can be achieved with lower peak airway pressures.

III. Lung Inflation and Volume

The lung inflation produced by HFJV and other techniques of high-frequency ventilation depends mainly on ventilatory frequency (Cartwright et al., 1984; Saari et al., 1984), end-expiratory pressure (Cartwright et al., 1984), and the inspiration to expiration time ratio (I/E) (Rouby et al., 1983). Higher values of these three variables are associated with an increased resting lung volume or functional residual capacity (FRC). Individual changes are closely related to the compliance of the respiratory system (Rouby et al., 1983). In most situations, mean airway pressure does not reflect lung volume, although a correlation exists between static recoil pressure and changes in lung volume (Saari et al., 1984).

In the clinical setting, lung volume or an index of alveolar pressure should be monitored to minimize the risk of overdistention, because central airway pressure does not correspond to peripheral pressure in the lung (Saari et al., 1984).

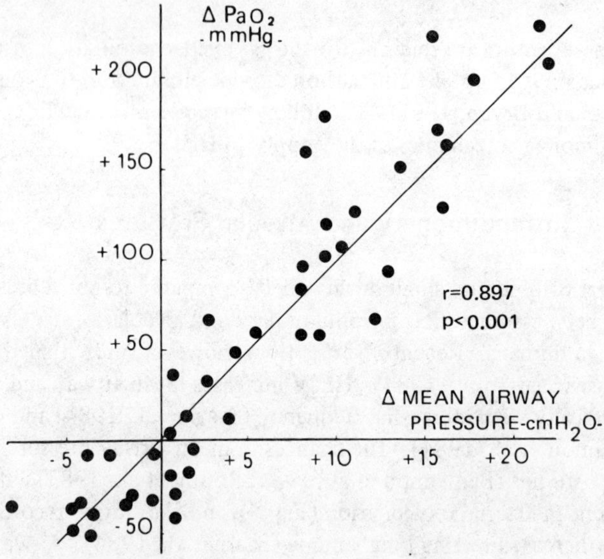

Figure 5 Relationship between changes in arterial oxygen tension and changes in mean airway pressure, observed between IPPV and HFJV. Data obtained in 15 patients ventilated during IPPV with a tidal volume of 15 ml/kg, a respiratory frequency of 15/min, and HFJV using a frequency of 100/min, with an I/E ratio between 0.25 and 0.67. Inspiratory oxygen concentration was constant at 100%. (From Rouby et al., 1983.)

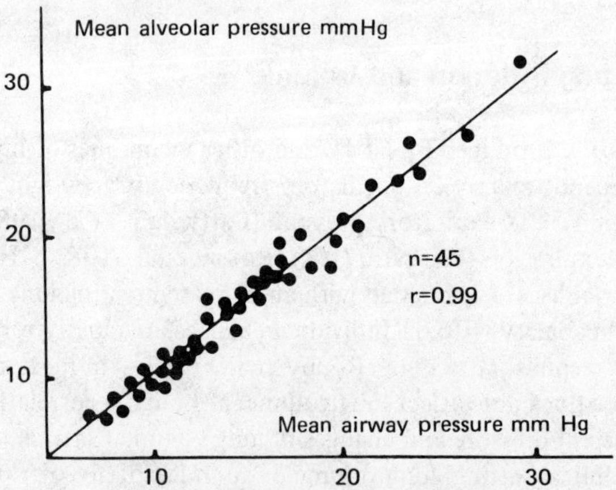

Figure 6 Relationship between mean alveolar pressure and mean airway pressure with increasing operating pressure of the HFJV source. Results obtained in 15 patients presenting with respiratory failure. (From Benhamou et al., 1984.)

IV. Functional Deadspace During HFJV

With decreasing tidal volume and increasing respiratory frequency, both "anatomical" and "physiological" deadspace volumes decrease in humans, while adequate blood gas values are maintained (Whitwam, 1984). The minimum values for physiological deadspace observed are approximately 1 ml/kg body weight, or 81-94 ml with a respiratory frequency of 80/min. In tracheotomized patients, these values can be even lower (Rossing et al., 1981) (i.e., below 45-100 ml), at ventilatory frequencies up to 900/min. Although the tidal volume can be decreased progressively above a frequency of 80/min, no further decrease in deadspace is seen, and the deadspace/tidal volume ratio (V_D/V_T) remains less than 1.0 (Whitwam et al., 1984). With high-frequency oscillation, this minimum deadspace concept may not apply, as very low tidal volumes do still allow sufficient CO_2 elimination (Slutsky et al., 1980).

The mechanisms of this reduction in deadspace volume during HFJV are not entirely clear. A better convection in the airways may contribute to a decreased anatomical deadspace. Changes in convection, distribution of ventilation, and enhanced diffusion may all be implicated in a diminished alveolar and total (physiological) deadspace (Brusasco et al., 1984; Schmid et al., 1981; Slutsky et al., 1980).

The clinical implications of these findings are interesting. There is clear evidence of a minimum or "functional" deadspace volume, reached at frequencies between 80 and 200/min in individual patients (Rossing et al., 1981; Whitwam, 1984) Above this frequency, carbon dioxide elimination cannot be improved further at constant tidal volume (Rossing et al., 1981). This may be due to a constant functional deadspace, or to an increasing mean or end-expiratory pressure in airways and alveoli, creating increased anatomical and/or alveolar deadspace.

V. Compliance

Conflicting results concerning the effects of HFJV on compliance and lung stability exist (Cartwright et al., 1984; Rouby et al., 1983; Weinmann et al., 1984). It is known from animal experiments that large tidal volumes deplete surfactant faster than small volumes, but high-frequency ventilation had similar effects to conventional ventilation on lung morphology, pressure-volume curves, and surface tension in recent studies (Weinmann et al., 1984). From these data it must be concluded that lung stability and compliance are not affected differently during conventional and high-frequency ventilation. However, opening and recruitment of collapsed areas at low lung volumes may be improved by ventilation at high frequencies, and large oscillatory pressure swings (Weinmann et al., 1984).

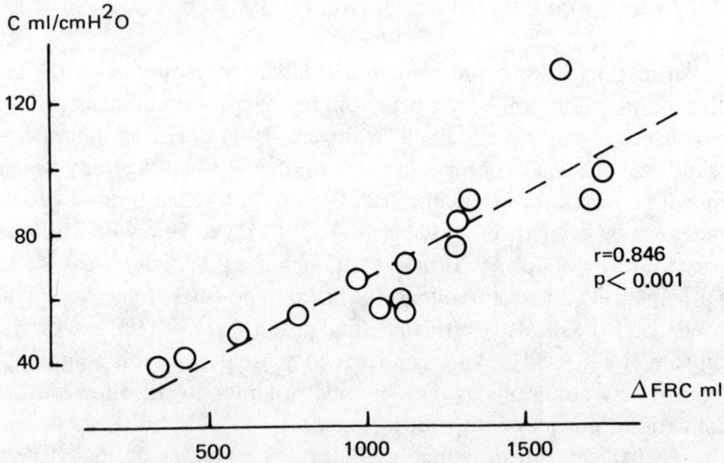

Figure 7 Relationship between static respiratory compliance (C) and changes in functional residual capacity (FRC) above apneic lung volume in 15 patients presenting with postoperative respiratory failure. The changes in FRC were obtained by switching from IPPV to HFJV, the I/E ratio being constant at 0.43 (From Rouby et al., 1983.)

In patients presenting with postoperative respiratory failure, static respiratory compliance can increase (Rouby et al., 1983) when lung volume increases with HFJV (Fig. 7). The changes in lung volume are secondary to and correlated with changes in mean airway and alveolar pressure. Therefore specific compliance, that is, compliance divided by mean end-expiratory lung volume or FRC, probably does not change with HFJV. On the other hand, the patient's individual compliance determines the change in lung volume with a given driving pressure, frequency, and I/E ratio (Rouby et al., 1983).

VI. Intrapulmonary Gas Distribution

Several studies have shown that high frequency ventilation improves intrapulmonary gas distribution (Brusasco et al., 1984; Schmid et al., 1981; Slutsky et al., 1980; Solway et al., 1984; Wattwil et al., 1983). The mechanisms involved are not entirely clear. However it seems likely that convective flow and mixing are enhanced, whereas diffusion is less altered in peripheral lung areas, but is increased in central airways (Solway et al., 1984).

These factors improve both oxygenation of arterial blood and CO_2 elimination. Current investigations will help us to understand and, it is hoped, control some of the mechanisms involved, allowing us to adjust the setting of the high-frequency ventilator for an optimal gas exchange (Froese and Bryan, 1981; Rossing et al., 1981).

References

Babinski, M., Smith, R. B., and Klain, M. (1980). High frequency jet ventilation for laryngoscopy. *Anesthesiology* **52**:178-180.

Benhamou, D., Ecoffey, C., Rouby, J. J., Fusciardi, J., and Viars, P. (1984). Impact of changes in operating pressure during high-frequency jet ventilation. *Anesth. Analg.* **63**:19-24.

Benjamin, B., and Gronow, D. (1979). A new tube for microlaryngeal surgery. *Anaesth. Intensive Care* **7**:258-263.

Benjaminsson, E., and Klain, M. (1981). Intraoperative dual-mode independent lung ventilation of a patient with bronchopleural fistula. *Anesth. Analg.* **60**:118-119.

Brusasco, V., Knopp, T. J., Schmid, E., and Rehder, K. (1984). Ventilation-perfusion relationship during high-frequency ventilation. *J. Appl. Physiol.* **56**:454-458.

Carden, E., and Vest, H. R. (1974). Further advances in anesthetic techniques for microlaryngeal surgery. *Anesth. Analg.* **53**:584.

Carlon, G. C., Ray, C. Jr., Klain, M., and McCormack, P. M. (1980). High-frequency positive-pressure ventilation in management of a patient with bronchopleural fistula. *Anesthesiology* **52**:160-162.

Carlon, G. C., Howland, W. S., Ray, C., Miodownik, S., Griffin, J. P., and Jeffrey, S. G. (1983). High-frequency jet ventilation–a prospective randomized evaluation. *Chest* **84**:551-559.

Cartwright, D. W., Willis, M. M., and Gregory, G. A. (1984). Functional residual capacity and lung mechanics at different levels of mechanical ventilation. *Crit. Care Med.* **12**:422-427.

El Baz, N., El-Ganzouri, A., and Ivankovich, A. (1983). High frequency positive pressure ventilation for major airway surgery. In *Perspectives in High Frequency Ventilation*. Edited by P. A. Scheck, U. H. Sjostrand, and R. B. Smith. The Hague, Martinus Nijhoff, pp. 216-226.

Froese, A. B., and Bryan, A. C. (1981). High frequency ventilation. (editorial). *Am. Rev. Respir. Dis.* **123**:249-250.

Guntupalli, K., Sladen, A., and Klain, M. (1981). High frequency jet ventilation (HFJV) in the prevention of a decrease in PaO_2 during suctioning. *Chest* **80**:381-382.

Klain, M., and Smith, R. B. (1977). High frequency percutaneous transtracheal jet ventilation. *Crit. Care Med.* **5**(6):280-287.

Klain, M., Miller, J., and Kalla, R. (1981). Emergency use of high frequency jet ventilation. *Crit. Care Med.* **9**(3):160.

Klain, M., Keszler, H., and Nordin, U. (1982a). Is jet ventilation without cuffed tube safe? *Anesth. Analg.* **61**(2):195-196.

Klain, M., Kalla, R., Sladen, A., Guntupalli, K., and Wald, M. (1982b). Weaning from respiratory support by high frequency jet ventilation. *Anesthesiology* **57**(3):A468.

Klain, M., Fine, J., Sladen, A., Guntupalli, K., Marquez, J., and Keszler, H. (1983). Clinical experience with high frequency ventilation. In *Perspectives in High Frequency Ventilation.* Edited by P. A. Scheck, U. H. Sjostrand, and R. B. Smith. The Hague, Martinus Nijhoff, pp. 233-239.

Marquez, J., Fine, J., Klain, M., Bennett, R., and Freeman, J. (1982). Clinical applications of high frequency jet ventilation in the operating room. *Anesthesiology* **57**:A464.

Miller, J., Iovino, W., Fine, J., and Klain, M. (1982). High frequency jet ventilation in oral and maxillofacial surgery. *J. Oral Maxillofac. Surg.* **40**:790-793.

Moulaert, P., and Rolly, G. (1983). High frequency jet ventilation for pulmonary resection. In *Perspectives in High Frequency Ventilation.* Edited by P. A. Scheck, U. H. Sjostrand, and R. B. Smith. The Hague, Martinus Nijhoff, pp. 227-232.

Pollard, B. J. (1968). Anesthesia for laryngeal microsurgery. *Anesthesia* **23**:534.

Rossing, T. H., Slutsky, A. S., Lehr, J. L., Drinker, P. A., Kamm, R., and Drazen, J. M. (1981). Tidal volume and frequency dependence of carbon dioxide elimination by high-frequency ventilation. *N. Engl. J. Med.* **305**:1375-1379.

Rouby, J. J., Fusciardi, J., Bourgain, J. L., and Viars, P. (1983). High-frequency jet ventilation in postoperative respiratory failure: Determinants of oxygenation. *Anesthesiology* **59**:281-287.

Saari, A. F., Rossing, T. H., Solway, J., and Drazen, J. M. (1984). Lung inflation during high-frequency ventilation. *Am. Rev. Respir. Dis.* **129**:333-336.

Scheck, P. A., Mallios, C., and Knegt, P. (1983). High frequency ventilation for laser surgery of the larynx. In *Perspectives in High Frequency Ventilation.* Edited by P. A. Scheck, U. H. Sjostrand, and R. B. Smith. The Hague, Martinus Nijhoff, pp. 204-211.

Schmid, E. R., Knopp, T. J., and Rehder, K. (1981). Intrapulmonary gas transport and perfusion during high-frequency oscillation. *J. Appl. Physiol.* **51**:1507-1514.

Slutsky, A. S., Drazen, J. M., Ingram, R. H. Jr., Kamm, R. D., Shapiro, A. H., Fredberg, J. J., Loring, S. H., and Lehr, J. (1980). Effective pulmonary ventilation with small-volume oscillations at high frequency. *Science* **209**:609-611.

Solway, J., Gavriely, N., Kamm, R. D., Drazen, J. M., Ingram, R. H. Jr., Khoo, M. C. K., Brown, R., and Slutsky, A. S. (1984). Intra-airway gas mixing during high-frequency ventilation. *J. Appl. Physiol.* **56**:343-354.

Spoerel, W. E., Narayanan, P. S., and Singh, N. P. (1971). Transtracheal ventilation. *Br. J. Anaesth.* **43**:932.

Wattwil, L. M., Sjöstrand, U. H., Borg, U. R., and Eriksson, I. A. (1983). Comparative studies of IPPV and HFPPV with PEEP in critical care patients: II. Studies on intrapulmonary gas distribution. *Crit. Care Med.* **11**:38-43.

Weinmann, G. G., Simon, B. A., and Mitzner, W. (1984). Lung compliance changes on high-frequency ventilation in normal dogs. *J. Appl. Physiol.* **56**:506-512.

Whitwam, J. G. (1984). Functional dead space during high frequency ventilation (Editorial). *Europ. J. Anaesth.* **1**:7-9.

9

Clinical Use of High-Frequency Jet Ventilation in Intensive Care

T. JAMES GALLAGHER

University of Florida
College of Medicine
Gainesville, Florida

High-frequency jet ventilation may play many important and contributory roles in ventilatory therapy. Although not all its aspects have been investigated, high frequency jet ventilation (HFJV) will become an essential tool of our day-to-day management of respiratory problems. Only by continued investigation and refinement of these devices can we hope to begin to use the machines and their capabilities most effectively.

Development, technical characteristics, and modalities of gas delivery of high-frequency ventilators should be clearly understood in order to appreciate their clinical applications. Each of these aspects, and the implications of the differences between high-frequency ventilators, have been discussed in detail in other chapters of this book.

For clinical applications, potential mechanical limitations of the ventilator and related safety considerations must be kept in mind. For instance, mechanical solenoids are subject to metal fatigue. At a rate of 100 breaths/min, the solenoid would open and close 144,000 times in each 24 hr. Depending upon the device and the manufacturer, life expectancies vary. One should be aware that some solenoids may fail sooner than expected. In general, spare parts and personnel competent to replace failing components should be available in all intensive care units where high-frequency ventilators are used.

I. Use of High-Frequency Jet Ventilation

When is it appropriate to use high-frequency jet ventilation in the intensive care unit and which patients might best benefit from this mode? Most published case reports suggest that patients were first placed on high-frequency jet ventilation when they could no longer be supported by conventional techniques. Interpreting information and obtaining data under these circumstances must be done very carefully. In most cases, the decision that a patient failed to respond to conventional respiratory support is based on arbitrary criteria.

Investigators employ different therapeutic end-points and different combinations of available mechanical respiratory support. Because the methodology is different, the decision that conventional methods have been exhausted may vary greatly from one institution to another. There are serious disadvantages in postponing institution of high-frequency jet ventilation until respiratory function has markedly deteriorated, for instance, in a patient with a progressive disease, for which no form of mechanical ventilation is satisfactory. One could reasonably argue that earlier utilization of high-frequency ventilation might have prevented progression of respiratory failure, but no mechanical device can reverse the course of patients whose lungs are damaged beyond salvage.

The several theoretical advantages of high-frequency jet ventilation over the more conventional techniques still have not been verified in controlled studies. This chapter will attempt to review the potential benefits of high-frequency ventilation and the available clinical evidence to support them.

II. Cardiac Performance

High-frequency jet ventilation generally delivers smaller tidal volumes than conventional devices, sometimes less than deadspace; therefore, peak airway pressures are also consistently lower (Carlon et al., 1983b) (Fig. 1). Reduction of airway pressure may provide several advantages. Venous return significantly improves when transpulmonary pressure is low and right ventricular ejection fraction enhanced (Figs. 2, 3). Right ventricular stroke work should also decrease with high-frequency jet ventilation, since reduction in airway pressure implies lower pulmonary artery pressure and vascular resistance. Right ventricular afterload decreases, facilitating maintenance of cardiac output.

III. Barotrauma

Peak inflation pressures developed during high-frequency jet ventilation are much lower than with conventional methods. Since pulmonary barotrauma appears to be related not only to high inflation pressures (Caldwell et al., 1970), but also to

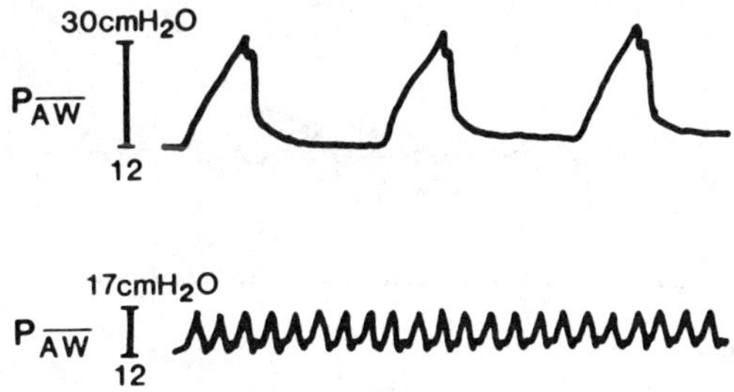

Figure 1 A comparison of airway pressure (P_{AW}) on conventional (top) and high-frequency jet ventilation (bottom). Note the marked decrease in peak inflation pressure and mean airway pressure with high-frequency jet ventilation. The amplitude under the curve indicates the tidal volume.

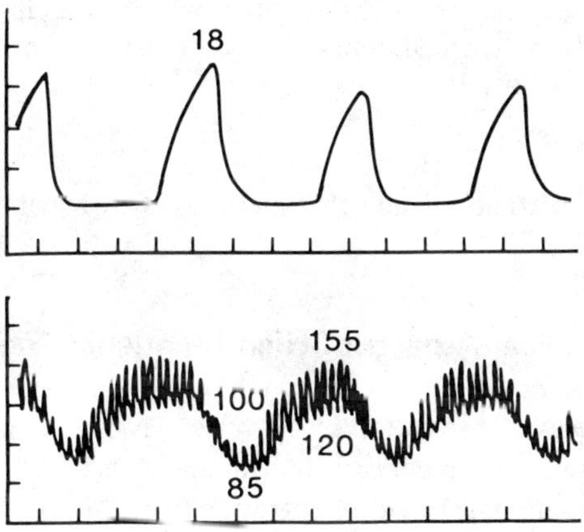

Figure 2 Conventional ventilation in an animal rendered hypovolemic. With each positive-pressure breath, blood pressure and cardiac output decrease.

delivery of large tidal volumes, minimization of both variables should reduce its incidence. To date, this theory has not been supported by well-documented studies, probably reflecting the low incidence of barotrauma as reported in most clinical studies of mechanical ventilation, including comparison of high-frequency with other techniques.

Other advantages of high-frequency ventilation may relate to the methods of gas movement in the airway, a phenomenon which is as yet little understood. The demonstrated ability to remove CO_2 and deliver O_2 at volumes lower than deadspace clearly indicates that significant intrinsic differences exist between

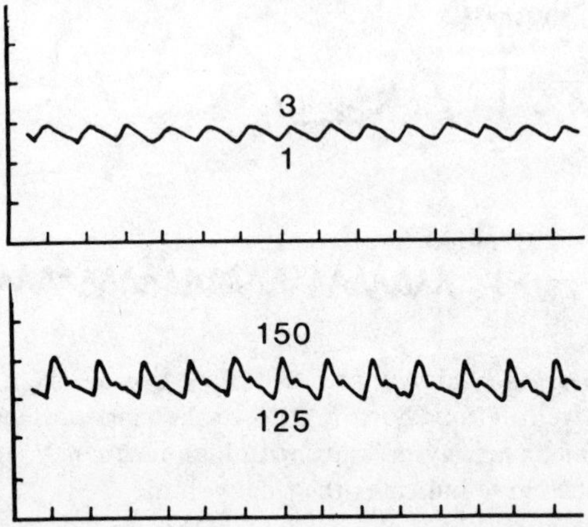

Figure 3 The same animal from Figure 2 is now placed on high-frequency jet ventilation. Note the marked stability in blood pressure, which indicates less depression of cardiac output.

high-frequency jet ventilation and other methods (Rossing et al., 1981) discussed at length elsewhere in this book.

IV. Mechanical Aspects of High-Frequency Ventilation

In pneumatic systems, the selection of the valve may greatly affect other functions, even though individual controls remain unchanged. When flow is diverted from one circuit to others, the entire operation of the device is affected. Usually, this problem develops at low driving pressures, most likely because gas flow is generally decreased. As stated earlier, high-frequency jet ventilators are among the few ventilators for adults that can operate at driving pressures of less than 50 psig, although higher pressures can also be used, if necessary. Driving pressure correlates linearly to flow rates and therefore tidal volume, which is a function of flow and inspiratory time. Therefore, driving pressure affects tidal volume and ultimately arterial P_{CO_2}. For small children, driving pressures of 10-20 psig are generally sufficient to provide adequate alveolar ventilation, while 35-50 psig may be required for adults. The less compliant the lungs, the higher the pressures (occasionally exceeding 50 psig) necessary to operate the machine.

In most cases, patients require a mixture of oxygen and air, provided by an air-oxygen blender. Blenders manufactured in the United States require operating pressures of 50 psig and are inaccurate at lower levels. Driving pressure to the jet ventilator therefore should be set between the blender and the device, not before the blender.

V. Frequencies

Most high-frequency jet ventilators operate at frequencies of 60-600 breaths/min. Although devices exceeding that frequency range can be obtained, they do not provide clinical advantages at this time. Frequency alone does not justify the definition of high-frequency jet ventilation, which is more accurately based on the presence of a jet injector and entrainment. Most systems operate effectively at frequencies of 80-300 breaths/min, and the optimal frequency varies for each device.

Each ventilator is uniquely characterized by its circuits, valves, injector, and other related parts. These factors determine the actual function of the equipment, precluding prediction of the best frequency range of new devices. Each ventilator should be tested and characterized in bench, laboratory, and clinical tests. For example, the Healthdyne and IDC units function best at frequencies between 100 and 200 breaths/min, while the Bird ventilator has an optimal frequency of approximately 250 breaths/min. Higher frequencies may preclude optimal function of the Venturi gating mechanism, a mechanical device that requires a finite time to operate effectively.

VI. Inspiratory Time

If inspiratory time (T_I) or I/E ratio remain unchanged, higher frequencies cause lower delivered tidal volume. This apparent paradox is related to the reduction of expiratory time. Expiration is ordinarily a passive maneuver, requiring more time than inspiration. At higher frequencies air trapping may develop, leading to an unexpected increase of positive end-expiratory pressure (PEEP). Clinically, $PaCO_2$ also may increase if higher pressure increases physiological deadspace.

Most high-frequency jet ventilators operate best with T_I 20 30% of the respiratory cycle. Within the actual time involved, at 100 breaths/min, a T_I 20% represents 120 msec. The longer the inspiratory time, the larger the tidal volume, but also the greater the risk of air trapping. At higher frequencies, expiratory time decreases. The briefer this nonmechanical passive maneuver, the more likely air trapping becomes. This will increase mean airway pressure and functional residual capacity. Deadspace-to-tidal volume ratio (Vd/Vt) will increase; most likely carbon dioxide levels will increase before oxygenation deteriorates.

VII. Tidal Volume

Accurate measurement of tidal volume is extremely difficult during clinical application of high-frequency jet ventilation. Commonly used devices, such as spirometers, contain too much deadspace, which causes inaccuracy. Other devices, such as pneumotachographs, have not proved useful because of inadequate frequency response. Still other reliable systems, such as a body box, are not applicable clinically.

As stated previously, driving pressure correlates linearly to tidal volume and airway pressure. Since the circuits of high-frequency jet ventilators often provide entrainment, a greater volume of gases will be delivered than that exiting from the injector cannula. The entrained volume depends on several factors. Up to a certain size, roughly equivalent to a 14-gauge intracath (1.62-mm internal diameter), the larger the diameter of the injector, the greater the entrained volume. Higher back pressure, which may occur with noncompliant lungs or high inspiratory pressure, decreases flow through the injector, the Venturi effect, and the amount of entrained gas. Flow from the jet is even pressure-dependent. The greater the airway pressure for a given ventilator setting, the more likely flow and tidal volume will decrease.

In our own institution, we ordinarily do not attempt to measure directly the tidal volume delivered. Instead, we are interested in verifying the presence of chest movements during high-frequency jet ventilation. We aim to obtain an amplitude displacement of the high-frequency breath between 8 and 20 cm H_2O, associated with visible chest expansion. This amplitude displacement represents the change in airway pressure with each breath from the baseline. While not directly correlated at a fixed drive pressure, the greater the amplitude, the larger the tidal volume. It has been our experience that the absence of any chest movement during high-frequency jet ventilation correlates with unacceptably high $PaCO_2$ and severe respiratory acidosis. Under these circumstances, an increase in frequency does not usually improve ventilation; this result is best achieved by increasing the pressure amplitude.

VIII. PEEP/CPAP

All high-frequency jet ventilators enable application of PEEP or continuous positive-airway pressure (CPAP). On some machines, this result is obtained by adding external devices, such as an Emerson water column. In other devices, a demand valve has been incorporated into the inspiratory circuit to maintain the desired level of PEEP or CPAP. If PEEP or CPAP were necessary to maintain oxygenation during conventional ventilation, this will generally be true with high-frequency jet ventilation as well. Additional PEEP or CPAP may be developed by air trapping, as already mentioned. Inadvertent PEEP is not usually clinically beneficial, since it reduces tidal volume and, thus, increases $PaCO_2$.

In systems with built-in demand valves, high PEEP or CPAP levels may hamper the performance of the ventilator. Flow may be redirected to the demand valve, which reduces pressure amplitude and gas volume delivered with each high-frequency breath, as is the case with the Bird high-frequency ventilator. Modifications of the control systems are necessary to restore tidal volume to its original levels.

IX. Airway Pressure

In the majority of high-frequency jet ventilators, airway pressure is monitored with the same type of manometer used on conventional machines. Ordinarily, they have been "snubbed" to some degree to prevent uncontrolled oscillation, which might occur if no damping were employed. As a result, the pressure gauge reflects an approximation of mean airway pressure that developed during high-frequency jet ventilation. These devices measure PEEP inaccurately. A rapidly responding strip chart recorder gives the most accurate measurements. An air-filled transducer system connects the recorder to the airway pressure line. PEEP or CPAP is read as the lowest pressure recorded during high-frequency ventilation. Newer machines are now available with oscilloscopic display of the airway pressure tracing. If calibration is done, the lowest pressure point observed on the oscilloscope during mechanical breathing will indicate the level of PEEP or CPAP employed.

X. Indications for Jet Ventilation

Utilization of HFJV during laryngeal surgery has been well documented in the last 15 years and is described elsewhere in this book.

The new area of development and research involves use of high-frequency jet ventilation in patients unable to maintain oxygenation and ventilation spontaneously.

A. Bronchopleural Fistula

Bronchopleural fistulae have been successfully treated with high-frequency jet ventilation (Carlon et al., 1981a; Mickell et al., 1983). Major clinical problems in patients with airway disruption include the inability to maintain alveolar ventilation. When hypercapnia develops, the usual maneuvers, such as increasing tidal volume or rate, do not successfully reduce $PaCO_2$. The higher pressures and greater frequencies employed with conventional techniques may keep the fistula patent, prevent healing, and impair cardiac performance. The lower pressures generated during high-frequency jet ventilation, on the other hand, result in a substantial reduction in air leaks (Pokora et al., 1983), which increases effective alveolar ventilation. Additionally, the marked reduction in airway pressures should facilitate healing of the lesion; although no experimental evidence has yet been provided.

Long-term high-frequency jet ventilation has been successful for bronchopleural fistula. We now highly recommend this technique for all forms of bronchopleural fistula.

B. Adult Respiratory Distress Syndrome

When high-frequency jet ventilation was first introduced in the United States, many believed that it could become the method of choice for treating adult respiratory distress syndrome (ARDS). At that time, little was understood about how the technique actually worked, but early reports suggested that it could surpass the effectiveness of conventional techniques, including positive end-expiratory pressure.

The evidence now accumulating does not confirm distinct advantages in using high-frequency jet ventilation for the treatment of ARDS. PEEP or CPAP, at levels comparable to those used during conventional ventilation, is still required to provide adequate oxygenation (Marchak et al., 1981; Rouby et al., 1983). A major difference, which may prove beneficial, is reduced peak inflation pressures on high-frequency jet ventilation.

Scattered reports in the literature indicate that some patients with ARDS not successfully treated on conventional techniques improved on high-frequency jet ventilation. Serious caution must be applied in interpreting these data. Often the levels of PEEP or CPAP employed to improve oxygenation were low compared with those used in other centers. Therefore, we cannot prove that patients would have failed to respond to more aggressive interventions on conventional therapy.

Because high back pressures reduce entrainment, patients with extremely poor lung compliance may also have impaired CO_2 elimination on high-frequency jet ventilation.

At least one manufacturer has developed a machine combining high-frequency jet ventilation with conventional techniques (Fig. 4). The device can deliver large-volume conventional breaths and, between them, high-frequency breaths up to 15 Hz. Any combination of large-volume breaths and high-frequency rates or volumes can be selected. CPAP or PEEP also can be added as needed.

We have utilized the combination of high-frequency jet ventilation and conventional ventilation in more than 50 patients with ARDS. Initial data are encouraging and suggest that oxygenation may be obtained at mean airway pressures and PEEP lower than required on conventional techniques. The higher mechanical minute ventilation enhances CO_2 elimination. We can postulate that the improvement in oxygenation may be related to recruitment of alveoli by large-volume conventional breaths. It is possible that the peak pressures generated on high-frequency ventilation are not sufficient to recruit all unstable alveolar units, which perpetuates ventilation/perfusion inequalities. Large-volume breaths may

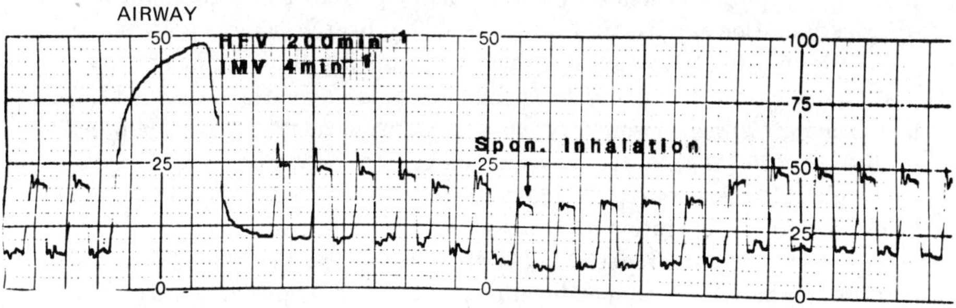

Figure 4 High-frequency ventilation (Bird) combined with conventional breaths. Notice the pause after the high-frequency interruption until the large pressure breath is delivered to the patient. This is followed by another pause before the resumption of high-frequency breaths. These large-volume breaths help recruit atelectatic airway units.

recruit these alveolar areas, which then remain expanded until the next large-volume breath. This mechanism can explain the overall improvement in gas exchange.

Other investigators have attempted to accomplish the same result by attaching the high-frequency jet ventilator circuit to the circuitry of a conventional ventilator. In other words, the entrained flow for high-frequency jet ventilation has been substituted with the ventilator circuitry commonly employed during controlled or intermittent mandatory ventilation. High-frequency jet ventilation continues throughout the entire conventional cycle, either superimposed on large mechanical breaths or by itself during exhalation or pauses. This approach has been associated with improved oxygenation and carbon dioxide clearance (see Chap. 5).

Proper manipulation of the controls of high-frequency jet ventilation requires understanding of the interaction between mechanical variables and clinical results. Inadequate oxygenation evidenced by a low PaO_2 or high venous admixture (Qsp/Qt) can be corrected by several methods. Higher PEEP/CPAP will increase mean airway pressure, which may improve matching of ventilation to perfusion. However, if mean airway pressure decreases venous return or increases pulmonary vascular resistance, cardiac function may decrease because of decreased preload or increased afterload. Prolonging inspiratory time will also increase mean airway pressure, which may improve PaO_2. Higher driving pressure will increase tidal volume, inspiratory flow, and thus mean airway pressure, which again possibly will improve oxygenation. Also, raising driving pressure will augment tidal volume and, thus, reduce $PaCO_2$. A significant increase in respiratory frequency favors air trapping, which in turn adds to airway pressure and, thus, improves oxygenation. However, this last maneuver will ordinarily cause hypercapnia.

Additional strategies are available when reducing $PaCO_2$ is the primary goal. A decrease in respiratory rate will increase tidal volume delivered with each breath and prolong the inspiratory phase. This may lead to an overall improvement of alveolar gas exchange. A reduction in mean airway pressure from decreasing PEEP or inspiratory time may improve deadspace-to-tidal volume ratio and ensure better ventilation-to-perfusion matching.

Contrary to some reports (Butler et al., 1980; Zwart et al., 1981), in our observations patients continued breathing during high-frequency ventilation. Neither clinical nor laboratory studies have verified the development of apnea. Spontaneous ventilation may continue because a degree of vagal stimulation persists or afferent impulses from the pulmonary stretch receptors, whose presence is generally accepted, become weaker on high-frequency ventilation.

The level of delivered FIO_2 will be inaccurate if the entrained gas is not kept at the same concentration as the jet flow. Ordinarily this is achieved by using the same blender. Attempts to ventilate the patient with an uncuffed endotracheal tube may also result in unpredictable FIO_2 levels, since room air may be entrained around the uncuffed tube.

The selection of the initial setting of a high-frequency jet ventilator in treating patients with ARDS depends largely on the device used. When manufacturers build ventilators that do not conform to uniform standards, it becomes extremely difficult to predict the flow characteristics of each device. Furthermore, delivery circuits, role of entrainment, and length and location of the injector also vary greatly from system to system, which clearly affects gas delivery characteristics of each high-frequency ventilator.

In adults, the machines operate best at pressures of 35-50 psig. This is usually sufficient in all machines to deliver tidal and minute volumes that can support alveolar ventilation. The worse the lung compliance, the greater the driving pressure necessary to deliver that tidal volume. The 20-30% inspiratory time discussed earlier ensures an I/E ratio from 1:2 to 1:4. This may permit enough time for adequate exhalation during the passive phase of respiration.

Since tidal volume cannot be measured directly, it is indispensable to have other methods to verify that ventilation is adequate. Clinical observation of chest movements remains important. One must not simply feel the presence of vibrations in the chest; there should be clear chest motion. The airway pressure excursion can also be utilized as a guide to adequacy of ventilation. With most devices, at driving pressures of 35 psig or greater, airway pressure excursions will vary between 8 and 20 cm H_2O.

These remarks only serve as initial guidelines to begin therapy; changes should then be made on the basis of blood gas values. PEEP/CPAP should be manipulated as necessary to ensure adequate oxygenation. Placement of a water column on the expiratory limb is an effective way to provide PEEP. Some machines have incorporated a demand valve system for spontaneous breathing into the inspiratory circuit. The demand valve may then be utilized to maintain the desired level of PEEP or CPAP.

The ideal method to wean patients from high-frequency jet ventilation has not been established unequivocally. An effective technique consists of incrementally decreasing driving pressure, and therefore mechanical minute volume. Spontaneous breathing will then increase to compensate for the reduced mechanical support. Once driving pressure falls below 20 psig and blood gas levels remain adequate, adult patients can probably be safely disconnected from the high-frequency apparatus. An alternative method for weaning from high-frequency ventilation relies on incremental reduction of ventilatory rate. Once this has decreased below 80 breaths/min, the patient may be safely transferred to a conventional ventilator, and weaning continues with further reduction of mechanical rate. This technique can cause problems since adult ventilators do not operate properly at rates of 60-80 breaths/min. The large volumes and pressures involved can significantly affect cardiac performance. For that reason we favor progressively decreasing driving pressure as the preferred weaning method.

C. Intracranial Pressure

High-frequency jet ventilation may also facilitate reduction of intracranial pressure with closed head injuries or other pertinent neurological complications. Several patients with high intracranial pressures (ICP) who have come to us have responded with a precipitous drop in ICP to high-frequency jet ventilation and no other change in therapy (Figs. 5, 6). Compared with conventional ventilation, the major effect of high-frequency jet ventilation is lower mean and peak airway pressures, and therefore intrathoracic pressure. Venous return from the head is thus facilitated. The reduction in intracranial blood volume results in lower ICP, especially when this latter variable has reached very high values. High-frequency jet ventilation has less of an effect when ICP is only 20-25 mmHg. Presumably, when ICP is very high, the brain lies on a steep portion of its pressure volume curve, and even small changes in blood volume induced by lower airway pressure may contribute to a significant reduction in ICP.

An additional benefit of high-frequency jet ventilation may come from improved cerebral perfusion pressure (CPP), since cardiac output and blood pressure may increase when airway pressure falls. It is also well known that conventional positive pressure breaths can cause transient, sharp elevations of intracranial pressures during the inspiratory phase. Since peak inflation pressure decreases with high-frequency jet ventilation, peaks of ICP are prevented or reduced and intracranial pressure is stabilized.

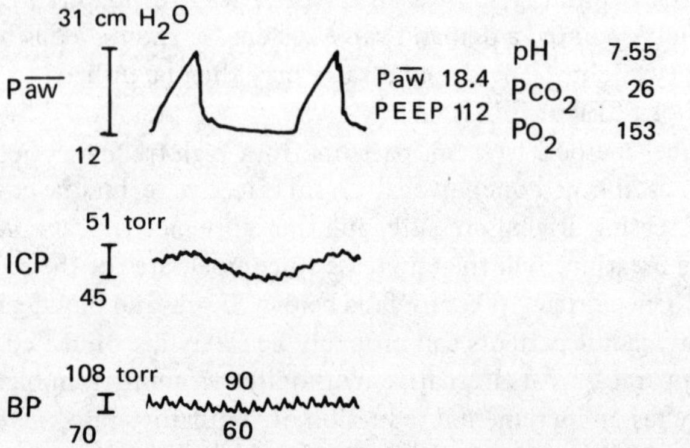

Figure 5 Airway pressure, intracranial pressure, and blood pressure of a patient with closed head injury. Note the high intracranial pressure despite hypocapnea.

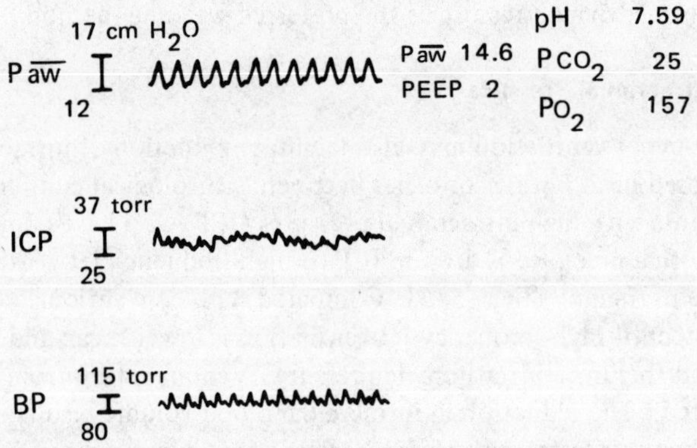

Figure 6 High-frequency ventilation was used for the patient in Figure 5. After 1 min and without any change in arterial carbon dioxide tension, intracranial pressure decreased significantly.

D. Airway Maintenance

High-frequency jet ventilation may have a role in emergency airway maintenance (Klain and Smith, 1977). Occasionally airway obstruction or lack of intubation skills prevents placement of a translaryngeal tube or tracheostomy. Under these conditions the only other appropriate method for securing the airway is a cricothyrotomy, a therapy of limited and temporary benefit. Added to high-frequency jet ventilation, cricothyrotomy can ensure good oxygenation and ventilation for an extended period of time. The technique, while simpler than tracheostomy, may not be suitable for paramedical personnel to perform.

E. Cardiopulmonary Resuscitation

High-frequency jet ventilation may prove beneficial during cardiopulmonary resuscitation (Swartzman et al., 1984). There are indications that simultaneous ventilation and chest compression may be most efficacious for maintaining perfusion during CPR. Synchronized chest compression raises intrathoracic pressure during cardiac compression. Transmural aortic pressure (vascular pressure - intrathoracic pressure) decreases as does left ventricular afterload. The net effect is improved cardiac output.

This method may also be used in patients not receiving CPR but with impaired cardiac performance (Carlon et al., 1981b). Jet ventilation may be synchronized with the electrocardiogram to increase airway pressure at the beginning of cardiac systole. The higher intrathoracic pressure ultimately would reduce transmural aortic pressure and left ventricular afterload and, thus, improve cardiac performance; few clinical and experimental data support this theory (Carlon et al., 1975, 1983a).

F. Differential Lung Ventilation

High-frequency jet ventilation also has been utilized for differential lung ventilation. Placement of a double-lumen tube and differential lung ventilation are generally reserved for patients with unilateral disease. The method permits selective delivery of high inflation pressures and high levels of PEEP to one lung only. Although very few data are available, the best use for high-frequency ventilation in unilateral lung disease may be reserved for the less diseased lung, which would receive a lower inflation pressure; thus, shunting of blood from uninvolved to involved areas, which worsens the ventilation-perfusion relationship, is minimized.

XI. Complications

Objective reviews of high-frequency jet ventilation must address some of the negative aspects of this technique.

There are instances in which high-frequency ventilation does not work. Patients satisfactorily responding to conventional ventilation have deteriorated when placed on high-frequency jet ventilation. At other times, high-frequency jet ventilation has failed to improve gas exchange, which also was inadequate on conventional ventilation. The reasons for these failures, which could not be rectified despite manipulation of all controls, remained mostly unclear. Some patients undoubtedly would have worsened beyond recovery on any ventilatory mode. In other cases, ventilator settings may not have been optimal to correct the underlying abnormality, since our understanding of the pathophysiology of respiratory failure and of high-frequency jet ventilation remains incomplete.

A major problem has been and remains humidification of gases during high-frequency jet ventilation. Some serious complications have occurred when insufficient humidification was provided. Thick, dry, caked secretions can obstruct the bronchial tree; at least one death has been partly associated with this problem.

Commercial humidifiers cannot work with high-frequency ventilators. The large compressible volume of these devices would greatly decrease the minute volume available to the patient. Attempts to humidify gas adequately have included entrainment of conditioned gases. The small and continuously changing volume of entrained gas makes this method unreliable. Other authors have recommended nebulization of water into the airway. Saline has been dripped into the gas stream emanating from the injector, to be fragmented into small particles. This system may not represent true humidification. Condensation developing in the airway may cause a risk of overhydration.

At least one manufacturer (Bird) has developed a method to humidify the jet gases, as well as entrained flow. The system appears to be quite adequate, and its small size minimizes compressible volume. Even these humidifiers can deliver large volumes of fluids, with the attendant risk of overhydration.

Many have questioned patients' acceptance of high-frequency jet ventilation. It has been our experience, as well as others', that some actually have preferred high-frequency over more conventional techniques, in particular after upper abdominal surgery. This probably relates to decreased abdominal expansion during ventilation, which reduces pain. The majority of patients appear indifferent when asked to compare high-frequency to other techniques. They may be too sick to have an appropriate response or simply may have no real basis for comparison. Chest-injured patients seem least accepting of the method. It may be that the continuous chest movement heightens their awareness of pain. As with most procedures, adequate explanations and reassurance dramatically increase patient acceptance.

Might generalized muscle fatigue develop during high-frequency jet ventilation? This was a common problem during the days of propeller-driven commercial aircraft. With the advent of jets and a marked decrease in the amount of vibrations, fatigue does not appear to be as great a factor. Patients receiving high-frequency ventilation are subjected continuously to vibrations. Although the problem has not been studied or documented, it should be considered when patients fail to wean after several days on high-frequency jet ventilation, in which case, sedation, the use of water beds, or similar methods should perhaps be considered.

At this time, we do not know whether high-frequency jet ventilation has any long-term detrimental effects. The most obvious would be the effect on the tracheal mucosa, subjected to the impact of high-velocity gases. Animal studies indicated that no real damage occurred after 24 hr of jet ventilation (Smith et al., 1981; Keszler et al., 1982). Since jet injector placement varies in relation to the carina, injury may be more or less severe.

We also have no indication of the long-term effects of high-frequency jet ventilation on pulmonary function. Do any changes take place because of the lack of cyclical lung expansion that normally occurs during conventional techniques? Are there changes in the amount of surfactant or its actions? Does continued maintenance of a stable, expanded functional residual capacity have any impact on surfactant? Are there any changes in pulmonary secretory function? All these questions remain unanswered.

XII. New Areas

Because of the almost instantaneous attainment of high flows during high-frequency jet ventilation, the technique may play a role in the treatment of other pulmonary problems, such as retained secretions and atelectasis. The high flow rates may represent a form of shock wave, which moves down the airway and favors internal vibrations. The cohesive forces of pulmonary secretions may become disrupted and result in smaller particulate material that is easier to expectorate. High flow rates also stimulate a cough reflex, further facilitating the removal of secretions.

In our own experience, these maneuvers have facilitated reexpansion of segmental atelectasis and removal of retained secretions. The treatment can be delivered through a mouthpiece to nonintubated patients and is administered frequently, usually every 2-4 hr. Since high pressures and velocities are needed to mobilize and remove secretions, tolerance must be developed slowly. This is best done by slowly increasing the driving pressure of the machine, until the desired results are obtained. Several treatments are usually required to reach the appropriate flow and pressure.

References

Butler, W. J., Bohn, D. J., Bryan, A. C., and Froese, A. B. (1980). Ventilation by high-frequency oscillation in humans. *Anesth. Analg.* **59**:577.

Caldwell, E. J., Powell, R. D., and Mullooly, J. P. (1970). Interstitial emphysema: a study of physiologic factors involved in experimental induction of the lesion. *Am. Rev. Respir. Dis.* **102**:516.

Carlon, G. C., Ray, C., Pierri, M. K. (1975). High frequency jet ventilation. *Chest* **68**:774.

Carlon, G. C., Kahn, R. C., Howland, W. S., Ray, C., and Turnbull, A. D. (1981a). Clinical experience with high frequency jet ventilation. *Crit. Care Med.* **9**:1.

Carlon, G. C., Miodownik, S., Ray, C., and Kahn, R. C. (1981b). Technical aspects and clinical implications of high frequency jet ventilation with a solenoid valve. *Crit. Care Med.* **9**:47.

Carlon, G., Pierre, M. K., Groeger, J., Howland, W., and Griffin, J. (1983a). Cardiac counterpulsation using high frequency jet ventilation. *Crit. Care Med.* **11**:244.

Carlon, G. C., Ray, C., Griffin, J., Miodownik, S., and Groeger, J. S. (1983b). Tidal volume and airway pressure on high frequency jet ventilation. *Crit. Care Med.* **11**:83.

Keszler, M., Klein, R., McClellan, L., Nelson, D., and Platt, M. (1982). Effects of conventional and high frequency jet ventilation on lung parenchyma. *Crit. Care Med.* **10**:514.

Klain, M., and Smith, R. B. (1977). High frequency percutaneous transtracheal jet ventilation. *Crit. Care Med.* **5**:280.

Marchak, B. E., Thompson, W. K., Duffy, P., Miyaki, T., Bryan, M. H., Bryan, A. C., and Froese, A. B. (1981). Treatment of RDS by high-frequency oscillatory ventilation: a preliminary report. *J. Pediatr.* **99**:287.

Mickell, J. J., and Doyle, H. J. (1983). Jet ventilation for air leak complicating "adult" respiratory distress syndrome (ARDS) in infants. *Pediatr. Res.* **17**: 383A.

Pokora, T., Bing, D., Mammel, M., and Boros, S. (1983). Neonatal high frequency jet ventilation. *Pediatrics* **72**:27.

Rossing, T. H., Slutsky, A. S., Lehr, J. L., Drinker, P. A., Kamm, R., and Drazen, J. M. (1981). Tidal volume and frequency dependence of carbon dioxide elimination by high-frequency ventilation. *N. Engl. J. Med.* **305**:1375.

Rouby, J. J., Fusciardi, J., and Bourgain, J. L. (1983). High-frequency jet ventilation in postoperative respiratory failure: determinants of oxygenation. *Anesthesiology* **59**:281.

Smith, R. B., Cutaia, F., Hoff, B. H., Babinski, M., and Belineau, J. (1981). Long term transtracheal high frequency ventilation in dogs. *Crit. Care Med.* **9**: 311.

Swartzman, S., Wilson, M. A., Hoff, B. H., Bunegin, L., Smith, R. B., and Sjosstrand, U. (1984). Percutaneous transtracheal jet ventilation for cardiopulmonary resuscitation: evaluation of a new jet ventilator. *Crit. Care Med.* **12**:8.

Zwart, A., Jansen, J. R. C., and Versprille, A. (1981). Suppression of spontaneous breathing with high frequency ventilation. *Crit. Care Med.* **9**:159.

10

High-Frequency Jet Ventilation
Miscellaneous Uses

HUGO KESZLER

University of Pittsburgh School of Medicine
Pittsburgh, Pennsylvania

As is often the case with new methods, high-frequency jet ventilation (HFJV) has evoked both exaggerated hopes and exaggerated fears. It has also suffered from a lack of generally accepted nomenclature and from the diversity of equipment used. Finally, incomplete understanding of how HFJV works has led to misunderstandings and controversies. The result of all these factors is that the whole potential of HFJV is often not utilized. Needless to say HFJV is not entirely free of risk, nor are some of the special uses described in this chapter. Known risks will be discussed; risk-benefit ratios must be assessed in each individual case.

I. Suctioning During High-Frequency Jet Ventilation

The effectiveness of HFJV is not dependent on a closed system, therefore, it is ideally suited for suctioning the airway without interrupting ventilation. This should be of considerable advantage, especially in patients who have a critically low PaO_2 and in those with copious secretions. We conducted an experimental study to confirm the effectiveness of HFJV during suctioning (Keszler and Klain, 1980). The study included 10 normal dogs (series 1) and 7 dogs made hypoxic by aspiration of 10 cc/kg of water (series 2). Both series were performed under endotracheal anesthesia with thiopental and pancuronium. Intraarterial pressures, arterial blood gases (ABGs), ECG, and CVP were monitored. A standardized suctioning procedure was carried out twice for 2 min, first during conventional ventilation (by Harvard animal ventilator) and after stabilization of ABGs and vital signs under HFJV at a rate of 100/min with the inspiration 30% of the cycle. FiO_2 in series 1 was 0.21, in series 2, FiO_2 was adjusted to keep the PaO_2 between 50 and 70 mmHg. Ventilation in both series and during both types of ventilation was adjusted to maintain a $PaCO_2$ of 35 ± 5 torr.

Results fully confirmed our expectations (Table 1). Blood gases deteriorated markedly during tracheobronchial toilet (TBT) without ventilation but not during TBT with HFJV. Cardiovascular changes (increase in blood pressure, drop in pulse rate and incidence of PVCs and PACs) were also much more marked in the absence of HFJV.

A clinical counterpart consisted of 15 postsurgical patients (Guntupalli et al., 1981b). HFJV with an FiO_2 of 1.0, a rate of 100-150/min, and inspiration 30% of the cycle was used. A PEEP of 2.5-10 cm H_2O was incorporated.

Driving pressure was adjusted to keep the $PaCO_2$ at or near the normal range. ABGs were obtained during a steady state prior to suctioning, after suctioning for 15 sec and 3 min after suctioning. HFJV was continued throughout this first study period. In a second study period, the same sequences were repeated but HFJV was discontinued during TBT.

Table 1 Results of Suctioning in Animals

	PaO_2 (mmHg)	$PaCO_2$ (mmHg)
Series 1 (10 dogs)		
Control: Harvard Pump	77.5 ± 3.6	34.6 ± 0.5
End of TBT (no effective vent)	45.5 ± 2.7	41.9 ± 0.8
Control: HFJV	79.7 ± 3.7	34.4 ± 1.1
End of TBT with HFJV	82.2 ± 4.5[a]	33.0 ± 1.0[a]
Series 2 (7 dogs)		
Control: Harvard Pump	63.8 ± 2.9	36.6 ± 1.5
End of TBT (no effective vent)	47.0 ± 2.8	51.9 ± 2.2
Control: HFJV	71.8 ± 2.7	38.2 ± 1.9
End of TBT with HFJV	71.8 ± 2.2	36.8 ± 1.7

[a]Significant difference at $p < 0.05$.
Values given as mean ± standard error.
Source: Modified from Keszler and Klain (1980).

Table 2 Arterial Blood Gases During Suctioning with and without HFJV

	HFJV during suctioning		No HFJV during suctioning	
	(Pa_{O_2}; mmHg)	(Pa_{CO_2}; mmHg)	(Pa_{O_2}; mmHg)	(Pa_{CO_2}; mmHg)
Presuction	404.2 ± 21.7	34.7 ± 9	417 ± 23.7	35.7 ± 9.7
Postsuction (15 sec)	389.4 ± 22.2	35.7 ± 9.2	327.6 ± 26.1	37.9 ± 9.8
Pa_{O_2} drop	14.8		89.4[a]	
Postsuction (3 min)	424.5 ± 21.1	35.4 ± 9.1	413.3 ± 23.0	36.0 ± 9.3

[a]Significant difference ($p < 0.001$) comparing Pa_{O_2} drop with and without HFJV.
Values given as mean ± standard error.
Source: Modified from Guntupalli et al. (1981b).

Results showed a significantly greater drop in Pa_{O_2} during suctioning without HFJV. The slight drop in the ventilated group is due to entrainment of room air during suctioning (Table 2).

Several methods that make ventilation possible during suctioning have been described but are rarely used, mainly because they are cumbersome. Recommendations for safe suctioning procedures invariably advise limiting suctioning time to 10-15 sec. In practice this is often not respected, especially if secretions are abundant. In our experimental series suctioning was prolonged to 2 min to underline the differences between groups. However, the clinical study quoted (Guntupalli et al., 1981b) showed a significant drop in Pa_{O_2} even after suctioning for only 15 sec if HFJV was interrupted during the procedure. This is even more remarkable because these patients had relatively normal lungs. The small drop in Pa_{O_2} observed during TBT with HFJV could have been prevented by suctioning through a T-tube carrying O_2, which was the method used in our experimental study. HFJV is a convenient and highly effective method of preventing deterioration of ABGs during suctioning. Judging from our experimental results, it would also largely prevent cardiovascular disturbance during TBT in sick patients.

II. Endotracheal Tube Change With HFJV

Desai et al. (1980) described a technique for changing tracheal tubes utilizing the Seldinger principle. While unnecessary in most patients it is extremely useful when reintubation is expected to be very difficult or if a delay in resuming ventilation could threaten the patient's life. Guntupalli et al. (1981a) carried the idea one important step further. To avoid interrupting ventilation during the tube change, they used a shortened #16 nasogastric tube as jet tube instead of a solid introducer. That enabled them to change a tracheal tube with interruptions in ventilation lasting only a few seconds. To create a terminal opening and facilitate connection to the ventilator, the nasogastric tube is cut at both ends. The remaining tube must be more than twice the length of the tracheal tube, and should be well-lubricated before introduction. We think it should be marked at a distance beyond which it must not be introduced: a point 5 cm above the carina. If the jet tube is introduced beyond the bifurcation there is a serious danger of barotrauma unless the ventilator is equipped with a reliable feedback mechanism that turns the gas stream off if the airway pressure at the tip of the jet tube exceeds safe limits. If such a ventilator is not available, we prefer to interrupt HFJV briefly while removing the old tube. The reason is that it is very difficult to make sure the jet tube is not withdrawn too far inadvertently unless it is fed into the old endotracheal tube during extubation. Instead of using the jet tube as a guide, it may be preferable to perform laryngoscopy and introduce the new tracheal tube alongside the jet tube.

III. HFJV and the Prevention of Aspiration

The ability of any method of artificial ventilation to prevent aspiration is of paramount importance. The only method in general use today is a cuffed endotracheal or tracheostomy tube. Although usually effective if properly used, the method itself may lead to serious complications. It also has many disadvantages, including the patient's inability to speak. Swallowing is often difficult. Discomfort may be a problem when the patient regains consciousness.

HFJV is a novel approach to the problem of avoiding aspiration. There are two methods of performing HFJV: transtracheal (by puncture) and transglottic ("endotracheal"), with a jet catheter or a special endotracheal tube inserted under laryngoscopy. Previously published clinical and experimental observations led us to believe that HFJV may prevent aspiration (Rock et al., 1976). First we explored the efficacy of HFJV administered transtracheally (Klain et al., 1981b, 1983). A jet catheter (14-gauge, 3/4 inch Angiocath with two side ports) was introduced by puncture between the first and second tracheal rings. A second thin, short plastic tube was used to monitor intratracheal pressures. In order to visualize the subglottis, an endoscope was inserted through a tracheostomy 5-6.5 cm below the site of the jet catheter. The head was propped up to allow effective filling of the dog's mouth with a mixture of its own saliva, saline, and indocyanine green (Cardio-Green). Observations consisted of endoscopy, watching for bubbling in the mouth, and measurement of endotracheal pressures. If aspiration did not take place, the frequency as well as the I/E ratio was changed. The frequencies tested were 60, 100, 200, and sometimes up to 500/min. The I/E ratios were 1:1, 1:2, and sometimes up to 1:5. The VS600 high-frequency jet ventilator was used for most experiments. Endoscopic observations and bronchoscopic films demonstrated convincingly that, under the conditions of our experiments, transtracheal HFJV prevents aspiration of fluid from the mouth if frequency does not decrease below 60/min and inspiration is not less than 33% of the cycle. Endotracheal pressures were always 1-2 torr higher than the corresponding fluid level in the mouth. If the ventilator was stopped, fluid would spill into the trachea. This usually occurred within 1-3 sec after the ventilator had been stopped. As soon as HFJV was started again not only did spilling stop but the fluid already spilled was pushed back into the larynx. With fluid of higher viscosity, the same occurred except that the process was slower (Klain et al., 1983). Normal Pa_{CO_2} and high Pa_{O_2} values were maintained and documented by intermittent sampling of ABG samples.

The prevention of aspiration is due to physical factors and not to anatomical structure. A valvular mechanism of the epiglottis and/or of the cords is definitely not involved because the cords are and remain in a semiabductor ("cadaver") position and the epiglottis never covers more than about two-thirds of the opening between the cords. Also, a thin layer of fluid is usually visible above the cords but below the epiglottis. If a valve mechanism were involved, it would not fail seconds after stopping HFJV. The physical factors that, we believe, explain our observations include the continuous flow of gas which acts as a pneumatic valve at the level of the cords and the small positive end-expiratory pressure (PEEP) effect of HFJV. Gas flow and PEEP are influenced by minute volume which in our experiments was between 10 and 17 liters/min. Physical factors that probably modify the Venturi effect of HFJV include the size and shape of the larynx and trachea. In dogs weighing 20 kg the larynx and trachea are similar in size to those in adult human patients. When the rate is slowed and/or exhalation prolonged, the intratracheal pressure and flow decrease to a level which allows the fluid to penetrate the larynx.

Some important questions could not be answered on the basis of the first series of experiments. We wanted experimental proof that aspiration could be prevented even in the presence of a translaryngeal catheter introduced into the trachea by laryngoscopy. We also wanted to find out if a head-up tilt of the table and fluctuations in intrathoracic pressure as produced by CPR or spontaneous ventilation would not cause aspiration even with otherwise effective HFJV.

Nineteen experiments were carried out on 15 mongrel dogs. The VS600 ventilator was again used. The following settings were tested: inspiratory time 30-70% of the cycle, rates 50-400/min, driving pressure 0.75-3.5 bar adjusted to maintain p_{CO_2} at 35 ± 5 mmHg. Methods of observation were the same as in the previous series and the results were again documented by film (Keszler et al., 1982). The experiments were carried out in two positions of the table: level and with 10° head-up tilt.

Of the total 19 experiments we used translaryngeal jet ventilation in 14 (group 1) and transtracheal jet ventilation in 5 experiments (group 2). For translaryngeal HFJV in group 1, two types of catheters were used: A custom made insufflation catheter 5-mm in external diameter, with four side ports (courtesy of National Catheter Corporation) and an insufflation catheter modified from a pediatric chest tube (Argyle, 16 Fr, 25 cm long) with a 14 gauge Angiocath inside. With both tubes, the effect of CPR on aspiration was also investigated.

In three of five experiments in group 2 with transtracheal ventilation through a 14-gauge Angiocath we tested the effect of modified spontaneous ventilation on aspiration. Spontaneous ventilation under light barbiturate anesthesia without muscle relaxant was considered 100% normal. The total of aspiration experiments with CPR was 12. Of these, three were with transtracheal HFJV. External cardiac compression (ECC) was performed in a manner known from previous experiments to provide adequate blood flow during CPR. In our aspiration experiments ECC was performed without actually stopping the heart.

The unpublished results showed that HFJV will prevent aspiration even under adverse conditions, that is, a head-up tilt, ECC, or spontaneous ventilation amounting to 50% of normal V_T, provided only one of these adverse factors is present and provided respiratory frequency and inspiratory time are appropriate. With inspiration 50% of the cycle and respiratory rate 140/min or more, aspiration did not take place even during CPR or about 50% of normal V_T spontaneous ventilation if the table was level. Seventy percent inspiratory time is even safer, if tolerated. In the absence of ECC or spontaneous ventilation, a 10° head-up tilt was usually tolerated without aspiration with rates of 100/min or more and inspiratory time 30% of the cycle. The presence of a jet catheter in the larynx did not increase the tendency to aspiration. This finding provided additional proof that a valve mechanism is not involved in the prevention of aspiration under HFJV. Certain barium mixtures have a high specific gravity, which is probably why some observers noted aspiration of barium during HFJV (Szele and Keenan, 1981; Calkins, personal communication). The protection afforded by HFJV is dependent on uninterrupted ventilation and adherence to certain parameters of inspiratory time and respiratory frequency. Protection may also fail if two adverse factors combine (e.g., head-up tilt plus CPR) or if vigorous inspiration occurs (e.g., before coughing).

Our views regarding the use of uncuffed tubes for HFJV in patients are based on the following assumptions:

1. During CPR, a head-up position will not normally be used, and cricothyroid membrane puncture followed by HFJV may be life-saving if intubation is difficult. Continuous suction in the mouth would probably further diminish the possibility of aspiration.

2. Unconscious patients are mostly nursed flat. The mouth is usually empty and the stomach should be kept empty by a nasogastric tube, if a cuffed tube is not being used.
3. Although coughing invites aspiration if the mouth is full, conscious patients will usually not cough unless their mouth is empty. Coughing actually provoked by aspiration is an exception.

The following suggestions are based on experimental evidence and clinical experience in patients under general anesthesia or following general anesthesia. At the present use of uncuffed catheters for HFJV should probably be limited to these categories:

1. Under general anesthesia, especially where indicated by the nature of the surgical procedure (e.g., endoscopy, surgery in the airway) or if endotracheal intubation is impossible for any reason.
2. For emergency ventilation, transtracheal ventilation may be the best choice under many circumstances. Especially if obstruction in the airway is suspected, one must watch chest expansions to make sure the foreign body is dislodged by HFJV without an excessive increase in intrathoracic pressure.
3. Transtracheal HFJV might be a good alternative to tracheostomy if the patient has been intubated for a week and is not quite ready for extubation. HFJV may make weaning easier and transtracheal ventilation will not interfere with speaking.

We must stress that a Venturi effect is more likely to occur in a narrow trachea. Therefore, our recommendations apply only to adults at any rate if elective use is contemplated. When using transtracheal ventilation, we must always make sure the jet orifice is in the trachea, not in a main bronchus or in soft tissues (risking the danger of barotrauma). Furthermore, whatever the circumstances, we must keep in mind that only matter above the jet orifice will be expelled up into the mouth. If aspiration has taken place before HFJV is started, the airway must be suctioned as soon as possible. This can be done without interrupting HFJV. The mouth must be empty during suctioning of the trachea and bronchi.

IV. Transtracheal HFJV for Emergencies Including CPR

Although cricothyroid membrane puncture was used by Caynut in 1920 for topical anesthesia and Jackson described cricothyroidotomy in 1921, the first report on transtracheal O_2 insufflation was published by Jacoby et al. in 1956. They insufflated 4 liters/min O_2 through a #18 needle for 5 to 66 min in five patients and recommended its use if intubation is impossible. They realized that intermittent insufflation and a larger needle to permit higher O_2 flows would be necessary for adequate CO_2 elimination. In 1967 Sanders recommended manual jet ventilation through a bronchoscope, and in 1971 Spoerel described manual jet ventilation through a #16 transtracheal needle. Since then numerous papers on emergency and elective transtracheal jet ventilation using either manual or mechanical devices have been published. A recent article summarizes many of these papers and also discusses complications of these procedures (Schwartzmann et al., 1984).

Cricothyroid membrane puncture for ventilation offers distinct advantages for emergency use in certain patients. It can be performed even in conscious patients without muscle relaxation. Inability to open the mouth and maxillofacial injuries are good indications as well as the inability to adequately visualize the larynx for any reason. In such a way sometimes traumatic attempts at intubation in emergency situations can be avoided. In cervical spine injuries neck hyperextension is eliminated. A local anesthetic can be used before puncture if the situation is not urgent. Because cricothyroid membrane puncture is usually easy, we can secure the airway and start ventilation in a short time. Manual jet ventilation is adequate for gas exchange but exact timing is not feasible. Mechanically triggered jet ventilators make it possible to adjust ventilation to desired parameters depending on circumstances and ABGs. We have stated previously that, as long as respiratory frequency is 100/min or higher and the inspiratory duration is at least 30%, we are able to prevent aspiration in dogs even under certain adverse conditions which do not, however, include CPR or attempts at spontaneous ventilation. Under these circumstances 50% inspiratory time and a rate of 140/min or more are safer. CPR experiments in six dogs showed similar ABGs and common carotid artery blood flows during alternating periods of HFJV and IPPV (Brader et al., 1981). During cardiopulmonary resuscitation it is not necessary to interrupt HFJV during cardiac compressions. Synchronization with the EKG is possible but it has no clear advantage. The favorable effect of HFJV on cardiac output is controversial.

The ability to administer drugs even before an IV line is established is a clear advantage but its efficacy is as yet less well established than administration into an endotracheal tube. We have shown by isotope scanning that cardioresuscitative drugs administered into the jet were not only dispersed within 12 sec in the periphery of the lungs but were also already in the cardiac pool (Klain et al., 1981).

Transtracheal ventilation should be considered beyond its use in emergency airway management. In view of the damage produced to the surface of the tracheal wall and to the function of normal mucociliary transport by endotracheal tubes, transtracheal ventilation may offer an alternative even for medium and long-term ventilation. The discomfort produced by a large, cuffed endotracheal tube often requires sedation or muscle relaxants to permit ventilatory support. Transtracheal ventilation would allow the conscious patient to be more comfortable, and even to speak and eat. Unfortunately, but not unexpectedly, cricoid membrane puncture and transtracheal ventilation have their share of risks and complications.

Membrane puncture has been used for many years for reasons other than airway management and ventilation: topical anesthesia, induced coughing (prevention of pulmonary postoperative complications, sampling of sputum), and bronchography. Thousands of punctures have been performed and although a few fatal complications have been described, serious complications must be extremely rare if proper technique is used. Complications include local infection, bleeding (both on the surface and into the airway), bradycardia, arrhythmias, and subcutaneous emphysema sometimes with spread to the mediastinum (especially if there is much coughing, grunting, or nose-blowing following the procedure). Coughing can also cause regurgitation and aspiration as well as breakage of the needle. Membrane puncture performed for jet ventilation can be expected to be associated with a higher complication rate because the needle is bigger and because if the gas mixture is inadvertently directed into the tissues, rapidly spreading emphysema will result. Furthermore, if there is any obstacle to expiration, barotrauma will occur.

Although the technique of membrane puncture is simple, I know from personal experience and observation that failures and unnecessary delays occur, especially in emergency situations. Haste, swelling of the neck, and distortion of the normal anatomy following radical neck surgery or radiation can all contribute to this.

Because complications do occur and because delays in performing successful puncture may lead to unnecessary loss of life, we recommend that the procedure be practiced by using it for local analgesia prior to intubation or for obtaining sputum for culture (in the intensive care unit). Before this is done, the anatomy must be mastered. (I have repeatedly seen the thyroid ligament mistaken for the membrane by mistaking the hyoid for the cricoid.) Contraindications for elective puncture include hemorrhagic diatheses, severe cough, a tendency to bronchospasm, a full stomach, and perhaps intracranial hypertension. If patients with these conditions are avoided, and if small short needles are used for elective puncture (unless done for ventilation), complications are very unlikely. Compression of the puncture site for a few minutes is also recommended. For jet ventilation whether manual and at low frequencies or rapid and mechanical, a 14- or 16-gauge catheter needle, 2½-3½ in. long, can be used. Catheters with two side holes are preferable because tissue emphysema and aspiration are less likely. These catheters are available from Sherwood and other manufacturers. Special catheters for jet ventilation are being developed but none are entirely satisfactory yet. Existing catheters are not suitable for long-term use because they can easily kink when patients start to use their auxiliary respiratory muscles or move their head. Especially for long-term ventilation, better-designed catheters which can be easily secured to the skin are necessary.

V. Controversial and Not Fully Explored Aspects of HFJV

The effectiveness of intratracheal instillation of drugs in cardiac arrest, described by Redding in 1967, has been confirmed by numerous experimental studies and some clinical observations. Our preliminary experiments with the injection of cardioactive drugs into the jet stream gave similar results (Klain et al., 1981), but many details remain to be worked out. These include optimal speed of injection, optimal volume, and the best diluent (saline or distilled water). It appears that the dosage is similar to the IV dosage but the effect is considerably prolonged. Bicarbonate and norepinephrine must not be given by intrapulmonary route, whether instillation or jet.

There is general agreement that humidification is mandatory for prolonged HFJV but not necessary for very short-term use. However some experimental work seems to show that HFJV without humidification may be safe for up to 24 hr, while our own experimental studies would set the limit at 1-2 hr (Nordin et al., 1982; Keszler et al., 1984). There is certainly no need to worry about humidification during emergency HFJV but we urge the use of humidification should the need for HFJV continue beyond 1-2 hr.

Asymmetrical (differential) lung ventilation is sometimes very desirable in asymmetrical lung disease. We explored the possibility of achieving asymmetrical ventilation with a single-lumen jet tube by directing the jet orifice to one or the other side (Keszler and Klain, 1982). The general problems of asymmetrical lung disease and its management with double-lumen tubes and other measures were well-presented in a recent paper (Kvetan et al., 1982). Our own efforts with a single-lumen tube (Keszler and Klain, 1982) showed that this approach is feasible, but fraught with considerable technical problems. We do, however, stress that even slightly asymmetrical placement of the orifice can cause considerable asymmetry in ventilation if the orifice is near the carina. This, if unwanted, can of course cause a drop in PaO_2. Therefore we must emphasize that keeping the tip of the jet tube 5 cm above the carina is important for routine HFJV, not only to prevent barotrauma but also to prevent inadvertent asymmetrical ventilation.

References

Brader, E., Klain, M., Safar, P., and Bircher, N. (1981). High frequency jet ventilation versus IPPV for CPR during ventricular fibrillation in dogs. *Crit. Care Med.* **9**:162.

Desai, S. P., and Fencl, V. (1980). A safe technique for changing endotracheal tubes. *Anesthesiology* **53**:267.

Guntupalli, K., Klain, M., and Sladen, A. (1981a). High frequency jet ventilation and tracheal tube reintubation. *Crit. Care Med.* **9**(3):190.

Guntupalli, K., Sladen, A., and Klain, M. (1981b). High frequency jet ventilation (HFJV) in the prevention of a decrease in Pa_{O_2} during suctioning. *Chest* **80**(3):391-382.

Jacoby, J. J., Hamelberg, W., Ziegler, C. H., Flory, F. A., and Jones, J. R. (1956). Transtracheal resuscitation. *JAMA* **162**:625.

Keszler, H., and Klain, M. (1980). Tracheobronchial toilet without cardiorespiratory impairment. *Crit. Care Med.* **8**(4):298-301.

Keszler, H., and Klain, M. (1982). Importance of position of jet orifice in high frequency jet ventilation. *Crit. Care Med.* **10**(3):234.

Keszler, H., Klain, M., Nordin, U., and Stool, S. (1982). High frequency jet ventilation prevents aspiration, part II. Scientific film, University of Pittsburgh.

Keszler, H., Nordin, U., Klain, M., and Stool, S. Short-term use of HFJV with and without humidification. To be submitted for publication.

Klain, M., Keszler, H., and Nordin, U. (1981). Intrapulmonary drug administration during high frequency jet ventilation (abstr.). 2nd World Congress on Emergency and Disaster Medicine, Pittsburgh.

Klain, M., Keszler, H., Stool, S., Rabinovitz, N., and Coulter, J. (1981b). Transtracheal high frequency jet ventilation prevents aspiration. Scientific film, University of Pittsburgh.

Klain, M., Keszler, H., and Stool, S. (1983). Transtracheal high frequency jet ventilation prevents aspiration. *Crit. Care Med.* **11**(4):309-310.

Kvetan, V., Carlon, G. C., and Howland, W. S. (1982). Acute pulmonary failure in asymmetric lung disease: Approach to management. *Crit. Care Med.* **10**: 114.

Nordin, U., Klain, M., and Keszler, H. (1982). Electron-microscopic studies of tracheal mucosa after high frequency jet ventilation. *Crit. Care Med.* **10**(3): 211.

Rock, J. J., Pfaeffle, H., Smith, R. B., Mendelow, H., and Klain, M. (1976). High pressure jet insufflation used to prevent aspiration and its effect on the tracheal mucosal wall. *Crit. Care Med.* **4**(2):135.

Schwartzman, S., Wilson, M. A., Hoff, B. H., Bunegin, L., Smith, R. B., and Sjostrand, U. (1984). Percutaneous transtracheal jet ventilation for cardiopulmonary resuscitation: Evaluation of a new jet ventilator. *Crit. Care Med.* **12**:8-13.

Szele, G., and Keenan, R. (1981). Does percutaneous transtracheal high frequency ventilation prevent aspiration? A word of caution. *Crit. Care Med.* **9**:163.

11

Theoretical Evaluation of High-Frequency Ventilation

WAYNE MITZNER and SOLBERT PERMUTT

The Johns Hopkins Medical Institutions
Baltimore, Maryland

EDITH R. SCHMID

University Hospital
Zurich, Switzerland

I. Theoretical Principles and Physiological Applications

Wayne Mitzner and Solbert Permutt

High-frequency ventilation (HFV) is the term used to describe adequate ventilation with tidal volumes which may be smaller than the anatomical dead space. In terms of classic respiratory physiology this concept may appear impossible, but when ventilatory frequency is rapid enough, many studies have clearly demonstrated its feasibility (Bohn et al., 1980; Butler et al., 1980; Mitzner et al., 1981; Slutsky et al., 1980). A variety of mechanisms have been proposed to account for this remarkable phenomenon. A rather complex regional pendeluft has been suggested by Lehr et al. (1980), irreversible flow patterns at airway bifurcations have been invoked by Haselton and Scherer (1980), and enhanced diffusion in the airways was suggested by Bohn et al. (1980) and worked out theoretically and experimentally by Fredberg (1980) and Slutsky et al. (1980). The concept of enhanced diffusion originates from Taylor's elegant work on the dispersion of an indicator in tubes under laminar and turbulent flow regimens (Taylor, 1953, 1954).

Before considering the mechanisms that explain gas exchange under conditions where the tidal volume is less than the dead space volume, it might be helpful to consider why the classic models are not adequate. Conventionally, the lung is divided into an alveolar compartment of uniform gas concentration where gas exchange with the blood takes place by diffusion, and a dead-space compartment in which no gas exchange occurs. Steady-state exchange is proportional to tidal volume minus dead-space volume, thus there is *no* steady-state gas exchange when the tidal volume equals the volume of the dead space. Dead-space volume is usually defined as the volume of the airways that contains only inspired gas, after a tidal exchange which has removed all alveolar gas from the previous expiration. The implicit assumption is also accepted that ambient gases during inspiration, and alveolar gases during expiration, traverse the dead space as a uniform front, where all gas molecules move with equal velocity. If this model were not correct, steady-state gas exchange could occur when tidal volume is less than dead space. Ironically, while there is complete agreement that gas does not move across the dead space with uniform velocity, many are surprised that effective steady-state gas exchange does occur under conditions in which tidal volume is considerably less than dead space.

The classic determination of dead space volume by the Fowler (1948) technique, in which the relation between the concentration of alveolar gas at the air outlet and volume expired is measured, quantifies the extent of the nonuniformity of velocities through the dead space. The magnitude of expired volume over which gas concentration is changing from atmospheric to alveolar provides no useful information in determining the volume of the dead space itself, but might allow a prediction of the effectiveness of HFV. Such an assumption is at the basis of a model of gas exchange during HFV which we propose. Our theory is based on the classic model of gas exchange, to which is added consideration of the effect of nonuniform velocities.

II. Model

The dead space can be divided into N compartments in series, each with a volume equal to the tidal volume, V. Let HFV start at the end of a normal inspiration. During the first expiration of HFV, alveolar gas moves into the compartment nearest to it (compartment 1), while at the same time previous gas is transferred from compartment 1 to 2, from 2 to 3, and so on. Compartment N transfers gas across the air outlet. Most of the gas transferred from compartment 1 to 2 during the first expiration will be inspired gas. If all gas molecules moved at a constant velocity from compartment 1 to 2, only inspired gas would be transferred from the first to the second compartment during the first expiration, and at the end of this expiration, the first compartment would contain pure alveolar gas. During the subsequent inspiration, if all gas moved at a constant velocity, the alveolar gas from compartment 1 would be returned to the alveoli, and compartment 1 would be filled with inspired gas that it had received from compartment 2. Thus, there would be no net transfer of alveolar gas, regardless of the number of times the cycle was repeated.

If, as happens, gas did not move through compartment 1 with a constant velocity, but some molecules moved faster and some slower than the mean gas velocity, some alveolar gas would reach beyond compartment 1 during the first expiration. Thus, at the end of the first cycle, the first compartment would contain gas at a mean concentration somewhat less than alveolar gas, and the second compartment would contain gas at a concentration somewhat greater than the inspired gases. Similarly, compartment 3 might contain some alveolar gas, but at lower concentration than 2, etc. If N is large, there would be no transfer of alveolar gas across the air outlet during the first expiration, but alveolar gas would be within the dead space at a decreasing concentration from the first to the Nth compartment.

During the first inspiration, a similar process would occur in relation to the inspired gas transferred from the Nth compartment to the N - 1th compartment, etc. At the end of the first complete cycle, there would be a smaller but finite amount of alveolar gas in the dead space, with decreasing concentration from the first to the Nth compartment.

Each succeeding cycle would proceed in the same way, except that now some of the alveolar gas that remained in the dead space after the previous cycle would move closer to the air outlet. At the end of each succeeding cycle, the gas concentrations in the compartment near the air outlet would become closer to alveolar gas concentration, but there would still be a decreasing concentration from the first to the Nth compartment. The alveolar gas transferred from the Nth compartment across the air outlet during each cycle did not reach it during a single cycle, but rather came to it from the alveoli through a series of successive transfers through the compartments in series between it and the alveoli.

As cycles continued, a steady state would be reached in which the concentration in each compartment would rise toward alveolar during each expiration and fall by exactly the same amount during inspiration. Each complete cycle would involve a constant exchange of alveolar gas from the Nth compartment to the ambient environment across the air outlet. Similarly, there would be a constant transference of inspired gas from the first compartment to the alveoli.

The detailed mathematical solution of the amount of gas exchange through such a series of compartments is presented elsewhere (Permutt et al., 1985). The solution is based on calculations of the changes in gas concentration within finite volume elements of the dead space at the beginning and end of each ventilatory stroke. To solve the resultant equations, we made the simplifying assumption that each discrete volume element acts as a compartment with a uniform concentration that varies with time during a complete ventilatory cycle. We have already divided the dead space into N compartments of volume = V, where V = tidal volume and

$NV = V_D$. We next divide each of these compartments into α subcompartments, where each subcompartment receives a well-mixed concentration from the adjacent compartment and passes a well-mixed concentration to another in the direction of flow. The total dead space thus contains αN compartments. The mathematical analysis mentioned above thus requires the solution of $2\alpha N$ simultaneous equations.

A. HFV When $V = V_D$

It is quite instructive to consider the special case when tidal volume is exactly equal to the volume of the dead space. In this case V_D is divided into α subcompartments. The number of compartments determines how the concentration of gas at the airway outlet varies during expiration. Figure 1 shows the theoretical prediction of gas concentration at the airway outlet during a continuous exhalation as a function of α, that is, the effective number of well-mixed subcompartments. Of course, during ventilation with $V = V_D$, the expiration would stop when the expired volume (V_E) equalled V_D (i.e., when $V_E/V_D = 1$), and inspiration would then commence. From looking at Figure 1, one can easily appreciate not only that a certain fraction of alveolar gas would pass through the dead space during a single expiration of $V = V_D$, but also that the amount that left the dead space would be a function of α. The greater the number of well-mixed subcompartments, the less gas will be transferred. Intuitively one can reason that, if there are more well-mixed compartments, the concentration profile or dispersion will be blunted.

How many subcompartments are needed to represent the dead space in the human lung? This can be simply determined by analyzing the N_2 concentration at the mouth during a standard Fowler dead-space maneuver. Such a curve taken from Bouhuys (1974) is shown in Figure 2. He shows curves done at both high and low flow rates and they are essentially the same. This finding suggests that α may not be very sensitive to changes in flow rate. Figure 2 also shows that the typical features of the human N_2 washout can be reproduced quite well with 9-10 compartments in series.

Figure 3 shows the expiratory washout curve for the specific case where $V = V_D$, and $\alpha = 9$. The shaded area represents the amount of alveolar gas that passes through the dead space during the first expiration of HFV. During the subsequent inspiration, a similar process would apply to ambient air passing into the alveoli. It is thus clear that even a single cycle with $V = V_D$ will provide some gas exchange, though it may be rather small. However, if the frequency of breathing is fast enough, there may be enough gas exchange to sustain normal blood gas levels.

In actual applications of HFV, there will, in fact, be an even greater gas exchange that would be predicted by Figure 3, where the dead space was assumed to be entirely devoid of any alveolar gas. After repeated cycling with $V = V_D$,

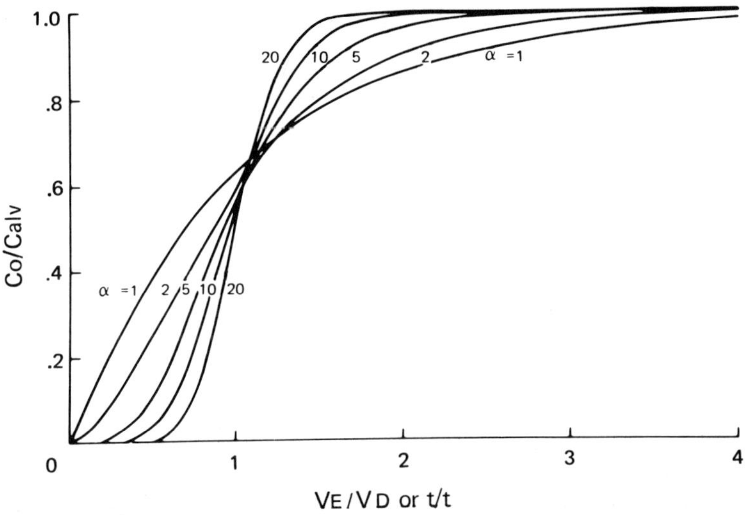

Figure 1 The ratio of the concentration of alveolar gas at the air outlet (Co) to the concentration of alveolar gas in the alveolar compartment (Calv) in relation to the ratio of the expired volume (V_E) to the dead-space volume (V_D), or the ratio of the time of expiration (t) to the mean transit time ($\overline{t}$) during a prolonged expiration at constant expiratory flow ($\dot{Q}$) with no alveolar gas in the dead space at the beginning of the expiration. The mean transit time $(\overline{t}) = V_D/\dot{Q}$. $V_E/V_D = t/\overline{t}$ at constant $\dot{Q}$. The isopleths are for different values of α where α = number of compartments in series into which V_D is divided.

however, the dead space is no longer washed of all alveolar gas after the inspiratory cycle; therefore during the subsequent expiration, the amount of alveolar gas which leaves will be equal to the shaded area in Figure 3 plus a substantial portion of the alveolar gas left in the dead space from the previous breaths. The theoretical difference in the concentration profile between the first complete cycle and the steady-state situation is shown in Figure 4, which shows the alveolar gas composition of the dead space at the end of inspiratory and expiratory cycles. It is clear that the fractional amount of alveolar gas is increased in each subcompartment during steady state. Quantitatively, gas exchange is 46% greater during steady-state than during the first cycle (shaded area of Fig. 3) (Permutt et al., 1985).

B. Gas Exchange When V is Much Less Than V_D

From the above discussions, it may already be apparent that it is not necessary to have $V = V_D$ to support gas exchange. From Figure 3, it is clear that, with V =

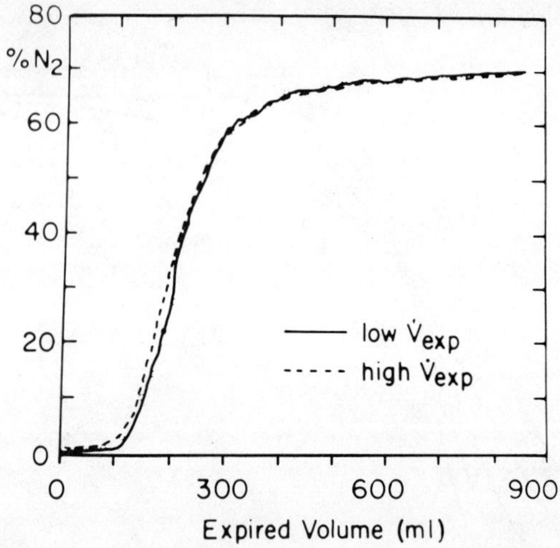

Figure 2 Single-breath N_2 curve at two different expiratory flow rates (low flow = 1.4 liters/sec; high flow = 5.7 liters/sec) (5). The open circles are the values that would arise from a dead space consisting of 9.32 compartments in series (α = 9.32); a mean transit time ($\bar{t}$) of 0.16 sec at a flow ($\dot{Q}$) of 1.4 liters/sec; and a volume (V_D) = $\dot{Q}/\bar{t}$ = 0.224 liters.

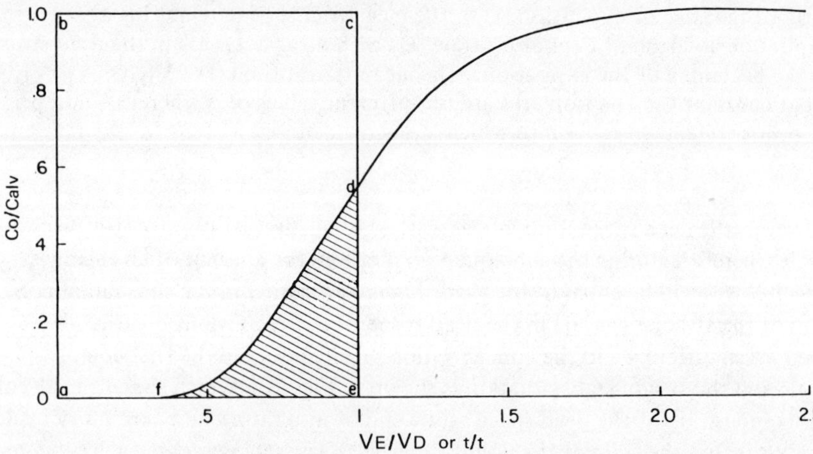

Figure 3 The relation between Co/Calv and either V_E/V_D or $t/\bar{t}$ during a prolonged expiration at constant flow for a dead space consisting of nine compartments in series (α = 9). The ratio of the shaded ares *def* to the rectangular area *abce* equals the ratio of alveolar gas transferred out of the dead space with respect to the amount of alveolar gas brought to the dead space, for a volume expired equal to the volume of the dead space ($V_E = V_D$).

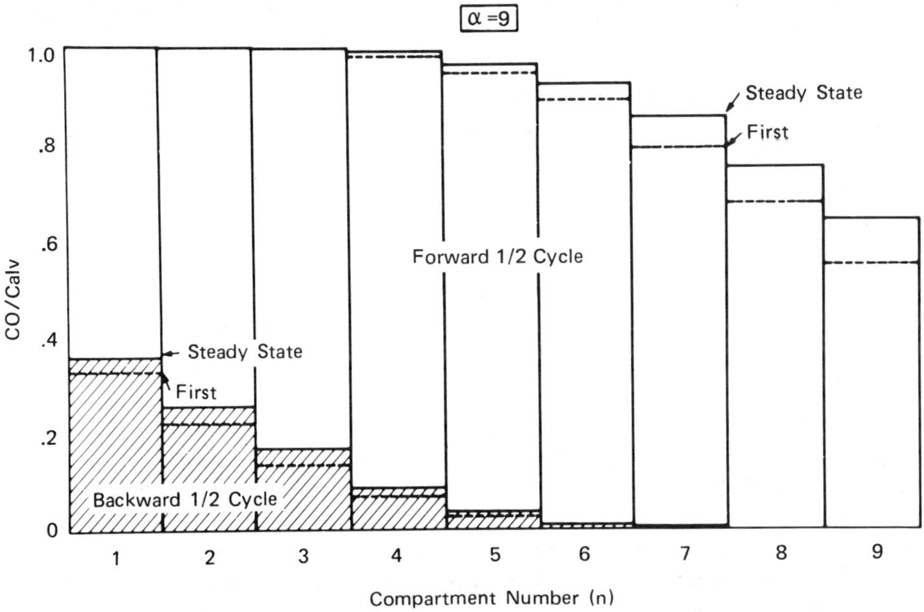

Figure 4 The concentration profiles in the dead space for HFV where $V = V_D$, for $\alpha = 9$. The concentration of alveolar gas in each compartment of a dead space consisting of nine compartments in series at the end of the forward half cycle (end expiration) and at the end of the reverse half cycle (end inspiration). Shown are both the steady-state concentrations and the concentrations present at the end of the first half cycle. Concentration at the outflow end of the dead space is assumed to be zero.

$1/3\ V_D$, almost no alveolar gas would transit the dead space during the first expiration. However, after the subsequent inspiration some alveolar gas would be retained in the dead space. During the following expiration, the alveolar gas would be further transported toward the airway outlet. If this process is repeated frequently, adequate alveolar ventilation can be maintained.

To analyze quantitatively the amount of gas exchange, it is convenient to use an index of the distribution of transit times of gas molecules through the dead space. From the previous discussion it can be derived that if there is a broad distribution of transit times, a fraction of the gases will move through the dead space very quickly, allowing ventilation with small tidal volumes. The broader the transit time distribution, the better the ventilation will be. Statistically, the broadness of a distribution function is expressed by the mean divided by the standard deviation. For transit times, the symbol for this coefficient of dispersion is $(\sigma_t/\bar{t})$.

On the basis of Figure 3, it might be expected that there should be a relationship between $\sigma_t/\bar{t}$ and α. Indeed this is so, and we have shown that ($\sigma_t/\bar{t} = 1/\sqrt{\alpha}$) (Permutt et al., 1985).

We have also demonstrated that, when tidal volume is very small is relation to the dead space (V less than 20% V_D), certain limiting conditions apply and a relatively simple formula for gas exchange can be derived. This formula, adapted for CO_2 exchange, states that:

$$\dot{V}CO_2 = f\,V^2(FaCO_2)(\sigma_t/\bar{t})^2/V_D$$

where f = frequency and $FaCO_2$ is alveolar CO_2 fraction. Thus, for very small tidal volumes, gas exchange should vary directly with frequency, the square of volume, and the square of the coefficient of dispersion of transit times through the dead space.

Unfortunately, despite the simplicity of this formula, it is accurate in a range of tidal volumes which are unlikely ever to have practical utility. Indeed, most applications of HFV utilize tidal volumes greater than one-third the dead space. The general formula for gas exchange in this range is slightly more complex and requires certain assumptions regarding the nature of the flow, that is, whether it is streamline or turbulent. For the purposes of the present discussion, we shall only consider the solution for streamline flow, since most of the available empirical data seem to fit this model.

The general solution for gas exchange with tidal volume close to the dead space (adapted for the special case of CO_2 exchange*) is given by the formula (Permutt et al., 1985):

$$\dot{V}CO_2 = 0.6(\sigma_t/\bar{t})fV_D(V/V_D)^P\,FaCO_2$$

where $FaCO_2$ = alveolar CO_2 fraction, V_D = dead space, f = frequency, V = tidal volume, $\sigma_t/\bar{t}$ = coefficient of dispersion of transit times throughout the whole dead space, and P = exponent to which tidal volume is raised.

It can be shown that P varies inversely with the square root of the coefficient of dispersion, and the formula for P is $P = 1 + 0.7/\sqrt{\sigma_t/t}$). In considering the above formula for $\dot{V}CO_2$, it is clear that the coefficient of dispersion plays a major role in determining how good the gas exchange will be during HFV. Not only does $\sigma_t/\bar{t}$ appear in the equation as a direct multiplier, but it also determines the sensitivity of gas exchange to variations in tidal volume. A prediction of this tidal volume variation can be estimated from the value of $\sigma_t/\bar{t}$ measured from the N_2 washout curve in Figure 2. For this curve, the coefficient of dispersion is 0.33,

---

*An analogous formula would exist for O_2 exchange, but the $FaCO_2$ would be replaced by the fractional O_2 difference between alveolar and ambient air. The formula for CO_2 exchange assumes ambient CO_2 to be zero.

and thus the exponent to which volume is raised in the equation is 2.2. If our model is applicable, we would predict that, even with tidal volumes close to the dead space, gas exchange during HFV should vary roughly with the product of frequency and tidal volume squared.

III. Test of Model

We have performed experiments in dogs to test the validity of our model during high-frequency ventilation (Weinmann et al., 1984). In this study we used a high-frequency ventilator which operated by interrupting flow from a high-pressure source with a rotating valve. Both entrainment and leakage during inspiration were prevented by a similar valve on the expiratory line. The I/E ratio was 1:1.8. It is worth noting that our model can be applied to any I/E ratio as long as one knows that magnitude of the inspiratory and expiratory dispersions. To the extent that they are different, an average dispersion per cycle can be determined (Permutt et al., 1985).

The experimental protocol required adjustments of frequency and tidal volume, with the aim of maintaining arterial P_{CO_2} constant in order to evaluate the relationship between frequency and tidal volume at constant $\dot{V}_{CO_2}$ and $F_{A_{CO_2}}$. After measuring the animals' dead space, we resolved the proposed equation for $\dot{V}_{CO_2}$, to determine the coefficient of dispersion which would best fit our data. Additional details of the experimental design have been presented elsewhere (Weinmann et al., 1984).

The relationship between frequency and tidal volume can be determined by rearranging the $\dot{V}_{CO_2}$ equation:

$$f = \dot{V}_{CO_2}/[K(V/V_D)^P]$$

where $K = 0.6(\sigma_t/\bar{t})V_D F_{A_{CO_2}}$, and $P = 1 + 0.7/\sqrt{\sigma/\bar{t}}$.

The experimental data resulted in a mean fractional concentration of CO_2 of 0.38 and a mean $\dot{V}_{CO_2}$ of 126 ml. The average value of the measured dead space was 102 ml.

Figure 5 shows the experimental data points and the best fit of the mean data, obtained by the least-squares method. The best fit was with a $\sigma_t/\bar{t}$ of 0.32, and a volume exponent of 2.2. For these values, the theoretical equation becomes: $f = 2.8/(V/V_D)^{2.2}$. This exact coincidence between observed and predicted exponent, based on the α determined from the N_2 washout, was somewhat accidental. Individual exponents on the tidal volume in each of three animals studied were 2.11, 2.11, and 2.49. Also shown in Figure 5 is the theoretical prediction based on the simple alveolar gas equation, $V_A = f(V - V_D)$ which, at constant alveolar ventilation, as was used in our study, is a straightforward hyperbolic relation between f and V.

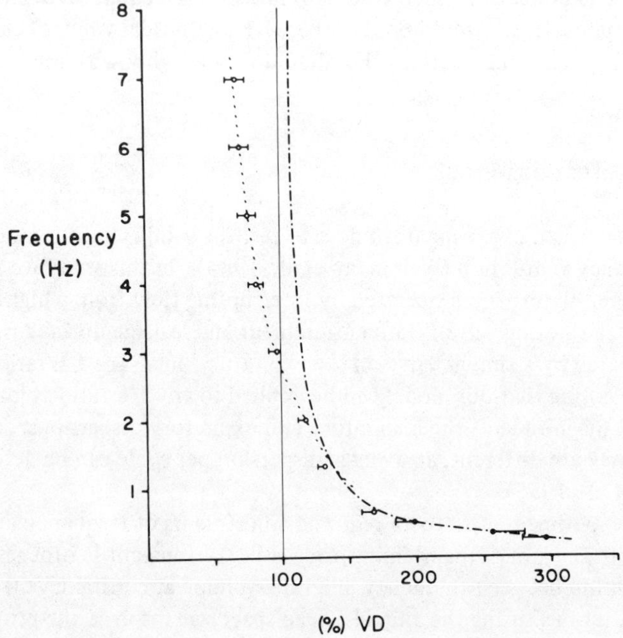

Figure 5 Frequency vs. volume (normalized as % V_D) required to maintain constant alveolar ventilation (shown as mean ± SEM). The frequency vs. tidal volume relationship calculated by the formula $f(V - V_D) = \text{constant}$, assuming a constant physiological dead space, asymptotes on V_D (dash/dotted curve). The deviation of this classic formula from the mean data points at low tidal volume is apparent. The theoretical f vs. V relationship calculated from our model of high-frequency ventilation (dotted curve) is given in the text.

The experimental data obtained thus provide strong support for our theoretical model, suggesting that tidal volume is more important that frequency in determining the efficacy of high-frequency ventilation. This fact may have important clinical implications. At low tidal volumes, any reduction of V must be balanced by large increases in frequency. For example, from the theoretical curve in Figure 5, it can be derived that when V is decreased from 65 to 50% of V_D, frequency must be approximately doubled from 7 to 14 Hz. While high frequencies by themselves are not necessarily harmful, the high concomitant flow rates may create technical difficulties in measurements of mean airway pressure (Simon et al., 1984) and estimation of lung volumes, and danger of accidental occlusion of the expiratory port and possibly drying the mucociliary lining. For these reasons, one must carefully consider the lowest acceptable tidal volume.

It may be possible to achieve the desired therapeutic end point with a slightly larger tidal volume and much lower frequency.

The model of classic gas exchange divides the lungs into two uniform compartments: alveolar and dead space. Our model merely adds the effects of nonuniform transit times across the dead space to the classic model. This effect is quantified by the ratio of the standard deviation to the mean of the transit times, also called the coefficient of dispersion. Interestingly, the conventional technique of determining the volume of the dead space (Fowler technique) also allows the coefficient of dispersion of the transit times to be determined.

The virtue of the classic model of gas exchange is its simplicity. Where it was inadequate, slight modifications were added, such as physiological dead space and alveolar dead space. These additional concepts have been developed within the original model. We suggest that the major features of steady-state gas exchange during HFV can be predicted from the volume of the dead space and the coefficient of dispersion of the transit times across the dead space. This simple model will probably be insufficient to explain all aspects of gas exchange during HFV, but we suggest that the discrepancies will arise only in detail and not in principle.

IV. Determinants of Pulmonary Gas Exchange

Edith R. Schmid

Since the pioneering observation of Lunkenheimer et al. (1972, 1973), a number of investigators have confirmed that high-frequency small-volume (less than anatomical dead space) oscillations (HFO) applied to the gas in the airways result in adequate pulmonary gas exchange (Bohn et al., 1980; Butler et al., 1980; Schmid et al., 1981; Marchak et al., 1981; Thompson et al., 1982; Kolton et al., 1982; Hamilton et al., 1983; Frantz et al., 1983; Rehder et al., 1983; Rehder and Crawford, 1983). Recent literature includes proposals of different mechanisms explaining gas transport and efficacy of gas exchange during HFO (Schmid et al., 1981; Kolton et al., 1982; Fredberg, 1980; Slutsky et al., 1980; Haselton and Scherer, 1980; Lehr, 1980; Khoo et al., 1982; Lee, 1983; Mitzner et al., 1985), as well as attempts to reconcile theoretical predictions with experimental observations (Slutsky et al., 1980, 1981, 1983; Rossing et al., 1981; Goldstein et al., 1981).

Although understanding of gas transport and gas exchange during HFO has increased, considerable unknowns still exist regarding the significance of different proposed mechanisms. Experimental data on the determinants of pulmonary gas exchange are limited and, in part, conflicting. This section reviews the current understanding of, and remaining areas of uncertainty about, factors governing pulmonary gas exchange during HFO.

V. Theoretical Concepts

Based on findings using a semiempirical analysis, Fredberg (1980) suggested that augmented gas transport in the central airways, akin to Taylor turbulent dispersion (1954), combined with molecular diffusion in the periphery of the lung could explain gas transport during HFO. This model was later modified by including the combined effects of laminar convection and molecular diffusion in the small airways (Slutsky et al., 1980). Analysis of these models quantitates axial gas transport during HFO using equations originally developed for molecular diffusion (Taylor, 1953, 1954) where the molecular diffusion coefficient (D_{mol}) is replaced by an effective diffusion coefficient, D_{eff} (Fredberg, 1980; Slutsky et al., 1980). Although based on effective duffusion the concept of augmented dispersion during HFO includes both diffusive enhancement of gas transport and convective dispersion due to turbulence and secondary flows at airway bifurcations (Slutsky et al., 1980).

Haselton and Scherer (1980) proposed a purely convective, nondiffusional *longitudinal* mass transfer mechanism based on differences in shape between inspiratory and expiratory velocity profiles at airway bifurcations. Flow visualization of tracer beads with negligible gravitational settling and coefficient of diffusion showed that forward and reverse flow at airway bifurcations resulted in deformation of flow profiles and net axial transfer of volume in both directions (Haselton and Scherer, 1980; Scherer, 1982, 1983). Longitudinal convective gas transport may also occur by direct alveolar ventilation of lung units with short path lengths, even if stroke volume is less than anatomical dead space (Khoo et al., 1982; Chang, 1983).

Augmented transport by convective gas transfer between *parallel* lung units may be inferred from cinematographic studies conducted by Lehr (1980). By observing the motion of excised dog lungs exposed to stroboscopic light, Lehr (1980) demonstrated phase differences in lung expansion between and within lobes, presumably due to differences in local time constants. In intact dogs, Schmid et al. (1981) examined regional distribution and clearance of ^{133}xenon and presented evidence that considerable interregional gas transport exists during HFO which is consistent with (but not necessarily dependent on) phase differences in regional lung expansion. It was postulated that interregional gas transport may be of sufficient magnitude to affect overall pulmonary gas transport and gas exchange during HFO (Schmid et al., 1980, 1981).

Importance of convective rather than diffusive gas transport in the upper airways during HFO was recently stressed by Knopp et al. (1983). They demonstrated similar time courses of washout between helium and sulfur hexafluoride (SF_6) in dogs during HFO at oscillation frequencies of 20-30 Hz, and concluded that gas mixing in the upper conducting airways is not significantly limited by molecular diffusion.

The theoretical quantitative analysis of gas transport presented by Slutsky et al. (1980) is based on augmented dispersion in turbulent (Fredberg, 1980) and laminar oscillatory flow and, more recently, was refined by including direct alveolar ventilation of lung regions with short path lengths (Khoo et al., 1982). It ignores, however, the effects of differences in shape between inspiratory and expiratory velocity profiles at airway bifurcations, and interregional mixing due to pendelluft or a pendelluftlike mechanism (Slutsky, 1981). Although the relative contribution of these latter mechanisms to overall pulmonary gas transport during HFO is currently unclear, they may provide a more comprehensive data base to describe gas transport during HFO. In addition, comparison of theoretical predictions with experimentally measured gas transport showed, as anticipated (Fredberg, 1980), that mathematical models based on the assumption that airways behave like rigid, noncompliant structures may not adequately describe gas transport during HFO, at least in the presence of lung disease, and may not account for species-related differences in the mechanical properties of the lung (Rossing et al., 1981; Goldstein et al., 1981; Slutsky et al., 1983).

According to current thinking, gas transport during HFO most probably represents a complex phenomenon including both diffusive and convective transport mechanisms (Lee, 1983; Chang, 1983). Mechanisms based on convective gas transport, such as convective mixing due to turbulence (Fredberg, 1980) and secondary motions at airway bifurcations (Fredberg, 1980; Scherer et al., 1975), augmented longitudinal gas transport induced by differences in the shape of inspiratory and expiratory velocity profiles (Haselton and Scherer, 1980; Scherer, 1982, 1983), direct alveolar ventilation (Khoo et al., 1982; Chang, 1983), and pendelluft, that is, gas transport between parallel lung units with different local time constants (Lehr, 1980) is probably more important in the conductive airways (Knopp et al., 1983). The relative significance of these different proposed gas transport mechanisms is unclear and may vary between different regions of the lung (Lee, 1983; Chang, 1983). Gas transport by molecular diffusion presumably occurs only at the alveolar level, just as with any other ventilatory mode (Knopp et al., 1983).

Development of models and comparison with experimental observations are important to define gas transport and gas exchange during HFO. Both agreement and disagreement of experimental findings with model predictions may help us in understanding the mechanisms underlying pulmonary gas transport and gas exchange during HFO. Recently, an important framework has been provided. Final clarification of the mechanisms governing gas transport and gas exchange during HFO, however, still lies ahead.

VI. Rate of CO_2 Elimination: Dependence on Frequency, Tidal Volume, and Lung Volume

A. Effect of Tidal Volume and Oscillation Frequency

At the high frequencies used with HFO, considerable problems complicate accurate measurements of tidal volume, that is, the volume actually delivered to the lung. Insufficient precision of conventional differential pressure transducers and flowmeters precludes systematic evaluation of the independent effects of oscillation frequency and tidal volume on pulmonary gas exchange (Froese and Bryan, 1981). More recently, hot-wire anemometers, ultrasonic flowmeters, and body plethysmography have been used to measure tidal volume. Controversy exists, however, about the reliability of plethysmography to determine tidal volume during HFO (Jones, 1983). Moreover, the considerable variations among the HFO systems used by different investigators almost preclude distinctions between circuit artifacts and physiological consequences.

To generate high-frequency oscillations, Bohn et al. (1980), and, subsequently, other investigators (Butler et al., 1980; Schmid et al., 1981), used a piston pump connected to a cuffed endotracheal tube. To minimize the loss of pressure oscillations, excess fresh gas and CO_2 escaped the system through a high-impedance bias flow tubing which was believed to behave like a low-pass filter, offering high impedance to high frequencies, but low impedance to low frequencies (Bohn et al., 1980). In this system, the gas volume actually delivered to the lung depends on the relative impedances of the respiratory system and the bias flow tubing. Hence, the volume delivered to the lung is not equal to the volume displaced by the piston and varies with frequency (Bohn et al., 1980; Schmid et al., 1981). The gas volume entering the lung may be further reduced by gas compression in the pump chamber. Under these experimental conditions, optimal oscillation frequencies in terms of CO_2 elimination may thus reflect a circuit artifact rather than a physiologic entity (Schmid et al., 1981; Froese and Bryan, 1981).

To circumvent this problem, Slutsky et al. (1980, 1981) altered the mechanics of the high-impedance bias flow system. Subsequently, the effects of changing oscillation frequency and tidal volume on the rate of CO_2 removal was quantified in anesthetized healthy dogs (Slutsky et al., 1980, 1981), conscious normal human volunteers (Goldstein et al., 1981), and in patients with respiratory failure requiring mechanical ventilation (Rossing et al., 1981). Consistent with predictions from models provided by Fredberg (1980) and Slutsky et al. (1980), the critical factor in determining CO_2 elimination in anesthetized dogs during HFO at oscillation frequencies of 4-30 Hz and with tidal volumes ranging between 20 and 85% of the estimated dead space volume was reported to be the amplitude of oscillatory flow given by the product of oscillation frequency and tidal volume (Slutsky et al., 1980) (Fig. 6A). In contrast to these findings, but in accordance with the observations of other investigators (Mitzner et al., 1985; Berdine et al., 1983;

Brusasco et al., 1983), the same group of authors later confirmed that both tidal volume and oscillation frequency had independent effects on CO_2 removal. For a given product of frequency multiplied by tidal volume, CO_2 elimination was greater with large tidal volumes and high frequencies (Slutsky et al., 1981) (Fig. 6B). This observation was attributed to convective purging of the equipment dead space and upper airways (Khoo et al., 1982; Slutsky et al., 1981). In anesthetized healthy dogs, no optimal frequency in terms of CO_2 elimination was found within the ranges studied (2-30 Hz) (Slutsky et al., 1980, 1981).

In contrast to theoretical predictions and experiments in dogs, Rossing et al. (1981) observed in patients with chronic respiratory failure, mainly due to neuromuscular disease, a critical oscillation frequency of 3-6 Hz above which (at constant tidal volume) CO_2 elimination did not further increase with increasing frequency. They speculated that variation in size and compliance of proximal airways and in resistance of peripheral airways, either species-related (Rossing et al., 1981) or due to small-airways disease (Slutsky et al., 1983) could account for this finding. A frequency-dependent progressive distention of the compliant upper airways, reducing the gas volume transmitted to peripheral airways, was also invoked to explain the lower CO_2 elimination observed at higher frequencies in nonintubated, healthy human volunteers, who were ventilated by HFO through a mouthpiece (Goldstein et al., 1981). Supportive evidence that compliance of upper airways may act as a shunt compliance in parallel with the peripheral airways (Mead, 1969) was provided from the finding of a similar frequency-dependent optimal CO_2 elimination in dogs after experimental peripheral bronchoconstriction (Rossing et al., 1982) and from a recent cineradiographic study on airway dynamics during HFO (Gavriely et al., 1982).

In conclusion, many investigators have shown that CO_2 elimination can be easily controlled during HFO. Assessment of its determinants depends critically on the reliability of the devices used to measure the volume actually delivered to the lungs. In contrast to early predictions (Fredberg, 1980; Slutsky et al., 1980), more recent studies indicate that CO_2 removal is not a simple function of the frequency-tidal volume product, irrespective of the individual values of frequency and tidal volume, but is more dependent (at constant oscillatory flow amplitude) on tidal volume. Assuming that tidal volume determinations are reliable, optimal oscillation frequencies, that is, those above which elimination of CO_2 is determined solely by tidal volume, may vary with species-related differences in the mechanical properties of the lung and with changes in airway dynamics in disease states. Additional investigations are needed to define the mechanisms that promote and limit CO_2 elimination during HFO.

B. Lung Volume and Ventilation Efficacy

The available reports on the influence of lung volume on ventilation efficacy during HFO are conflicting. Based on the augmented dispersion theory of pulmonary

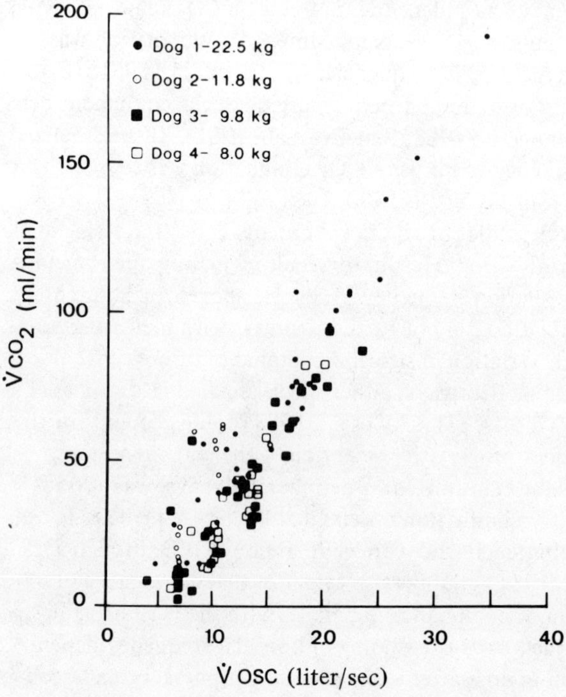

Figure 6A

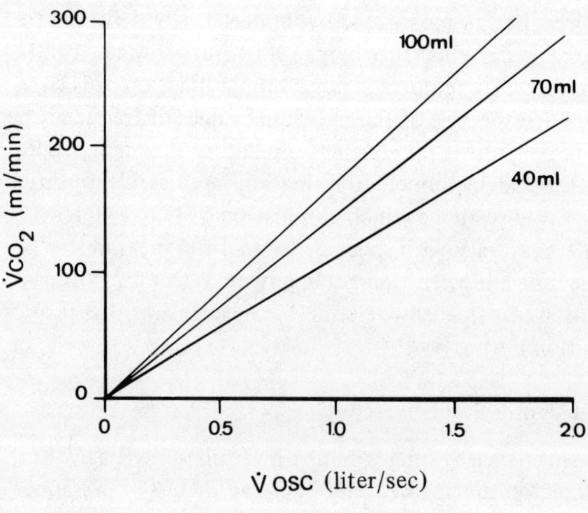

Figure 6B

gas transport during HFO, Fredberg (1980) predicted that CO_2 elimination at any given oscillatory flow amplitude should be independent of lung volume at lung volumes equal to or greater than functional residual capacity, provided that the lung expands isotropically. A lung volume-dependent decrease of linear velocities in the airways was postulated to cancel the effect of increasing cross-sectional area on the diffusional resistance to CO_2 flux (Fredberg, 1980; Slutsky et al., 1981). Consistent with this theory, an increase in lung volume was reported to have little effect on CO_2 removal in anesthetized, paralyzed dogs (Slutsky et al., 1981). Other investigators observed in dogs a significant negative correlation between the longitudinal transfer rates of a tracer gas (^{133}xenon) and functional residual capacity, suggesting that the turnover rate of ^{133}Xe was inversely proportional to lung volume Brusasco et al., 1983). CO_2 elimination in conscious human volunteers with normal lungs was demonstrated to increase with increasing lung volume (Goldstein et al., 1981) which is inconsistent with both these observations.

Although different experimental conditions and study protocols (Goldstein et al., 1981; Froese and Bryan, 1981), species-related differences in the pattern of lung expansion, and expiratory flow limitation (Goldstein et al., 1981) may be invoked to explain, to some extent, these apparently conflicting results, more information is needed to establish the effect of lung volume on ventilation efficacy. The relations that apply in the diseased lung, where inhomogeneities in regional lung expansion may alter the distribution of flow oscillations (Fredberg, 1980) remain unanswered.

VII. Effect of Mean Airway Pressure and Lung Volume on Oxygenation

The majority of studies conducted to examine the efficiency of pulmonary gas exchange during HFO addressed the question of CO_2 elimination and its determinants; reports regarding the factors determining oxygen exchange are, however, limited (Bryan, 1983).

Current understanding proposes two mechanisms to explain how HFO af-

Figure 6 (A) CO_2 elimination ($\dot{V}CO_2$, ml/min) in dogs, plotted as a function of oscillatory flow amplitude $\dot{V}_{osc}$ (liters/sec) (from Slutsky et al. (1980), by copyright 1980. Reproduced with permission of the American Association for the Advancement of Science). (B) Mean experimental results for CO_2 elimination ($\dot{V}CO_2$, ml/min) vs. oscillatory flow amplitude ($\dot{V}_{osc}$, liters/sec) at constant tidal volume (100 ml, 70 ml, and 40 ml) in dogs (reproduced from Slutsky et al. (1981). *J. Clin. Invest.* **68**:1475-1484, by copyright permission of The American Society for Clinical Investigation). ($\dot{V}_{osc}$ (liters/sec), equals the product of oscillation frequency X tidal volume).

fects oxygenation. On the one hand, adequate oxygenation in the presence of experimentally induced lung disease (Thompson et al., 1982; Kolton et al., 1982; Hamilton et al., 1983; Wright et al., 1981), as well as adult (Butler et al., 1980) or infant respiratory distress syndrome (Marchak et al., 1981; Frantz et al., 1983) appears to be a function of recruitment and maintenance of alveolar volume (Kolton et al., 1982), as is the case with conventional positive-pressure ventilation (Ashbaugh et al., 1969; Herman and Reynolds, 1973). Theoretical considerations (Bohn et al., 1980) and experimental data (Schmid et al., 1981; Brusasco et al., 1984) also support the theory that, during HFO, homogenization of alveolar gas concentrations due to interregional and intraregional gas mixing within the lung might contribute to the efficiency of oxygenation, which is at variance with conventional mechanical support. This latter mechanism is discussed in Sec. VIII.

Adequate oxygenation during HFO has been demonstrated in laboratory animals with healthy lungs (Bohn et al., 1980; Schmid et al., 1981; Rehder et al., 1983; Lunkenheimer et al., 1977) and with preexisting (Rehder et al., 1983) or experimentally induced lung disease (Thompson et al., 1982; Kolton et al., 1982; Hamilton et al., 1983; Wright et al., 1981), even if HFO was applied for prolonged periods of time (Rehder et al., 1983; Froese and Bryan, 1981). Oxygenation was satisfactorily maintained in anesthetized patients undergoing orthopedic procedures (Rehder and Crawford, 1983), in patients requiring mechanical ventilation following major vascular surgery or for treatment of respiratory failure (Butler et al., 1980), and in neonates with respiratory distress syndrome (Marchak et al., 1981; Frantz et al., 1983) and pulmonary interstitial emphysema (Frantz et al., 1983). Oscillation frequencies varied among investigators and ranged between 5 and 40 Hz in experimental animals (Lunkenheimer et al., 1972; Bohn et al., 1980; Kolton et al., 1982; Hamilton et al., 1983; Rehder et al., 1983), 12 and 18 Hz in adult humans (Butler et al., 1980; Rehder and Crawford, 1983), and 5 and 20 Hz in infants treated for respiratory failure (Marchak et al., 1981; Frantz et al., 1983). A significant positive correlation was reported between mean intratracheal airway pressure and arterial oxygen tension (Pa_{O_2}) in dogs (Thompson et al., 1982) and rabbits (Wright et al., 1981) after oleic-acid-induced lung injury and in neonatal respiratory distress syndrome (Marchak et al., 1981; Frantz et al., 1983). During randomized ventilation using either HFO or conventional mechanical ventilation, Thompson et al. (1982) found similar values for Pa_{O_2} (at comparable arterial CO_2 tensions and cardiac output) when mean intratracheal pressures were matched between the two modes of ventilation, indicating that HFO (at the conditions of this study) was equally effective, but not superior to, conventional positive-pressure ventilation in maintaining oxygen exchange. The authors concluded that oxygenation during both HFO and conventional mechanical ventilation showed the same strong dependence on mean airway pressure and, as implicated, mean lung volume.

Comparison of the efficiency of oxygenation during HFO and conventional mechanical ventilation at matched mean tracheal pressures may, however, not be conclusive. Similar proximal mean airway pressures may not necessarily reflect similar mean lung volumes with the two modes of ventilation. On HFO, the value of mean airway pressure may depend on the location of its measurement (Schmid et al., 1981; Simon et al., 1984). Mean airway pressure recorded with a side-hole catheter varies considerably between measurement sites within the lumen of the endotracheal tube and the airways (Schmid et al., 1981). Lateral mean airway pressure inside the endotracheal tube was lower than mean tracheal and endobronchial pressures measured distally to the endotracheal tube tip (Schmid et al., 1981) or at the alveolar level (Simon et al., 1984), presumably as a consequence of increased gas velocities (Bernoulli effect) (Schmid et al., 1981; Simon et al., 1984) and, in part, of different inspiratory and expiratory impedances of the airways (Simon et al., 1982). Hence, proximal mean airway pressure may underestimate alveolar pressure and, thus, mean lung volume.

Factors other than the measurement location may contribute to the dissimilarity of mean lung volumes between HFO and conventional mechanical ventilation at similar mean intratracheal airway pressures. Marchak et al. (1981) reported that higher mean airway pressures were required during HFO than during conventional positive-pressure ventilation in providing comparable arterial oxygen tensions in neonates with respiratory distress syndrome. These authors postulated that activation of respiratory muscle tone due to chest-wall vibrations (Gillespie et al., 1980) in the unanesthetized, nonparalyzed state may have led to a decrease in chest-wall compliance, possibly explaining the need for higher airway pressures to achieve the same lung volume (Marchak et al., 1981). Kolton et al. (1982) systematically studied the effect of varying mean airway pressures and their relationship to mean lung volumes during HFO at 15 Hz and conventional mechanical ventilation in rabbits with lung injury following oleic acid infusion or pulmonary saline lavage. They confirmed previous findings reported by Thompson et al. (1982), that below a critical alveolar opening pressure, mean lung volumes and oxygenation were similar with both modes of ventilation. Matching of mean airway pressures above opening pressure, or HFO preceded by a sustained inflation, however, resulted in higher mean lung volumes during HFO, associated with a dramatic improvement in arterial oxygenation (Fig. 7). In contrast, sustained inflations preceding conventional positive-pressure ventilation had no effect on lung volume and oxygenation. Adjustment of mean lung volumes during conventional mechanical ventilation to the postinflation values measured during HFO required much higher mean airway pressures with the accompanying risk of pulmonary barotrauma. It was concluded that recruitment of air space provided by a sustained inflation is maintained during HFO by positioning and holding the lung on the steeper deflation limb of its pressure-volume curve. In contrast, the large phasic pressure swings inherent to conventional mechanical ventilation may lead to derecruitment of alveolar volume during expiration despite the application of positive end-expiratory pressure.

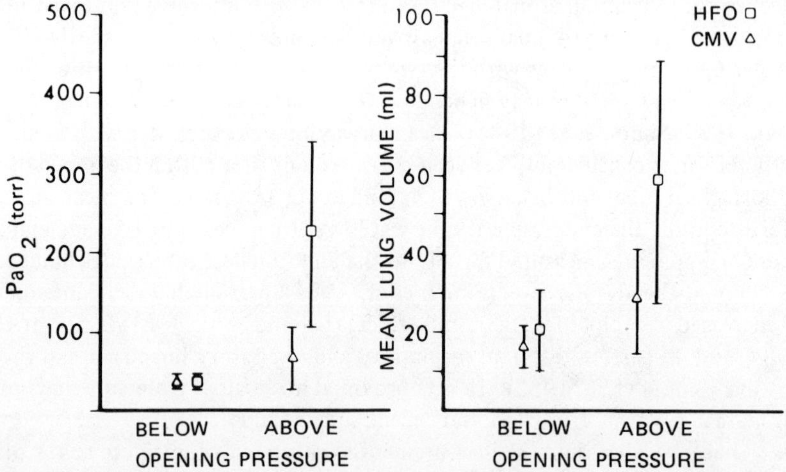

Figure 7 Comparison of arterial oxygen tension (PaO_2, torr) (left panel) and mean lung volume (ml) (right panel) during high-frequency oscillation (HFO) and conventional mechanical ventilation (CMV) at matched mean airway pressure (MAP) in rabbits with lung injury following pulmonary saline lavage. At matched MAP below opening pressure, there was no difference in PaO_2 and mean lung volume between HFO and CMV. At matched MAP above opening pressure, higher PaO_2 values and mean lung volumes were achieved during HFO than CMV (from Kolton et al., 1982), by copyright permission of the International Anesthesia Research Society.

Hence, recruitment and maintenance of air space determine oxygenation in pulmonary disease states during both HFO and conventional mechanical ventilation. At similar mean airway pressures, absence of large phasic pressure changes during HFO enables, in contrast to positive-pressure ventilation at conventional respiratory frequencies, one to maintain a greater fraction of lung volume recruited and, hence, to improve oxygenation and decrease the risk of pulmonary barotrauma (Kolton et al., 1982; Hamilton et al., 1983). This finding, although based on observations in two defined models of lung injury, may be substantial in designing protocols for future comparative clinical studies in adult and neonatal respiratory distress syndrome. Definition of reliable estimates of alveolar pressure during HFO is of crucial importance in avoiding pulmonary overdistention due to false reliance on proximal airway pressure determinations (Simon et al., 1984; Breen et al., 1984).

VIII. Interregional Gas Mixing and Ventilation-Perfusion Relationship

Additional information regarding the factors determining gas transport and gas exchange during HFO is provided from studies applying radioactive tracer techniques with ^{133}xenon (Brusasco et al., 1983, 1984; Forkert and Burks, 1980; Schmid et al., 1980, 1981; Stark et al., 1980). One might argue that transport of ^{133}Xe may not be quantitatively representative of the transport of respiratory gases, either individually or as a composite mixture. If transport is significantly influenced by molecular diffusion or a diffusionlike process, each type of gas would be affected by its specific diffusivity (Schmid et al., 1981). Pulmonary washout of gases with different molecular weights was, however, similar during HFO, indicating that molecular diffusion was not rate-limiting (Knopp et al., 1983; McEvoy et al., 1982). Hence, ^{133}Xe transport during HFO may be considered representative of the transport of other gases (Schmid et al., 1981).

Assessment of intrapulmonary gas distribution by radioactive tracer techniques revealed that gas transport during HFO differs substantially from that observed during conventional mechanical ventilation (Schmid et al., 1981; Brusasco et al., 1983). Regional pulmonary ^{133}Xe clearance rates during HFO at 15 and 30 Hz were similar in different regions of dog lungs at lung volumes equal to or greater than functional residual capacity (Schmid et al., 1981). This is in contrast to conventional mechanical ventilation, in which dependent lung regions are cleared faster than nondependent regions (Schmid et al., 1980). Regional ^{133}Xe distribution was also more uniform in paralyzed kittens (Stark et al., 1980) and in seated human subjects with normal lungs (Forkert and Burks, (1980). Following induction of large perfusion-dependent differences in the vertical distribution of ^{133}Xe concentrations, ventilation by HFO abolished the concentration gradients and equalized pulmonary ^{133}Xe distribution by interregional mixing (Schmid et al., 1980, 1981) (Fig. 8). In contrast, no interregional gas transport was detected during conventional mechanical ventilation (Schmid et al., 1981).

In conclusion, total transport of gas to a lung region during HFO is a function of not only longitudinal gas motion from the mouth to a specific lung region, but also of interregional gas transport (Schmid et al., 1981; Brusasco et al., 1983). This mechanism has been invoked to explain the inappropriateness of a parallel ventilation-perfusion ($\dot{V}_A/\dot{Q}$) model, as is assumed with the technique of inert gas elimination, to predict gas exchange efficiency during HFO (Robertson et al., 1982).

Interregional gas transport during HFO may occur by rebreathing of common dead-space gas via the airways or by collateral ventilation (Schmid et al., 1981). Asynchronous filling and emptying of lung regions with different local

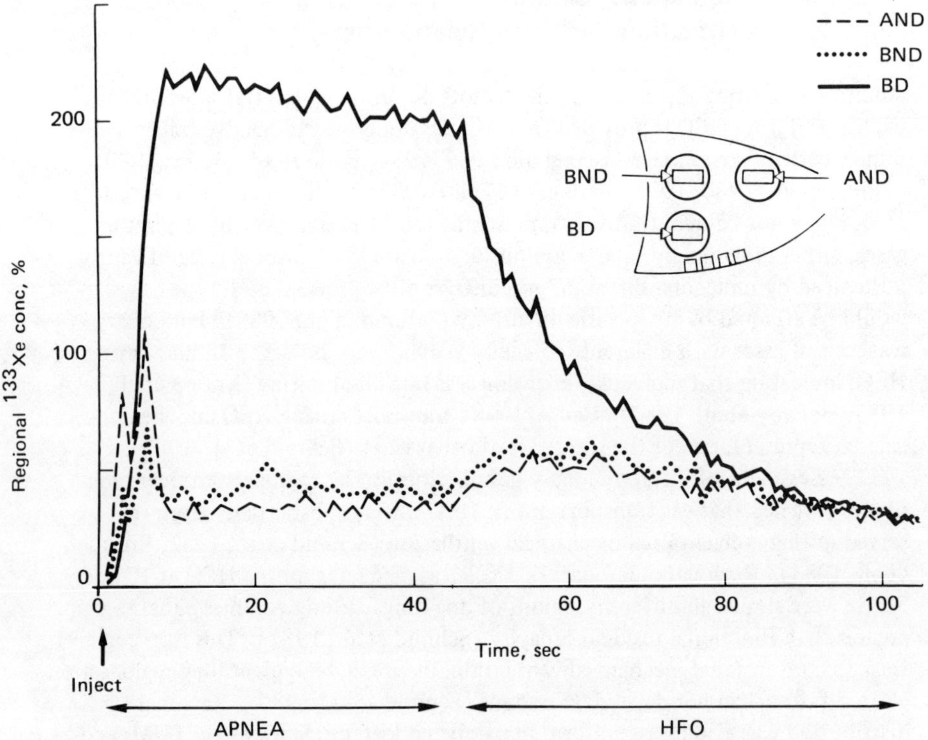

Figure 8 Regional ^{133}Xe concentrations after intravenous (right atrial) bolus injection of ^{133}Xe during apnea, followed by regional ^{133}Xe clearances during HFO at 30 Hz in one dog lying supine. AND, apical nondependent; BND, basal nondependent; BD, basal dependent lung regions. Note transient increase in ^{133}Xe concentrations in AND and BND lung regions with the onset of HFO, indicating a flux of ^{133}Xe to these regions (adapted from Schmid et al., 1981).

time constants (Lehr, 1980) may contribute to interregional gas transport. The relative significance of these mechanisms is currently unclear. During apnea, the vertical gradient in regional ^{133}Xe concentrations remained fairly constant as compared to HFO (Fig. 8), indicating that cardiogenic mixing and redistribution of ^{133}Xe via pulmonary blood flow contribute only little to interregional gas mixing during HFO (Schmid et al., 1981).

Interregional (and intraregional) mixing may significantly affect pulmonary gas exchange during HFO. Interregional gas transport may decrease the effect of $\dot{V}_A/\dot{Q}$ inhomogeneities on gas exchange (Schmid et al., 1981). Ross and Farhi (1960) demonstrated that rebreathing of common dead-space gas has a buffering action in limiting the range of possible alveolar gas compositions. In the presence of uniform alveolar gas concentration, the effect of the $\dot{V}_A/\dot{Q}$ relationship on pulmonary gas exchange does not need to be considered (Ross and Farhi, 1960). Thus, interregional mixing, if of sufficient rate and magnitude, should minimize the effect of $\dot{V}_A/\dot{Q}$ variance on gas exchange by reducing regional differences in alveolar gas concentrations (Schmid et al., 1981).

Indirect evidence that interregional mixing may be important in determining efficiency of pulmonary gas exchange during HFO has come from a recent study examining regional longitudinal gas transfer rates during HFO (Brusasco et al., 1983). By analyzing in supine dogs the initial part of regional pulmonary wash-in of ^{133}Xe (which can be assumed to be only minimally affected by interregional gas mixing), Brusasco et al. (1983) found longitudinal distribution of gas transport to be nearly uniform for frequencies of 5-57 Hz and tidal volumes from 9 to 64% of the anatomical and equipment dead space volume. At 5 Hz and with tidal volumes approaching the dead-space volume, longitudinal gas transport was nonuniform with higher gas transfer rates to the dependent than nondependent lung regions. The gravitation-oriented vertical gradient in pulmonary blood flow distribution is preserved during HFO (Schmid et al., 1981; McEvoy et al., 1982). Accordingly, if no interregional mixing occurred, $\dot{V}_A/\dot{Q}$ matching and pulmonary gas exchange could be less satisfactory during HFO than during conventional mechanical ventilation in which regional distribution of both $\dot{V}_A$ and $\dot{Q}$ is not uniform (Schmid et al., 1980). It was postulated that pulmonary gas exchange might be more efficient during HFO at lower oscillation frequencies and with tidal volumes approaching the dead space volume than during HFO at higher frequencies and smaller tidal volumes (Brusasco et al., 1983).

Using continuous intravenous infusions of ^{133}Xe, Brusasco et al. (1984) derived in supine dogs $\dot{V}_A/\dot{Q}$ matching along the vertical axis from the ratio of ^{133}Xe concentrations in basal nondependent (BND) and basal dependent (BD) regions of the lung. The study was performed during steady-state eucapnic-isocapnic ventilation on conventional mechanical ventilation at 12 breaths/min and on HFO at 6, 15, and 30 Hz. The ratios of regional ^{133}Xe concentrations along the vertical axis (C_{BND}/C_{BD}) were similar during conventional mechanical ventilation and during HFO at 15 and 30 Hz (Fig. 9), indicating similar $\dot{V}_A/\dot{Q}$ distributions. Accordingly, arterial oxygen tensions were similar during conventional mechanical ventilation and HFO at 15 and 30 Hz (Fig. 9). During HFO at the lower oscillation frequency (6 Hz), C_{BND}/C_{BD} was closest to unity (Fig. 9), indicating a nearly uniform distribution of regional $\dot{V}_A/\dot{Q}$. In accordance with this observation, arterial oxygen tensions were highest during HFO at 6 Hz. One might speculate, on the basis of these data, that interregional mixing during HFO at 15 and 30 Hz was sufficient to reduce $\dot{V}_A/\dot{Q}$ imbalance, resulting from a nearly uniform distribution of longitudinal gas transport associated with nonuniform pulmonary blood flow distribution. The net result was a $\dot{V}_A/\dot{Q}$ distribution simi-

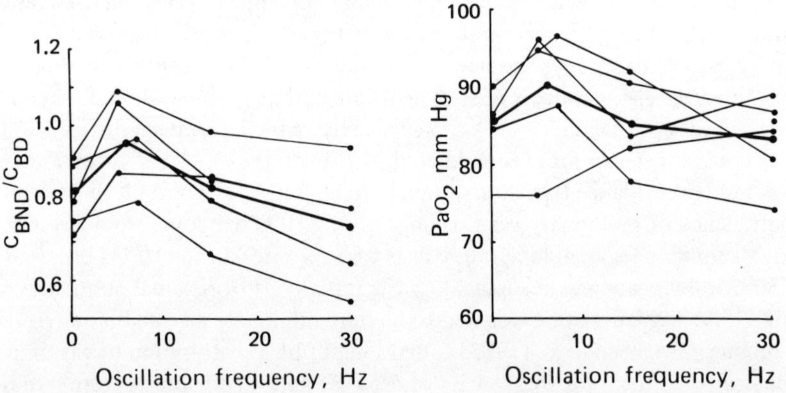

Figure 9 Ratio of ^{133}Xe concentrations in basal nondependent and basal dependent lung regions (C_{BND}/C_{BD}) (left panel) and arterial oxygen tension (PaO_2, mmHg (right panel) during conventional mechanical ventilation (values at zero oscillation frequency) and high-frequency oscillation (HFO) at 6, 15, and 30 Hz for five dogs lying supine. Heavy lines denote mean values. For lung regions (BND, BD) see chest wall scheme in Figure 8. C_{BND}/C_{BD} was consistently closest to unity during HFO at 6 Hz, indicating most uniform distribution of regional ventilation-perfusion ratio along vertical axis. PaO_2 was highest during HFO at 6 Hz in 4 of 5 dogs (adapted from Brusasco et al. (1984)).

lar to that observed during conventional mechanical ventilation. The nearly uniform $\dot{V}_A/\dot{Q}$ and more efficient oxygenation during HFO at 6 Hz may reflect a combination of more favorable matching of regional longitudinal gas transfer rates and blood flow distribution, and interregional mixing (Brusasco et al., 1984).

Hence, interregional gas transport may be an important determinant of the efficiency of oxygen exchange during HFO. Quantitation of interregional gas mixing and definition of its determinants could be of importance for optimizing $\dot{V}_A/\dot{Q}$ balance and pulmonary gas exchange during HFO.

IX. Summary and Conclusions

Pulmonary gas exchange can be maintained during HFO with tidal volumes smaller than the combined anatomical and equipment dead space volumes. The mechanisms determining this efficiency are as yet incompletely understood. The observed dependence of CO_2 elimination on oscillation frequency and tidal volume may, to some extent, be predicted from theoretical models coupling augmented dispersion (Fredberg, 1980; Slutsky et al., 1980) with convective direct alveolar ventilation of lung units with short path lengths (Khoo et al., 1982). The mechanical properties of the lung significantly modify efficacy of ventilation during HFO. Oxygen exchange shows a strong dependence on recruitment and maintenance of lung volume in pulmonary disease states (Kolton et al., 1982). Due to the minimal pressure changes during HFO, a greater fraction of lung volume once recruited can be maintained, resulting in improved oxygenation with decreased risk of pulmonary barotrauma (Kolton et al., 1982; Hamilton et al., 1983). Interregional and intraregional redistribution of gas (Schmid et al., 1980, 1981; Lehr, 1980) may explain the efficacy of oxygenation during HFO, despite a less favorable matching of longitudinal gas transport and pulmonary perfusion at higher oscillation frequencies.

Although both theoretical and experimental studies have shed some light on the determinants of pulmonary gas exchange during HFO, further investigation is needed to define the mechanisms underlying its efficacy. Controlled evaluation of the physiological variables governing gas exchange during HFO requires exact statement of equipment specifications and further definition and development of appropriate monitoring techniques.

References

Ashbaugh, D. G., Petty, T. L., Bigelow, D. B., and Harris, T. M. (1969). Continuous positive pressure breathing (CPPB) in adult respiratory distress syndrome. *J. Thorac. Cardiovasc. Surg.* **57**(1):31-41.

Berdine, G. B., Lehr, J. L., and Drazen, J. M. (1983). Ethane washout by high frequency (2-40 Hz) low volume (20-100 ml) ventilation (HFV) in excised dog lungs (abstr.). *Fed. Proc.* **42**(4):763.

Bohn, D. J., Miyasaka, K., Marchak, B. E., Thompson, W. K., Froese, A. B., and Bryan, A. C. (1980). Ventilation by high-frequency oscillation. *J. Appl. Physiol.* **48**:710-716.

Bouhuys, A. (1974). The anatomical dead space. In *Breathing.* New York, Grune and Stratton, pp. 42-58.

Breen, P. H., Ali, J., and Wood, L. D. H. (1984). High-frequency ventilation in lung edema: effects on gas exchange and perfusion. *J. Appl. Physiol.* **56** (1):187-195.

Brusasco, V., Knopp, T. J., and Rehder, K. (1983). Gas transport during high-frequency ventilation. *J. Appl. Physiol.* **55**(2):472-478.

Brusasco, V., Knopp, T. J., Schmid, E. R., and Rehder, K. (1984). Ventilation-perfusion relationship during high-frequency ventilation. *J. Appl. Physiol.* **56**(2):454-458.

Bryan, A. C. (1983). Historic and future development of high frequency oscillation (abstr.). *J. Biomed. Engin.* **11**:59.

Butler, W. J., Bohn, D. J., Bryan, A. C., and Froese, A. B. (1980). Ventilation by high frequency oscillation in humans. *Anesth. Analg.* **59**:577-584.

Chang, H. K. (1983). Bases théoriques de la ventilation par oscillation à haute fréquence. In *Ventilation à Haute Fréquence.* Edited by J. L. Bourgain, A. Lienhart, and P. Viars. Paris, Librairie Arnette, pp. 65-83.

Forkert, L., and Burks, J. E. (1980). The regional distribution of gas during high frequency oscillations (abstr.). *Physiologist* **23**:177.

Fowler, W. S. (1948). Lung function studies. II. The respiratory dead space. *Am. J. Physiol.* **154**:405-416.

Frantz, I. D. III, Werthammer, J., and Stark, A. R. (1983). High-frequency ventilation in premature infants with lung disease: Adequate gas exchange at low tracheal pressure. *Pediatrics* **71**(4):483-488.

Fredberg, J. J. (1980). Augmented diffusion in the airways can support pulmonary gas exchange. *J. Appl. Physiol.* **49**:232-238.

Froese, A. B., and Bryan, A. C. (1981). High frequency ventilation (editorial). *Am. Rev. Respir. Dis.* **123**(3):249-250.

Gavriely, N., Solway, J., Loring, S., Ingram, R. H. Jr., Brown, R., Slutsky, A., and Drazen, J. (1982). Airway dynamics during high frequency ventilation (HFV). A cineradiographic study (abstr.). *Physiologist* **25**(4):282.

Gillespie, D. J., Rodarte, J. R., and Hyatt, R. E. (1980). Respiratory mechanics during ventilation by high frequency oscillation (HFO) (abstr.). *Physiologist* **23**(4):1.

Goldstein, D., Slutsky, A. S., Ingram, R. H., Westerman, P., Venegas, J., and Drazen, J. (1981). CO_2 elimination by high frequency ventilation (4 to 10 Hz) in normal subjects. *Am. Rev. Respir. Dis.* **123**(3):251-255.

Hamilton, P. P., Onayemi, A., Smyth, J. A., Gillan, J. E., Cutz, E., Froese, A. B., and Bryan, A. C. (1983). Comparison of conventional and high-frequency ventilation: Oxygenation and lung pathology. *J. Appl. Physiol.* **55**(1): 131-138.

Haselton, F. R., and Scherer, P. W. (1980). Bronchial bifurcations and respiratory mass transport. *Science* **208**:69-71.

Herman, S., and Reynolds, E. O. R. (1973). Methods for improving oxygenation in infants mechanically ventilated for severe hyaline membrane disease. *Arch. Dis. Child.* **48**:612-617.

Jones, L. S. (1983). High frequency ventilation in immature infants (special conference report). *Pediatrics* **71**(2):280-287.

Khoo, M. C. K., Slutsky, A. S., Drazen, J. M., Solway, J., Gavriely, N., and Kamm, R. D. (1982). An improved model of gas transport during HFV (abstr.). *Physiologist* **25**(4):283.

Knopp, T. J., Kaethner, T., Meyer, M., Rehder, K., and Scheid, P. (1983). Gas mixing in the airways of dog lungs during high-frequency ventilation. *J. Appl. Physiol.* **55**(4):1141-1146.

Kolton, M., Cattran, C. B., Kent, G., Volgyesi, G., Froese, A. B., and Bryan, A. C. (1982). Oxygenation during high-frequency ventilation compared with conventional mechanical ventilation in two models of lung injury. *Anesth. Analg.* **61**:323-332.

Lee, J. S. (ed.) (1983). Transport mechanisms of high frequency ventilation. *J. Biomed. Engin.* **11**:59-62.

Lehr, J. (1980). Circulating currents during high frequency ventilation (abstr.). *Fed. Proc.* **39**:576A.

Lunkenheimer, P. P., Rafflenbeul, W., Keller, H., Frank, I., Dickhut, H. H., and Fuhrmann, C. (1972). Application of transtracheal pressure oscillations as a modification of "diffusion respiration." *Br. J. Anaesth.* **44**:627.

Lunkenheimer, P. P., Frank, I., Ising, H., Keller, H., and Dickhut, H. H. (1973). Intrapulmonaler Gaswechsel unter simulierter Apnoe durch transtrachealen periodischen intrathorakalen Druckwechsel. *Anaesthesist* **22**:232-238.

Lunkenheimer, P. P., Ising, H., Frank, I., Scharsich, M., Welham, K., and Dittrich, H. (1977). Enhancement of CO_2-elimination by intrapulmonary high frequency pressure alternation during "apneic oxygenation," *Adv. Exp. Med. Biol.* **94**:599-603.

McEvoy, R. D., Davies, N. J. H., Mannino, F. L., Prutow, R. J., Schumacker, P. T., Wagner, P. D., and West, J. B. (1982). Pulmonary gas exchange by high-frequency ventilation. *J. Appl. Physiol.* **52**(5):1278-1287.

Marchak, B. E., Thompson, W. K., Duffty, P., Miyaki, T., Bryan, M. H., Bryan, A. C., and Froese, A. B. (1981). Treatment of RDS by high-frequency oscillatory ventilation: A preliminary report. *J. Pediatr.* **99**(2):287-292.

Mead, J. (1969). Contribution of compliance of airways to frequency-dependent behavior of lungs. *J. Appl. Physiol.* **26**(5):670-673.

Mitzner, W., Ngeow, Y. K., and Caguicla, N. (1981). Optimization of high frequency ventilation (abstr.). *Fed. Proc.* **40**:384.

Mitzner, W., Permutt, S., and Weinmann, G. (1985). Gas transport during high-frequency ventilation: Theoretical model and experimental validation. *Ann. Biomed. Engin.* (in press).

Permutt, S., Mitzner, W., and Weinmann, G. (1984). A model of high frequency ventilation. *J. Appl. Physiol.*

Rehder, K., and Crawford, M. (1983). Hochfrequente Druckoszillations-beatmung (HFV) beim anaesthesierten Menschen (abstr.). *Anaesthesist* **32** (Suppl.):52.

Rehder, K., Schmid, E. R., and Knopp, T. J. (1983). Long-term high frequency ventilation in dogs. *Am. Rev. Respir. Dis.* **128**(3):476-480.

Robertson, H. T., Coffey, R. L., Standaert, T. A., and Truog, W. E. (1982). Respiratory and inert gas exchange during high-frequency ventilation. *J. Appl. Physiol.* **52**(3):683-689.

Ross, B. B., and Farhi, L. E. (1960). Dead-space ventilation as a determinant in the ventilation-perfusion concept. *J. Appl. Physiol.* **15**(3):363-371.

Rossing, T. H., Slutsky, A. S., Lehr, J. L., Drinker, P. A., Kamm, R., and Drazen,

J. M. (1981). Tidal volume and frequency dependence of carbon dioxide elimination by high-frequency ventilation. *N. Engl. J. Med.* **305**(23):1375-1379.

Rossing, T. H., Slutsky, A. S., Ingram, R. H. Jr., Kamm, R. D., Shapiro, A. H., and Drazen, M. M. (1982). CO_2 elimination by high-frequency oscillations in dogs–effect of histamine infusion. *J. Appl. Physiol.* **53**(5):1256-1262.

Scherer, P. W. (1983). Gas transport in branched airways during high frequency ventilation (abstr.). *J. Biomed. Engin.* **11**:60.

Scherer, P. W., and Haselton, F. R. (1982). Convective exchange in oscillatory flow through bronchial-tree models. *J. Appl. Physiol.* **53**(4):1023-1033.

Scherer, P. W., Shendalman, L. H., Greene, N. M., and Bouhuys, A. (1975). Measurement of axial diffusivities in a model of the bronchial airways. *J. Appl. Physiol.* **38**(4):719-723.

Schmid, E. R., Knopp, T. J., and Rehder, K. (1980). Interregional mixing during high frequency oscillation (HFO) (abstr.). *Physiologist* **23**:166.

Schmid, E. R., Rehder, K., Knopp, T. J., and Hyatt, R. E. (1980). Chest wall motion and distribution of inspired gas in anesthetized supine dogs. *J. Appl. Physiol.* **49**:279-286.

Schmid, E. R., Knopp, T. J., and Rehder, K. (1981). Intrapulmonary gas transport and perfusion during high-frequency oscillation. *J. Appl. Physiol.* **51** (6):1507-1514.

Simon, B., Weinmann, G., and Mitzner, W. (1984). Mean airway pressure and alveolar pressure during high frequency ventilation. *J. Appl. Physiol.* **57**:1069-1078.

Slutsky, A. S. (1981). Gas mixing by cardiogenic oscillations: A theoretical quantitative analysis. *J. Appl. Physiol.* **51**(5):1287-1293.

Slutsky, A. S., Drazen, J. M., Ingram, R. H. Jr., Kamm, R. D., Shapiro, A. H., Fredberg, J. J., Loring, S. H., and Lehr, J. (1980). Effective pulmonary ventilation with small volume oscillation at high frequency. *Science* **209**: 609-610.

Slutsky, A. S., Kamm, R. D., Rossing, T. H., Loring, S. H., Lehr, J., Shapiro, A., Ingram, R. H. Jr., and Drazen, J. M. (1981). Effects of frequency, tidal volume, and lung volume on CO_2 elimination in dogs by high frequency (2-30 Hz), low tidal volume ventilation. *J. Clin. Invest.* **68**:1475-1484.

Slutsky, A. S., Kamm, R. D., and Drazen, J. M. (1983). A review of experimental and theoretical studies in high frequency ventilation. In *Perspectives of High-Frequency Ventilation.* Edited by P. A. Scheck, U. H. Sjostrand, and R. B. Smith. Boston, Martinus Nijhoff, pp. 59-70.

Stark, A. R., Frantz, I. D. III, Fredberg, J. J., Dorkin, H. L., and Jackson, A. C. (1980). Physiologic studies and lung scans during ventilation with high frequency low pressure oscillations (abstr.). *Am. Rev. Respir. Dis.* **121** (Suppl.):304.

Taylor, G. I. (1953). Dispersion of soluble matter in solvent flowing slowly through a tube. *Proc. R. Soc.* **A219**:186-203.

Taylor, G. I. (1954). The dispersion of matter in turbulent flow through a pipe. *Proc. R. Soc.* **A223**:446-468.

Thompson, W. K., Marchak, B. E., Froese, A. B., and Bryan, A. C. (1982). High frequency oscillation compared with standard ventilation in pulmonary injury model. *J. Appl. Physiol.* **52**(3):543-548.

Weinmann, G., Mitzner, W., and Permutt, S. (1984). Physiologic dead space during high frequency ventilation in dogs. *J. Appl. Physiol.* **57**:881-887.

Wright, K., Lyrene, R. K., Truog, W. E., Standaert, T. A., Murphy, J., and Woodrum, D. E. (1981). Ventilation by high-frequency oscillation in rabbits with oleic acid lung disease. *J. Appl. Physiol.* **50**(5):1056-1060.

12

High-Frequency Oscillatory Ventilation
Technical Development and Experimental Evaluation

R. DOUGLAS McEVOY

Royal Adelaide Hospital
Adelaide, South Australia

Few subjects in respiratory physiology have generated as much interest as high-frequency oscillatory ventilation (HFOV). The catalyst was a short report (Bohn et al., 1979) and subsequent paper by Bohn et al. (1980) demonstrating that normal gas exchange could be maintained with tidal volumes substantially smaller than anatomical dead space using exceedingly high ventilatory frequencies. It appears that similar observations were made earlier by other investigators (Lunkenheimer et al., 1972; Bunnell et al., 1978) but had passed largely unnoticed.

The surge of experimental work that followed these early reports arose largely from the wish to understand mechanisms of gas exchange, but also from the hope that HFOV would improve survival in patients with severe respiratory failure. A considerable body of practical and theoretical information has since accumulated on ventilator design and function.

The experimental evaluation of HFOV has occurred in three main areas: gas exchange mechanisms, nonventilatory physiological effects, and application to lung disease. The first topic has attracted a great deal of attention and recent work has brought to light some exciting new concepts of gas transport (Fredberg, 1980; Haselton and Scherer, 1980; Slutsky et al., 1980; Lehr, 1980; Lehr et al., 1982; McEvoy et al., 1982b). These and other aspects are covered in detail elsewhere in this book and they will therefore be mentioned only as they relate to ventilator design and operation. The other two areas will be discussed in detail.

I. Technical Development

Many different ventilators and techniques have been used to deliver HFOV. In some instances new devices have been hastily constructed by researchers anxious to obtain a workable system in the least possible time. More often, ventilators have been specifically designed to gain better control of variables such as tidal volume (Vt) and mean airway pressure (Paw) or alternatively, to develop new ways of coupling oscillations to the respiratory system. It is beyond the scope of this review to describe each ventilator used experimentally or clinically. Instead I will focus on some technical problems they have in common. A classification of HFOV methods will follow and, lastly, a review of information on the effects of variables such as respiratory frequency (fr) and Vt on ventilator function.

A. Technical Problems Common to Most Oscillatory Ventilators

The internal compressible volume and impedance of a ventilator are relatively unimportant at physiological frequencies, but during HFOV they may become critical determinants of the system's efficiency. If either is too large, a great deal of the piston displacement can be wasted on gas compression, in which case overheating may occur. Endotracheal tube dimensions contribute substantially to ventilator resistance (Gavriely et al., 1982b) and may be important in this regard.

Some of the earlier oscillatory ventilators appeared to have an optimal gas exchange frequency (Bohn et al., 1980; McEvoy et al., 1982b). For a time this was attributed to intrinsic mechanical properties of the lung or chest wall (Bohn et al., 1980). Subsequently, comparisons of actual delivered tidal volumes with those predicted from piston displacement indicated that the observation was simply a manifestation of gas compression at high frequencies (Wright et al., 1981) (Fig. 1).

Gas moving at high velocity may entrain particulate material. Ngeow and Mitzner (1982) found that solid lime dust was entrained if the CO_2 absorbed in their HFOV circuit was placed near the gas mainstream. It is a reasonable concern that lubricants used in piston or rotating valve pumps might suffer a similar fate.

The volume of fresh gas delivered to the upper airway during HFOV can be large. A dog ventilated with a Vt of 60 ml at 20 Hz could have a tracheal minute ventilation of approximately 72 liters. Even if this gas is partly conditioned, the potential exists for considerable dehydration of the upper airway. Current humidification systems may be able to condition bias-flow gas adequately before it enters the airway, but this assumption has not been verified experimentally.

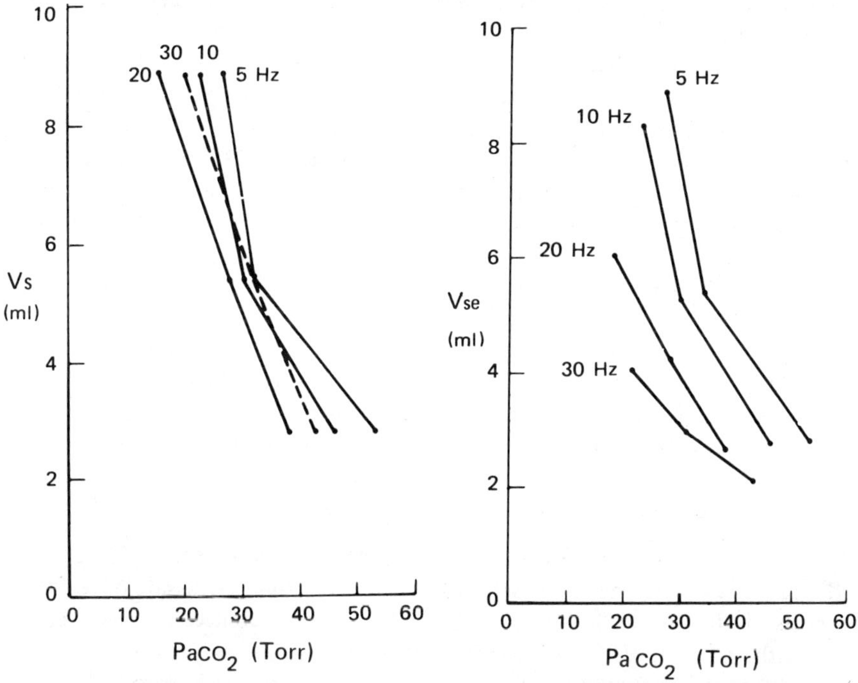

Figure 1 In the left panel, piston stroke volume, Vs, is plotted against arterial carbon dioxide tension, $PaCO_2$, for various oscillator frequencies. Gas exchange appears to be optimal at 20 Hz for all Vs. A similar plot of effective tidal volume, Vse (i.e., the volume of the gas actually delivered to the airway) against $PaCO_2$ does not elicit an optimal frequency (right panel). In these experiments, Vse was measured proximal to the bias exhaust. The explanation for the different results is that excessive gas compression occurred in the ventilator and/or its connections at high frequencies (reproduced by permission from Wright et al., 1981).

Accurate measurement of airway pressure, Vt, and fr during HFOV is exacting and sometimes difficult (Froese and Bryan, 1981). Standard respiratory pressure transducers are generally capable of following pressure fluctuations to 20 Hz or more but their linearity should be checked (Jackson and Vinegar, 1979). Low-compliance tubing of suitable internal diameter should be used for connections, and a side-hole configuration used to measure airway pressure since the use of end-hole catheters will lead to substantial errors. Interpretation of airway pressure measurements has been complicated by recent observations, in isolated rabbit lung, that alveolar pressure may exceed tracheal pressure at or near the resonant frequency of the lung (Allen et al., 1983). The findings seriously challenge the concept that large peak-to-peak pressure oscillations in the trachea would progressively attenuate in the lower airway and be lowest in the alveoli, and may reduce the value of tracheal pressure measurements. Pneumotachographs, routinely used for respiratory flow measurement, were not specifically designed to function at very high frequencies, but may be calibrated to provide reliable flow and tidal volume data during HFOV (Jackson and Vinegar, 1979; Slutsky et al., 1981). Measurement of ventilation frequency need not be difficult, and can be obtained from expanded pressure tracings, or with a variable frequency stroboscopic light focused on a moving component of the oscillator.

Finally, some problems may be connected to the presence of rapidly moving parts. Most of them (excessive noise, component failure) can be prevented by good engineering design, but the risk of serious injury to either operator or patient should not be underestimated. Suitable alarms are necessary to monitor for airway pressure or loss of fresh gas supply. Automatic flow interruption and open venting of the airway should occur with high pressure conditions.

B. Categorization of High-Frequency Oscillators

Six different methods of oscillatory ventilation are shown schematically in Figure 2. This classification has been devised merely to facilitate discussion of technical aspects of HFOV and does not imply fundamental differences between ventilators with respect to their physiological implications.

Whole-body oscillatory excitation (Fig. 2A) has received relatively little attention. Two methods have thus far been used. The first was discovered serendipitously during the course of experiments testing for adverse effects of infrasound (Johnson, 1973). It was noted that dogs placed inside an oscillating (1-8 Hz) chamber (Fig. 2A) became apneic, but were apparently well-ventilated by small chest-wall oscillations induced by the system. The second method used a vibrating plate to shake the whole body and thus, presumably, oscillate the diaphragm. However, it only partially met the ventilatory requirements of anesthetized cats (Bitterman et al., 1983). At this stage, both techniques are highly experimental and untested in humans. Nevertheless, as with other methods that attempt to impart oscillatory motion to the respiratory system from the outside (Fig. 2E), they may prove useful when airway intubation is either undesirable or impossible.

The second type of ventilator (Fig. 2B) is a closed system in which a piston pump (Ngeow and Mitzner, 1982) or vibrating membrane (Lunkenheimer et al., 1972, 1973) induces oscillatory motion to airway gases. Soda lime absorbs CO_2 and a flow of oxygen is added, to meet metabolic needs. The advantage of this technique is that the entire stroke volume is delivered to the airway and humidification problems are minimized. The main problems include:

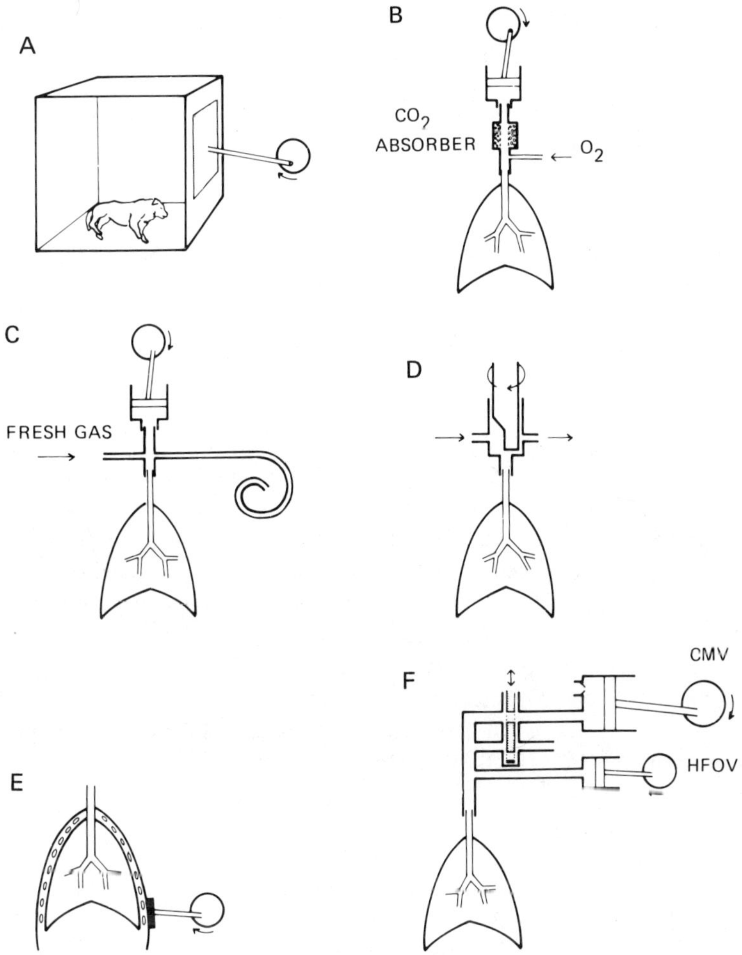

Figure 2 Schematic representation of six different types of HFOV. (A) Whole-body oscillation administered either in a dynamic pressure chamber or by whole-body mechanical vibration. (B) A "closed" system in which CO_2 is absorbed and O_2 added to meet metabolic demand. (C) Bias flow oscillator circuit. As with B, the pump may be a piston-cylinder combination, loudspeaker cone, or other vibrating membrane. The bias-flow circuit can utilize a long, low-impedance exhaust or high-impedance tube with positive source and negative sink pressures. It may be directed down the airway rather than across the airway opening. (D) Rotating valve that interrupts a high pressure gas source. (E) oscillations coupled to the thorax either by a vibrating disc or a pressure cuff. (F) HFOV, combined with CMV, as shown, or spontaneous ventilation.

1. Need to replace exhausted soda lime
2. Entrainment of soda lime dust
3. Overheating due to the exothermal soda lime-CO_2 reaction
4. Need to match O_2 delivery and O_2 uptake exactly.

Ngeow and Mitzner (1982) have designed a circuit that largely overcomes these difficulties: the CO_2 absorber material has been removed from the main gas flow; a heat exchange and dust filter have been added; a simple O_2 pressure demand valve circumvents the difficulty of maintaining a precise O_2 flow. The only remaining problems are the need regularly to replace the exhausted soda lime and the absence of an alternative circuit allowing spontaneous breathing.

In the third type of ventilator (Fig. 2C), fresh gas is supplied to the airway opening by a bias-flow system of variable design (Bohn et al., 1980; Slutsky et al., 1981; Butler et al., 1980). Several investigators (McEvoy et al., 1982b; Butler et al., 1980; Schmid et al., 1981) have used a long, relatively low-impedance bias exhaust tube. Its high inertance produces a "low-pass filter" effect: High-velocity pump oscillations are directed toward the airway, while the low-velocity bias flow moves relatively unimpeded toward the exhaust. The major drawback is that the efficiency of the "filter" varies with pump frequency and airway impedance.

To overcome this difficulty, Slutsky et al. (1981) developed a circuit that directs all the pump's stroke volume to the airway. It employs very high impedance bias tubing and a positive-pressure source and negative-pressure sink for the fresh gas. The system has been used successfully for short periods in experimental animals (Slutsky et al., 1980, 1981; Rossing et al., 1982) and humans (Goldstein et al., 1981; Rossing et al., 1981). A fail-safe pop-off pressure valve is essential for this system.

The fourth type of HFOV (Fig. 2D) is similar to jet ventilation. A high-pressure gas source is interrupted by a valve rotating at variable, but high, frequency (Fletcher et al., 1982; Fletcher and Epstein, 1982). A negative pressure at the exhaust port may be needed to avoid excessive gas trapping and lung distention.

External oscillation of the lungs (Fig. 2E) has been used successfully in the isolated-perfused rat lung (Ward et al., 1983) and anesthetized dogs (Zidulka et al., 1983). Intubation is avoided and, in contrast with HFOV applied to the airway (McEvoy et al., 1982a), this method appears to enhance mucus clearance (Gross et al., 1983; King et al., 1983).

The final category (Fig. 2F) combines HFOV with either spontaneous breathing (Calverley et al., 1983) or CMV (Harf et al., 1983; Okamoto, 1981; El-Baz et al., 1983). Preliminary reports suggest that it is effective in assisting ventilation and may reduce ventilation-perfusion inequality (Calverley et al., 1983; Harf et al., 1983; Okamoto, 1981).

C. Determining Optimal HFOV

A major difficulty in trying to determine the relative importance of variables such as fr, Vt, Paw, bias flow, and oscillatory waveform is that considerable uncertainty still exists about basic gas exchange mechanisms during HFOV. Early experimental work indicated that a linear relationship exists between oscillatory flow, $\dot{V}$osc (the product of fr and Vt), and CO_2 elimination (Slutsky et al., 1980, 1981), implying that at any Vt, increasing fr would increase effective alveolar ventilation. Recent studies in humans and dogs with normal lungs (Goldstein et al., 1981; Ngeow and Mitzner, 1982) and with increased peripheral airway resistances (Rossing et al., 1981, 1982) do not, however, fully support this. They have found instead that beyond a "critical" frequency, which may vary between experimental subjects and be influenced by tidal volume, gas exchange is no longer enhanced by higher frequencies. A possible explanation is that, at very high frequencies, a significant part of Vt is wasted in upper airway distention (Slutsky, 1983).

Data on the effects of Paw in normal lungs also appear somewhat contradictory. Early experimental evidence (Slutsky et al., 1981) supported theoretical predictions (Slutsky et al., 1980) that gas transport during HFOV would be virtually independent of lung volume (or Paw), but more recent data in dogs (Mitzner et al., 1981a) and humans (Goldstein et al., 1981) show instead improved gas exchange efficiency with increasing Paw. Most investigators agree that increasing Paw improves gas exchange in the presence of diffuse lung injury (Wright et al., 1981; Thompson et al., 1982).

The bias flow configuration can be used in two different ways to support gas exchange during HFOV. If fresh gas moves across the airway opening (Butler et al., 1980), it will lower CO_2 concentration at the airway opening by a simple flushing action. On the other hand, bias flow directed down the airway (Bohn et al., 1980) will move the fresh gas front toward the alveoli, further improving the effectiveness of HFOV (Gavriely et al., 1982a).

Numerous studies have examined the effects of different ventilatory wave forms and inspiratory/expiratory ratios in CMV and jet ventilation (2-5 Hz), but the consequence of these gas delivery modalities has not yet been fully explored for HFOV (5 Hz). Preliminary data suggest that, in the frequency range of 4-7 Hz, shortening inspiratory time substantially increases gas exchange efficiency (Paloski et al., 1981). No information is available on the effects of different wave forms (square, sinusoidal, etc.), but one report suggests that even in a mixture of different frequencies, "noise," may represent an effective means of augmenting gas transport (Clarke et al., 1983).

III. Experimental Evaluation

A. Nonventilatory Effects of HFOV

Control of Breathing

Several groups have shown that spontaneous breathing is inhibited during high-frequency ventilation (Johnson, 1973; Thompson et al., 1981; Man et al., 1983; Wozniak et al., 1983; England et al., 1983; Banzett et al., 1983). In the first systematic study of the subject (Thompson et al., 1981) sustained apnea was induced in anesthetized dogs by applying HFOV to the upper airway at a Paw of approximately 6 cm H_2O. Spontaneous breathing resumed in 9 of 11 animals after either unilateral or bilateral vagotomy. The authors argued that, although lung volume was increased in their experiments, apnea was unlikely to have resulted simply from the Hering-Breuer inflation reflex since adaptation would have occurred during the relatively long course of their experiments. They believe, instead, that pulmonary stretch receptor stimulation by HFOV was responsible for the vagally mediated reflex. Since two dogs failed to resume breathing after vagotomy, the authors considered that inhibitory influences might also originate from chest-wall mechanoreceptors. However, more recent studies, in which HFOV was administered by chest-wall compression, suggest that chest-wall receptors are probably not involved (Zidulka et al., 1983). An alternative explanation for the failure of two animals to resume breathing after vagotomy (Thompson et al., 1981) is that the output from respiratory centers may remain inhibited for several minutes after vagal in afferent activity is blocked (Man et al., 1983).

Subsequent studies in dogs have confirmed that pulmonary stretch receptors are stimulated by HFOV (Man et al., 1983; Wozniak et al., 1983) and that, although the vagally mediated reflex is potentiated by increases in lung volume (Man et al., 1983; Banzett et al., 1983), the response is not simply a consequence of static lung inflation. HFOV-induced apnea can occur at resting lung volume but lesser degrees of expiratory lengthening are more often observed.

The strength of the reflex is apparently related to a number of factors, in addition to lung volume. For instance, HFOV-induced apnea can be disrupted by increasing of the chemical drive to breathe (Thompson et al., 1981; Banzett et al., 1983), by both light and very deep levels of anesthesia (Banzett et al., 1983), and by thermal panting (Banzett et al., 1983). Sleep state also has a marked influence. The reflex could not be elicited in chronically tracheostomized dogs when they were either fully awake or in phasic REM sleep, whereas it was elicited during quiet wakefulness and non-REM sleep (England et al., 1983).

Mucociliary Transport

Evidence suggests that the HFOV delivery method may be important in determining its effect on lung mucociliary transport. In anesthetized, intubated dogs,

McEvoy et al. (1982a) showed a significant reduction in the clearance of radioactive label from intrapulmonary airways, during 4 hr of HFOV, compared to CMV (Fig. 3). In their experiments, oscillatory gas flow was generated by a piston pump and directly administered to the upper airway. Excessive mucus was present in the central airway, after 4 hr of HFOV, and its rapid retrograde movement, induced by the high-velocity gas flows of HFOV (Fig. 4), was one possible reason for the reduced radioactive tracer clearance. Work of Armengol et al. (1981a) also suggested that tracheal HFOV may adversely affect tracheal mucus transport. In contrast, HFOV administered by chest-wall compression may enhance both peripheral (Gross et al., 1983) and central airway (King et al., 1983) mucus clearance.

Pulmonary and Systemic Circulations

Regional pulmonary blood flow distribution was not disturbed by HFOV (McEvoy et al., 1982b; Schmid et al., 1981; Gioia et al., 1981b) (Fig. 4). However, in these studies measurements were restricted to only a few oscillatory frequencies (10, 16, 20, and 30 Hz). Different results might conceivably be obtained at rates close to the resonant frequency of the lungs when alveolar pressure may be high (Allen et al., 1983).

Recent experiments conducted in isolated, perfused sheep lungs indicate that HFOV may attenuate hypoxic vasoconstriction by releasing prostacyclin from the lung (Gregory et al., 1983). If confirmed in other species, and in in vivo experiments, these findings will have important implications for the clinical use of HFOV.

Most investigators have found that cardiac output is unchanged during HFOV, compared with CMV at the same Paw (Bohn et al., 1980; McEvoy et al., 1982b; Thompson et al., 1982). There is, however, one brief report of cardiac output reduction with HFOV (Armengol et al., 1981b) and another of progressive metabolic acidosis, systemic hypotension, and bradycardia (Lunkenheimer et al., 1972, 1973). Systemic blood-flow distribution is not changed by HFOV (Gioia et al., 1981a).

Surfactant Metabolism and Lung Stability

Lung pressure-volume curves were unchanged in normal animals after 4-9 hr of HFOV (Frantz et al., 1982; Gillespie et al., 1980). In two studies, the quantity of alveolar surfactant was the same after short periods (1-4 hr) of CMV and HFOV (Ward et al., 1983; Frantz et al., 1982). Our investigations confirmed the absence of deterioration of lung pressure-volume relationships during 4 hr of HFOV in rabbits (unpublished data, Mannino, McEvoy, Hallman, 1981), but surfactant turnover, in the same animals, was considerably affected (Mannino et al., 1982). Disatu-

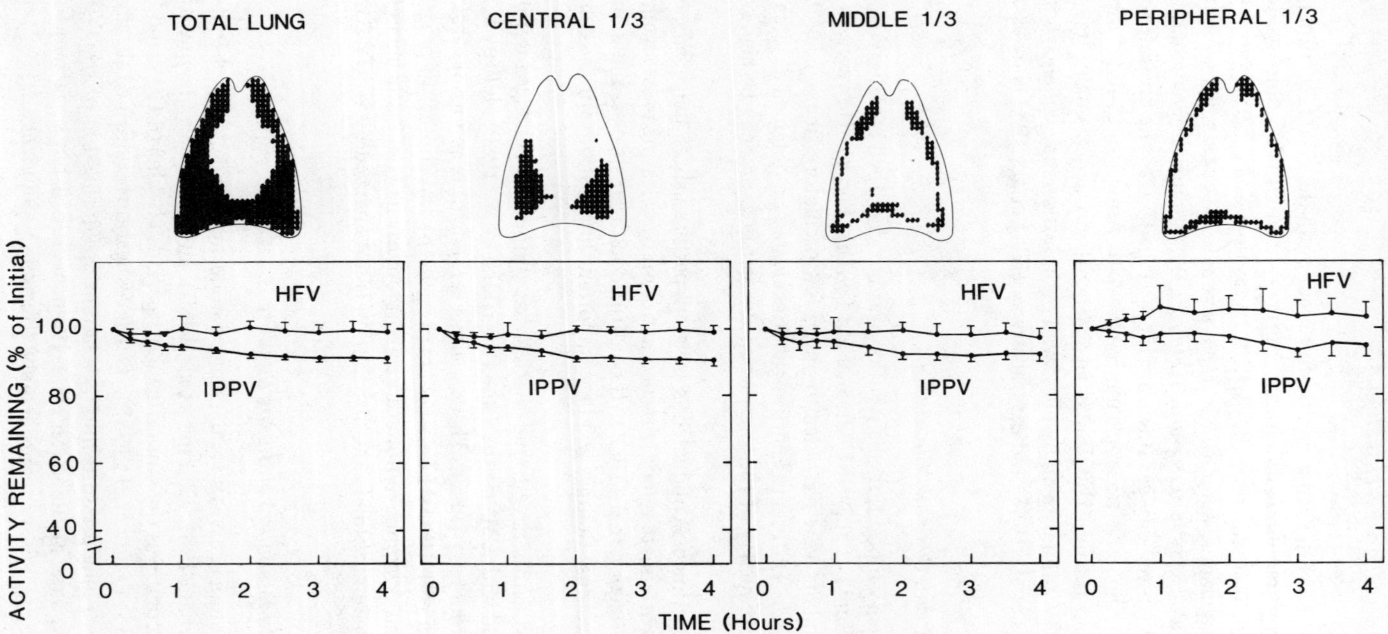

Figure 3 The clearance of radioactive label from airways in three different lung regions is compared with oscillatory ventilation (HFV) and conventional positive-pressure ventilation (IPPV). There was no significant clearance of isotope during HFV, whereas significant clearance occurred in all regions with IPPV (reproduced by permission from McEvoy et al., 1982a).

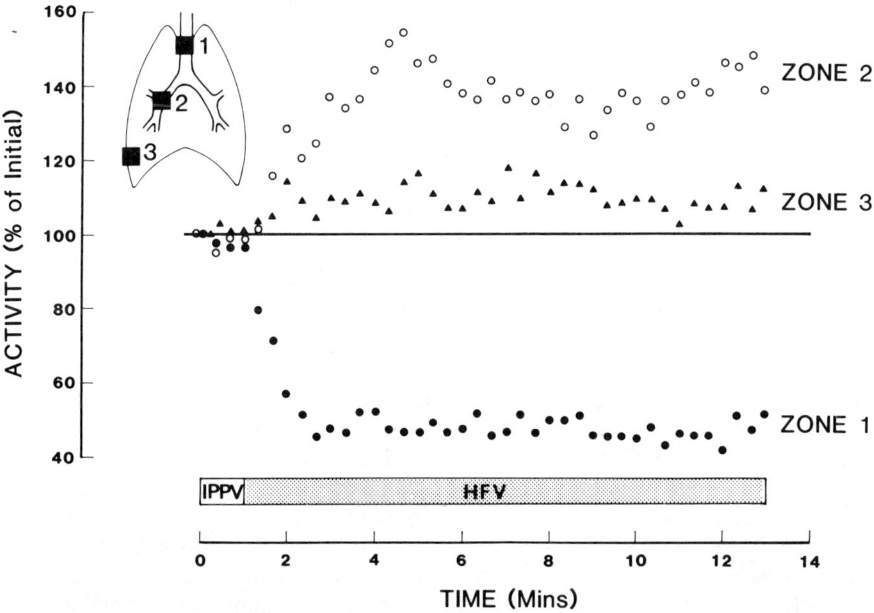

Figure 4 Disposition of a bolus of radioactive tracer, placed on the posterior wall of the trachea (ZONE 1) during oscillatory ventilation (HFV). Within 1 min of initiation of HFV, the tracer moved into the distal airway. It should be noted that this study was performed after 4 hr of HFV. At that time, visual inspection of the central airway revealed excessive secretions. (Reproduced by permission from McEvoy et al., 1982a.)

rated alveolar phosphatidylcholine (DPC, the major active component of surfactant) was reduced after 4 hr of HFOV, compared with CMV-supported and spontaneously breathing animals, while lamellar body DPC was increased. Additional data on surfactant kinetics suggested that these results were due to a greatly increased exchange of DPC between alveoli and pneumocytes (lamellar bodies) (Mannino et al., 1982), rather than a decrease in surfactant release. The significance of this finding is as yet undetermined, but it may indicate that HFOV helps to preserve surfactant function.

Lung Fluid Balance

Preliminary reports indicate that lung lymph flow is reduced during HFOV, compared to CMV and spontaneous breathing (Bland et al., 1980; Mitzner et al., 1981b). Since total lung water is not changed (Frantz et al., 1982) and lymphatic

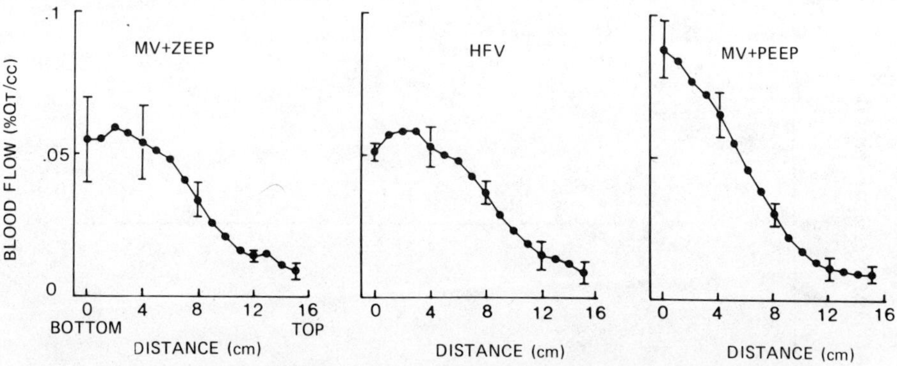

Figure 5 Topographical distribution of pulmonary blood flow plotted for conventional mechanical ventilation (MV) at 0 and 15 cm H_2O end-expiratory pressure (ZEEP and PEEP, respectively) and oscillatory ventilation (HFV). The blood flow distributions were obtained during each intervention by injections of differently labeled radioactive microspheres in three animals. The normal distribution (left panel) shows the typical increase in blood flow from the top to the bottom of the lung with a small decrease in flow in the most dependent portion (ZONE IV). This pattern is undisturbed by HFV (middle panel), but altered markedly and predictably by PEEP (reproduced by permission from McEvoy et al., 1982b).

protein concentration increases (Bland et al., 1982), flow reduction must be the result of decreased fluid filtration.

Other Physiology and Lung Morphology

Camporesi et al. (1982) have demonstrated reflex relaxation of tracheal smooth muscle during HFOV. The strength of such a response may be crucial to gas exchange efficiency in HFOV, since the capacitance of the upper airway may be an important factor determining the percentage of Vt reaching peripheral airways (Rossing et al., 1982).

Lung morphology at both light and ultrastructural level was found to be normal after 4-5 hr of HFOV (Frantz et al., 1982; Frank et al., 1975).

B. The Use of HFOV in Lung Disease

The introduction of positive-pressure mechanical ventilators for routine clinical use in the 1950s and 1960s represented a major advance in the management of severe lung disease (Tyler, 1983), but the new support modality was also accompanied by significant complications (Geer, 1980). Many lung diseases are characterized by large regional differences in compliance and resistance, which may result in severe maldistribution of ventilation during spontaneous breathing. Attempts to treat these abnormalities uniformly with conventional mechanical ventilators, which duplicate physiological frequencies and tidal volumes, are probably illogical and may be dangerous. High airway pressures are often required and complications that may follow include: pneumothorax, pneumomediastinum, and interstitial emphysema (Geer, 1980); reduced cardiac output; and, in neonates, bronchopulmonary dysplasia (Northway, 1977).

A number of researchers have suggested that these problems might be overcome by using devices that deliver higher ventilatory frequencies and smaller tidal volumes, such as HFOV. It was generally believed that high pressure fluctuations at the airway opening in HFOV would rapidly taper in distal airways, perhaps resulting in less barotrauma (Butler et al., 1980). In addition, theoretical studies (Fredberg, 1980) predicted that a major component of gas exchange in HFOV would occur by "augmented diffusion," in which case limitations imposed by abnormal lung mechanics may be less important.

Research has since focused on investigating the role of HFOV in the treatment of diffuse lung injury. One experimental model which has been closely studied is oleic acid-induced pulmonary edema. Early experiments in dogs (Thompson et al., 1982; Meredith et al., 1982) and rabbits (Wright et al., 1981) indicated that adequate oxygenation and CO_2 elimination were possible with HFOV, if mean airway pressures were similar to those generated during CMV (Thompson et al., 1982). However, when constant, positive Paw was maintained during HFOV, progressive hypoxemia sometimes developed (Wright et al., 1981). Similar results were obtained in a baboon model of respiratory distress syndrome (deLemos et al., 1983; Coalson et al., 1983). Intermittent sighs improved gas exchange, but increased the incidence of air leaks (Coalson et al., 1983)

A group of researchers subsequently reconsidered the oleic acid model, extending their observations to a method of producing hyaline membrane disease by repeated alveolar lavage. They looked more critically at the interaction between Paw, mean lung volume, and gas exchange during CMV and HFOV. They specifically drew attention to the marked hysteresis of the lung pressure volume relationship in both disease models and based on their findings, developed a strategy for the use of HFOV (Kolton et al., 1982). When mechanical ventilation was first instituted, as many atelectatic lung units as possible were recruited with a sustained 10-15-sec inflation at 30 cm H_2O of transpulmonary pressure. The lung was then allowed to deflate to a resting Paw 5-10 cm H_2O above critical opening pressure. With this technique, HFOV sustained excellent oxygenation and CO_2 elimination. In contrast, application of CMV at the same Paw, following sustained inflation, resulted in progressive hypoxemia. The investigators argued that the difference was related to progressive collapse of alveoli, when the lungs were subject to wide pressure and volume changes on CMV, whereas on HFOV the lung remained essentially in a position of static inflation. The theory was supported by measurements of lung volume at constant mean airway pressure on HFOV and

CMV. The investigators significantly noted that a progressive increase in PaO_2 occurred on HFOV. Although firm proof could not be obtained, they hypothesized that the finding was related to progressive recruitment of lung units or redistribution of pulmonary edema. The observation gains additional importance, considering that lung injury progressed throughout the experiments. The same investigators conducted further experiments (Hamilton et al., 1983) with a hyaline membrane disease model. After a sustained inflation, animals on HFOV maintained a high PaO_2 without sighs for 20 hr. More significantly, CMV-supported animals developed diffuse hyaline membranes after only 5 hr of ventilation, while animals on HFOV did not.

The significance of these findings for the treatment of diffuse lung injury in neonates and adults is not known. Nevertheless, these data provide justification for systematic, controlled studies in humans (deLemos et al., 1982).

On HFOV, fluid flux across the lung may be reduced. Mayers et al. (1982) postulated that this event might be particularly beneficial in diffuse lung injury, but could not find differences in lung water between two groups of dogs with oleic acid-induced respiratory failure, randomized to either CMV or HFOV.

There is less information on the effectiveness of HFOV in the treatment of other types of lung diseases. Theoretical considerations suggested that HFOV may result in better distribution of ventilation among lung units with uneven time constants and early results in two patients with COPD supported this contention. (Butler et al., 1980).

Additional information was obtained by comparing HFOV and CMV in a model of asthma produced by methacholine aerosol inhalation (Kaiser et al., 1982). This technique creates a population of low V/Q lung units and a small right-to-left intrapulmonary shunt which can be demonstrated by multiple inert gas elimination. HFOV decreased the size of the population of alveoli with low V/Q within 1 hr, consistent with a more homogeneous distribution of ventilation. However, total alveolar ventilation may have been reduced: Prior to aerosol challenge, $PaCO_2$ values had been matched in HFOV and CMV-treated animals by carefully adjusting ventilator settings. Following induction of asthma, $PaCO_2$ values during HFOV were higher than during CMV.

Rossing et al. (1982) measured CO_2 elimination in dogs supported for short periods with HFOV, both before and after histimine infusion. They found that peripheral airway constriction did not affect CO_2 elimination at low $\dot{V}osc$, but CO_2 elimination was reduced at high $\dot{V}osc$. It was postulated that peripheral airway constriction impeded gas penetration into terminal lung units at high $\dot{V}osc$, while increasing the proportion of tidal volume wasted in distention of the upper airway. Other data support this contention (Slutsky, 1983).

The same model of peripheral airway constriction has been studied by Weinmann et al. (1982) with specific reference to the effects of CMV and HFOV on hemodynamic and gas exchange functions. In contrast to the results obtained by Kaiser et al. (1982) with methacholine-induced airway constriction, they were unable to demonstrate any improvement in ventilation-perfusion matching during HFOV, but substantial differences exist between the two models.

Finally, data have been presented on the use of HFOV in the treatment of bronchopleural fistula (Hoff et al., 1981; Mayers et al., 1983) and major airway obstruction (Schmoller et al., 1983). As with high-frequency jet ventilation, HFOV appears highly effective in controlling gas exchange with large fistulae (Hoff et al., 1981; Mayers et al., 1983), particularly in the presence of diffuse lung disease (Mayers et al., 1983). Preliminary results in animals with major airway obstruction are far less encouraging (Schmoller et al., 1983). It should, however, be noted that, in those experiments, the obstruction was placed at the proximal end of a double-lumen bronchial catheter. Gas exchange may be substantially different with partial obstruction of a main bronchus.

III. Conclusion

A number of independent researchers have shown that pulmonary gas exchange can be maintained by high-frequency, low-volume gas oscillations. Devices that provide HFOV vary widely in design. Some apply the gas oscillation directly to the airway; others administer vibration to the chest wall or whole body. No single technique has emerged as clearly superior to another and the field is in rapid evolution. It is conceivable that different ventilatory techniques will prove suited to different clinical situations. Currently there are too many design variations and too few data on gas exchange mechanisms for us to reach firm conclusions on practical application of HFOV. Evidence on the effects of fr, $\dot{V}$t, and Paw is either incomplete or contradictory. HFOV poses unique technical problems related to rapid movement of gas and mechanical components which require an innovative approach to ventilator design.

A number of interesting physiological questions are raised by HFOV. The most obvious addresses the mechanism of gas exchange, when tidal volume is smaller than anatomical deadspace. Physiologists have also been offered a unique opportunity to reexamine the significance of normal and abnormal lung movement on fluid transport, chemical mediator release, surfactant metabolism, and mucus transport.

To the clinician, HFOV is potentially useful as an alternative method of mechanical ventilation in patients with severe lung disease, particularly where conventional positive-pressure ventilators may be ineffective or contraindicated. While some attempts to use HFOV in experimental lung disease have been disappointing, Kolton et al. (1982) demonstrated that good results can be achieved if the unique pathophysiological features of a disease are carefully examined, and management strategy is based on specific properties of HFOV, such as the ability to maintain the lung at a constant volume.

Safety of the technique remains an important issue. Careful microscopic and ultrastructural examination of the lungs after several hours of HFOV has shown no evidence of architectural change, and gas exchange is well-preserved. However, a number of subtle changes have been identified in the vascular response to hypoxia, fluid transport, and mucociliary clearance. It is not clear whether these changes will limit the clinical usefulness of HFOV; further controlled trials of HFOV in normal and diseased lungs are needed.

References

Allen, J. L., Keefe, D. H., Fredberg, J. J., Glass, G. M., and Frantz, I. D. (1983). Alveolar pressures and pulmonary impedance during high frequency oscillation in excised rabbit lungs (abstr.). *Pediatr. Res.* **17**(4):370A).

Armengol, J. A., Man, S. F. P., Logus, J. W., Man, G. C., and King, E. G. (1981a). Effects of high frequency oscillatory ventilation on canine tracheal mucus transport (abstr.). *Crit. Care Med.* **9**(3):192.

Armengol, J. A., Wells, A., Man, G. C. W., and King, E. G. (1981b). Hemodynamic and blood gas effects of high frequency oscillatory ventilation (abstr.). *Crit. Care Med.* **9**(3):192.

Banzett, R., Lehr, J., and Geffroy, B. (1983). High frequency ventilation lengthens expiration in the anesthetized dog. *J. Appl. Physiol.* **55**(2):329-334.

Bitterman, H., Kerem, D. H., Shabtai, Y., Gavriely, N., and Palti, Y. (1983). Respiration maintained by eternally applied vibration and tracheal insufflation in the cat. *Anesth. Analg.* **62**:33-38.

Bland, R. D., Raj. J. H., Hazinski, T. A., Sedin, G. E., and Goldberg, R. B. (1982). Lung fluid balance during vibratory ventilation in lambs (abstr.). *Pediatr. Res.* **16**:280A.

Bohn, D. J., Butler, W., Froese, A. B., and Bryan, A. C. (1979). Ventilation by high frequency oscillation (abstr.). *Fed. Proc.* **38**(3):951.

Bohn, D. J., Miyasaka, K., Marchak, B. E., Thompson, W. K., Froese, A. B., and Bryan, A. C. (1980). Ventilation by high frequency oscillation. *J. Appl. Physiol.* **48**(4):710-716.

Bunnell, J. B., Carlson, K. H., and Shannon, D. C. (1978). High frequency positive pressure ventilation in dogs and rabbits (abstr.). *Am. Rev. Respir. Dis.* **117**:289.

Butler, W. J., Bohn, D. J., Bryan, A. C., and Froese, A. B. (1980). Ventilation by high-frequency oscillation in humans. *Anesth. Analg.* **59**:577-584.

Calverley, P. M. A., Chang, H. K., Wight, D., Vartian, V., Gross, D., and Zidulka,

A. (1983). High frequency chest wall compression assists ventilation and improves gas exchange in normal man (abstr.). *Am. Rev. Respir. Dis.* **127** (4):238.

Camporesi, E. M., Salzano, J. V., and Martel, D. (1982). Airway smooth muscle tone during high frequency ventilation (abstr.). *Fed. Proc.* **41**(4):1358.

Clarke, J. R., Kerem, D., Flynn, E. T., Bradley, M. E., and Homer, L. D. (1983). Wide-band versus discrete excitation during high frequency oscillation (abstr.). *Physiologist* **26**(4):A-35.

Coalson, J. J., Kuehl, T. J., Ackerman, N. B., Escobedo, M. B., Stoddard, R. A., Minnick, L. A., Null, D. M., Robotham, J. L., and DeLemos, R. A., (1983). Air leak syndrome in premature baboons on high frequency ventilation (abstr.). *Am. Rev. Respir. Dis.* **127**(4):211.

deLemos, R. A., Null, D. M., and Meredith, K. S. (1982). High frequency ventilation: Panacea or problem? *Pediatrics* **69**(2):240.

deLemos, R. A., Kuehl, T. J., Null, D. M., Escobedo, M. B., Ackerman, N. B., Minnick, L. A., Stoddard, R. A., Bell, R. E., Yoder, B. A., Coalson, J. J., and Robotham, J. L. (1983). Ventilatory strategy for high frequency ventilation (HFV) of baboons with hyaline membrane disease (HMD) (abstr.). *Pediatr. Res.* **17**(4):310.

El-Baz, N., Faber, L. P., and Doolas, M. D. (1983). Combined high frequency ventilation for management of terminal respiratory failure. A new technique. *Anesth. Analg.* **62**:39-49.

England, S. J., Sullivan, C., Bowes, G., Onayemi, A., and Bryan, A. C. (1983). State related alterations of respiration during high frequency ventilation. (abstr.). *Fed. Proc.* **42**(4):739.

Fletcher, P. R., Epstein, M. A., and Epstein, R. A. (1982). A new ventilator for physiologic studies during high frequency ventilation. *Respir. Physiol.* **47**: 21-37.

Fletcher, P. R., and Epstein, R. A. (1982). Constancy of physiological dead space during high-frequency ventilation. *Respir. Physiol.* **47**:39-49.

Frank, I., Noack, W., Lunkenheimer, P. P., Ising, H., Keller, H., Dickhuth, H. H., Rafflenbeul, W., and Jacobson, M. (1975). Light and electron microscopic investigations of pulmonary tissue after high frequency positive pressure ventilation. *Anesthetist* **24**:171-176.

Frantz, I. D., Stark, A. R., Davis, J. J., Davies, P., and Kitzmiller, T. J. (1982). High frequency ventilation does not affect pulmonary surfactant, liquid or morphologic features in normal cats. *Am. Rev. Respir. Dis.* **126**:909-913.

Fredberg, J. J. (1980). Augmented diffusion in the airways can support pulmonary gas exchange. *J. Appl. Physiol.* **49**(2):232-238.

Froese, A. B., and Bryan, A. C. (1981). High frequency ventilation. *Am. Rev. Respir. Dis.* **123**:249-250.

Gavriely, N., Solway, J., Slutsky, A. S., Kamm, R. D., Shapiro, A. M., and Drazen, J. M. (1982a). Effect of endotracheal tube on CO_2 elimination by small volume high frequency ventilation in dogs (abstr.). *Am. Rev. Respir. Dis.* **125**(4):232.

Gavriely, N., Solway, J., Slutsky, A. S., Loring, S., Ingram, R. H., and Drazen, J. M. (1982b). Mechanical impedance of endotracheal tubes during high frequency, small tidal volume ventilation (abstr.). *Fed. Proc.* **41**(5):1627.

Geer, R. T. (1980). Mechanical ventilation. In *Pulmonary Diseases and Disorders.* Edited by A. P. Fishman. New York, McGraw Hill, pp. 1607-1617.

Gillespie, D. J., Rodarte, J. R., and Hyatt, R. E. (1980). Respiratory mechanics during ventilation by high frequency oscillation (abstr.). *Physiologist* **23** (4):1.

Gioia, F. R., Harris, A. P., Parker, S. D., Traystman, R. J., and Rogers, M. C. (1981a). Peripheral organ blood flow changes with high frequency oscillation (abstr.). *Physiologist* **24**(4):7.

Gioia, F. R., Rinehart, G., and Rogers, M. C. (1981b). Distribution of pulmonary blood flow accompanying high frequency ventilation (abstr.). *Crit. Care Med.* **9**(3):164.

Goldstein, D., Slutsky, A. S., Ingram, R. H., Westerman, P., Venegas, J., and Drazen, J. (1981). CO_2 elimination by high frequency ventilation (4-10 Hz) in normal subjects. *Am. Rev. Respir. Dis.* **123**:251-255.

Gregory, T. J., Wetzel, R. C., Gordon, J., and Gurtner, G. H. (1983). High frequency ventilation attenuates hypoxic pulmonary vasoconstriction (abstr.). *Fed. Proc.* **42**(33):595.

Gross, D., O'Brien, C., Wight, D., Rosenthall, L., Zudulka, A., and King, M. (1983). Enhanced peripheral mucus clearance with high frequency chest wall compression (abstr.). *Physiologist* **26**(4):A-35.

Harf, A., Legall, R., and Chang, H. K. (1983). Mechanical ventilation with superimposed high frequency oscillation (abstr.). *Am. Rev. Respir. Dis.* **127**(4): 253.

Hamilton, P. P., Onayemi, A., Smyth, J. A., Gillan, J. E., Cutz, E., Froese, A. B., and Bryan, A. C. (1983). Comparison of conventional and high frequency ventilation: oxygenation and lung pathology. *J. Appl. Physiol.* **55**(1):131-138.

Haselton, F. R., and Scherer, P. W. (1980). Bronchial bifurcations and respiratory mass transport. *Science* **204**:69-71.

Hoff, B. H., Wilson, E., Smith, B., Bennett, E., and Philips, W. (1981). Intermittent positive pressure ventilation and high frequency ventilation in dogs with experimental bronchopleural fistulae. *Crit. Care Med.* **11**(8):598-602.

Jackson, A. C., and Vinegar, A. (1979). A technique for measuring frequency response of pressure, volume and flow transducers. *J. Appl. Physiol.* **47**: 462-467.

Johnson, D. L. (1973). Various aspects of infrasound. In *Colloque International sur les Infra-sons.* Edited by L. Pimonow. Paris, Centre National de la Recherche Scientifique, pp. 337-358.

Kaiser, K. G., Davies, N. J. H., Rodriguez-Rosin, R., Bencowitz, H., and Wagner, P. D. (1982). Efficiency of high frequency ventilation in the presence of extensive ventilation/perfusion mismatching (abstr.). *Am. Rev. Respir. Dis.* **125**(4):233.

King, M., Phillips, D., Gross, D., Vartian, V., Chang, H. K., and Zidulka, A. (1983). Enhanced mucus clearance with high frequency chest wall compression. (abstr.). *Am. Rev. Respir. Dis.* **127**(4):166.

Kolton, M., Captran, C. B., Kent, G., Volgyesi, G., Froese, A. B., and Bryan, A. C. (1982). Oxygenation during high frequency ventilation compared with conventional mechanical ventilation in two models of lung injury. *Anesth. Analg.* **61**:223-232.

Lehr, J. (1980). Circulating currents during high frequency ventilation (abstr.). *Fed. Proc.* **39**(3):576.

Lehr, J. L., Drazen, J. M., Westerman, P. A., and Zatz, S. L. (1982). Regional expansion of excised dog lungs during high frequency ventilation. *Fed. Proc.* **41**(5):1747.

Lunkenheimer, P. P., Frank, I., Rafflenbeul, W., Dickhut, H. H., Keller, H., and Fuhrmann, C. (1972). Application of transtracheal pressure oscillations as a modification of "diffusion respiration" (letter). *Br. J. Anaesth.* **44**:627.

Lunkenheimer, P. P., Frank, I., Ising, H., Keller, H., and Dickhut, H. H. (1973). Intrapulmonaler gaswechsel unter simulierter apnoe durch transtrachealer, periodischen intrathorakaler druckwechsel. *Anesthetist* **22**:232-237.

McEvoy, R. D., Davies, N. J. H., Hedenstierna, G., Hartman, M. T., Spragg, R. G., Wagner, P. D. (1982a). Lung mucociliary transport during high frequency ventilation. *Am. Rev. Respir. Dis.* **126**:452-456

McEvoy, R. D., Davies, N. J. H., Mannino, F. L., Prutow, R. J., Schumacker, P. T., Wagner, P. D., and West, J. B. (1982b). Pulmonary gas exchange during high frequency ventilation. *J. Appl. Physiol.* **52**(5):1278-1287.

Man, G. C. W., Man, S. F. P., and Kappagoda, G. T. (1983). Effects of high frequency oscillatory ventilation on vagal and phrenic nerve activities. *J. Appl. Physiol.* **54**(2):502-507.

Mannino, F. L., McEvoy, R. D., and Hallman, M. (1982). Surfactant turnover in high frequency oscillatory ventilation (abstr.). *Pediatr. Res.* **16**:356A.

Mayers, I., Sandoval, J., Breen, P. H., Oppenheimer, L., and Wood, L. D. H. (1982). The effect of high frequency oscillatory ventilation on extravascular lung water (abstr.). *Fed. Proc.* **41**(4):1247.

Mayers, I., Breen, P. H., Long, G. R., and Wood, L. D. H. (1983). Canine bronchopleural fistula in low pressure pulmonary edema: High frequency oscillatory ventilation versus intermittent positive pressure ventilation (abstr.). *Am. Rev. Respir. Dis.* **127**(4):103.

Meredith, K., Walsh, W., Ackerman, N., Stoddard, R., Bell, R., Null, D., and Delemos, R. (1982). High frequency oscillatory ventilation as the initial ventilatory mode in diffuse alveolar disease (abstr.). *Pediatr. Res.* **16**:356.

Mitzner, W., Ngeow, Y. K., and Caguicla, N. (1981a). Optimization of high frequency ventilation (abstr.). *Physiologist* **24**(4):384.

Mitzner, W., Sylvester, J. T., and Permutt, S. (1981b). Effects of ventilation on lymph flow from the isolated perfused lamb lung (abstr.). *Physiologist* **24**(4):54.

Ngeow, Y. K., and Mitzner, W. (1982). A new system for ventilating with high frequency oscillation. *J. Appl. Physiol.* **53**(6):1638-1642.

Northway, W. H. (1979). Observations on bronchopulmonary dysplasia. *Pediatrics* **95**(5):815-819.

Okamoto, K. (1981). Superimposition of a high frequency jet oscillation on the convention mechanical ventilation. *Jpn. J. Anesth.* **30**(9):911-919.

Paloski, W. H., Barie, P. S., Mullins, R. J., and Newell, J. C. (1981). Effects of asymmetric waveforms on CO2 elimination during high frequency ventilation (abstr.). *Physiologist* **24**(4):7.

Rossing, T. H., Slutsky, A. S., Lehr, J. L., Drinker, P. A., Kamm, R., and Drazen, J. M. (1981). Tidal volume and frequency dependence of carbon dioxide elimination by high frequency ventilation. *N. Engl. J. Med.* **305**:1375-1379.

Rossing, T. H., Slutsky, A. S., Ingram, R. H., Kamm, R. D., Shapiro, A. H., and Drazen, J. M. (1982). CO2 elimination by high frequency oscillations in dogs—effects of histamine infusion. *J. Appl. Physiol.* **53**(5):1256-1262.

Sohmid, E. R., Knopp, T. J., and Rehder, K. (1981). Intrapulmonary gas transport and perfusion during high frequency oscillation. *J. Appl. Physiol.* **51**(6):1507-1514.

Schmoller, T., Schumacker, P. T., Wagner, P. D., and West, J. B. (1983). Effects of high frequency ventilation on gas exchange during partial obstruction of the left lung (abstr.). *Fed. Proc.* **42**(4):993.

Slutsky, A. S. (1983). Film demonstrating rapid oscillatory distentions of central airways. In *Proceedings of International Symposium on High Frequency Ventilation.* New York, Memorial Sloan-Kettering Cancer Center, pp. 7-8.

Slutsky, A. S., Drazen, J. M., Ingram, R. H., Kamm, R. D., Shapiro, A. H., Fredberg, J. J., Loring, S. H., and Lehr, J. (1980). Effective pulmonary ventilation with small-volume oscillations at high frequency. *Science* **209**:609-611.

Slutsky, A. S., Kamm, R. D., Rossing, T. H., Loring, S. H., Lehr, J., Shapiro, A. H., Ingram, R. H., and Drazen, J. M. (1981). Effects of frequency, tidal volume and lung volume on CO2 elimination in dogs by high frequency (2-30 Hz) low tidal volume ventilation. *J. Clin. Invest.* **68**:1475-1484.

Thompson, W. K., Marchak, B. E., Bryan, A. C., and Froese, A. B. (1981).

Vagotomy reverses apnea induced by high frequency oscillatory ventilation. *J. Appl. Physiol.* **51**(6):1484-1487.

Thompson, W. K., Marchak, B. E., Froese, A. B., and Bryan, A. C. (1982). High frequency oscillation compared with standard ventilation in pulmonary injury model. *J. Appl. Physiol.* **52**(3):543-548.

Tyler, D. C. (1983). Positive end-expiratory pressure: A review. *Crit. Care Med.* **11**(4):300-308.

Ward, H. E., Power, J. H. T., and Nicholas, T. E. (1983). High frequency oscillations via the pleural surface: An alternative mode of ventilation? *J. Appl. Physiol.* **54**(2):427-433.

Weinmann, G., Simon, B., and Mitzner, W. (1982). Lung stability and gas exchange on conventional ventilation and high frequency ventilation during normal and abnormal lung states (abstr.). *Fed. Proc.* **41**(5):1747.

Wozniak, J. A., Davenport, P. W., and Kosch, P. C. (1983). The response of pulmonary afferents to high frequency oscillatory ventilation (abstr.). *Fed. Proc.* **42**(4):1016.

Wright, K., Lyrene, R. K., Truog, W. E., Standaert, T. A., Murphy, J., and Woodrum, D. E. (1981). Ventilation by high frequency oscillation in rabbits with oleic acid lung disease. *J. Appl. Physiol.* **50**(5):1056-1060.

Zidulka, A., Gross, D., Minami, H., Vartian, V., and Chang, H. K. (1983). Ventilation by high frequency chest wall compression in dogs with normal lungs. *Am. Rev. Respir. Dis.* **127**:709-713.

13

Clinical Applications of High-Frequency Oscillation in Children and Adults

NEEL B. ACKERMAN, JR.*
ROBERT A. deLEMOS

Wilford Hall U.S. Air Force Medical Center
San Antonio, Texas

NABIL M. I. EL-BAZ

Rush Medical College
Rush Presbyterian-St. Luke's Medical Center
Chicago, Illinois

I. Clinical Use of High-Frequency Oscillation in Neonates

Neel B. Ackerman, Jr. and Robert A. deLemos

In 1967 Scotter and co-workers, in a series of agricultural studies of gas diffusion into soil, noted that oxcillatory gas flow enhanced gas dispersion into soil and other porous materials. These observations, coupled with those of Lunkenheimer et al. (1973) that adequate ventilation could be maintained for long periods in anesthetized paralyzed dogs by oscillating a loudspeaker diaphragm at the airway, at rates up to 50 Hz, led to the current interest in high-frequency oscillatory ventilation (HFOV).

After Lunkenheimer et al.'s observations, many investigators demonstrated the efficacy of a variety of piston or diaphragm sinusoidal gas flow generators in maintaining normal oxygenation and ventilation in experimental animals and humans using tidal volumes less than anatomical dead space. (Kolton et al., 1982b;

The opinions expressed herein are those of the authors and are not necessarily those of the Department of the Air Force or the Department of Defense.

**Present affiliation:* U.S. Air Force School of Aerospace Medicine, Brooks Air Force Base, San Antonio, Texas.

Slutsky et al., 1980; Thompson et al., 1982; Kuehl et al., 1984; Butler et al., 1980; Marchak et al., 1981; Rossing et al., 1981). The possibility of high-frequency ventilation with small tidal volumes incited great interest both among respiratory physiologists and clinicians. This innovative new technique, it was thought, might reduce many of the complications of assisted ventilation, especially in the premature infant.

In spite of dramatic improvement in the survival of premature infants with hyaline membrane disease who were treated with positive-pressure ventilation and continuous positive airway pressure (PPV/PEEP), patients in many institutions continue to experience ventilator-associated pulmonary complications. Although the precise roles of baroinjury and oxygen toxicity in bronchopulmonary dysplasia have not been determined, most investigators believe that high airway pressures play a significant role in the production of airway injury.

If the airways function as a series of rigid tubes of decreasing diameter, downstream pressures would be expected to fall as respiratory frequency increases or tidal volume decreases. Thus, observations that HFOV could result in adequate oxygenation and ventilation in a variety of short-term animal and human experiments led to the enthusiastic belief that this novel ventilatory technique might lessen the risk of pulmonary baroinjury (Kolton et al., 1982b; Thompson et al., 1982; Kuehl et al., 1984; Butler et al., 1980; Marchak et al., 1981; Slutsky et al., 1981; James, 1983).

This chapter will explore the clinical and experimental evidence for the use of HFOV in the newborn and older child with respiratory disease that requires ventilatory support.

II. Equipment Design Considerations

An oscillator displaces gas equally in an antegrade and retrograde manner and, in essence, delivers no net forward flow. Unlike high-frequency jet ventilation or high-frequency positive pressure ventilation, no net bulk flow of gas occurs. A source of fresh or bias gas must be introduced between the oscillator and the lung to compensate for the metabolic removal of oxygen by the patient. A mechanism is also required to remove carbon dioxide excreted into the ventilator circuit. Finally, a mechanism to control the mean ventilatory pressure and the waveform amplitude is necessary.

The oscillations can be delivered by a piston pump or by a variety of diaphragmlike devices. Delivered volumes may be regulated mechanically or electronically. The mechanically regulated piston oscillators are most often preferred for research purposes, where precise knowledge of oscillatory volume is desirable. Electronically controlled oscillators are more useful in clinical situations where frequent and rapid adjustments in volume are often needed and specific measurement of oscillatory volume is less critical.

The need to add bias flow to HFOV systems complicates ventilatory circuit design. While a few workers have designed systems that add oxygen and remove CO_2 as they are respectively consumed and produced, the engineering, operation, and maintenance of these systems make them unwieldy in clinical situations (Ngeow and Mitzner, 1982). Consequently, most investigators have developed systems in which fresh gas flow is added in excess of the metabolic demands of the subject being ventilated. This requires either constant removal of gas or creation of an "open" circuit. Although some ventilators allow a constant, controlled vacuum to remove excess gas, the most common option is an "open" circuit, obtained by adding a low-pass filter. This consists of a length of tubing of variable resistance which limits gas egress during the positive oscillatory phase and allows passive gas flow during other phases of the cycle.

Most oscillators rely on an open delivery system with the mean airway pressure (and mean lung volume) determined by the relationships between bias flow, resistance through the exhalation limb, and lung compliance and resistance. Both the rate of bias flow and its position of entry in the delivery circle as well as the delivered oscillatory tidal volume, will influence CO_2 elimination ($\dot{V}CO_2$) and mean lung volume (Rossing et al., 1981; Slutsky et al., 1981; Goldstein et al., 1981; Ngeow and Mitzner, 1982; Rieke et al., 1983). Although there is some evidence that placement of the bias flow port directly into the endotracheal tube increases $\dot{V}CO_2$ significantly in adults, this configuration may result in inadvertent lung overdistention in infants and small animals (Rossing et al., 1983). Humidification of inspired gas is relatively easy during HFOV since only the bias flow gas need pass through the humidifier. Consequently, the same humidification devices can be used that are employed with conventional positive-pressure ventilators. Finally, it should be noted that, unlike conventional positive-pressure ventilators, relatively minor changes in delivery circle design in oscillatory devices may result in substantial changes in ventilator function. Thus, each change should be followed by in vivo testing to assess its effect.

III. Effect of Ventilatory Adjustments on Ventilation and Oxygenation

Mean airway pressure (MAP) and lung volume are determined by a combination of bias flow rate, lung compliance and resistance, and the resistance to gas egress in the system. In subjects with diffuse alveolar injury or edema and large intrapulmonary shunts, oxygenation is related to mean lung volume and MAP (Kolton et al., 1982b; Thompson et al., 1982; Kuehl et al., 1984; Marchak et al., 1981; Saari et al., 1984; Brusasco et al., 1984). With most oscillators, adjustment of either the bias flow rate or a variable resistance at the exhalation port will allow manipulation of the MAP to obtain an optimal alveolar/arterial PO_2 ratio (a/A ratio). At higher flow rates or in situations where resistance to gas egress is high, a long I/E ratio may result in an inadvertent increase in lung volume, particularly at the higher frequencies (Saari et al., 1984). This may pose a significant problem in small infants with hyaline membrane disease, in whom high resistance across the endotracheal tube and airways predispose to lung overdistention as compliance improves during the recovery period. At any given frequency, $\dot{V}CO_2$ is a function of oscillatory amplitude or tidal volume. While it is difficult to measure delivered tidal volume precisely in open systems, an increase in diaphragm or piston excursion at the same frequency usually results in a corresponding increase in $\dot{V}CO_2$.

There is considerable debate about the optimal frequency during HFOV. At frequencies under 4-5 Hz there is an increase in $\dot{V}CO_2$ with increasing ventilatory rate *provided* V_t *is constant* (Rossing, 1983). Above 5 Hz, optimal frequencies appear related to the resonance characteristics of both the oscillator and the lung. For practical purposes, the optimal frequency depends upon the therapeutic goal. If the clinical endpoint is the lowest possible pCO_2, then a frequency below 5 Hz is probably desirable. If HFOV is used to prevent or treat barotrauma, the aim should be to minimize peak airway pressure, which is accomplished by using the highest respiratory frequency that results in acceptable PCO_2 (Dorkin et al., 1983). In general, ventilator adjustment during HFOV at any given frequency is similar to adjustment of conventional ventilators, with Vt affecting $\dot{V}CO_2$ and the MAP determining the optimal a/A ratio. The choice of frequency depends upon the therapeutic goals.

IV. Choice of a High-Frequency System: Comparison Between HFOV and HFPPV in Infants and Children

Several types of HFV systems are currently being evaluated for use in infants and children. The oscillator has particular applicability because piston size (and thus delivered tidal volume) is not a critical problem in the small patient, and ventilation can be accomplished via a standard endotracheal or tracheostomy tube. Adjustment of mean airway pressure is relatively simple and problems of tracheal injury, humidification, and inadvertent pulmonary overdistention are less common than with other high-frequency techniques. All other nonoscillator high-frequency devices use some variation of mechanical flow interruption to gate delivery of gas under pressure. Tidal volume delivered is dependent on the gas flow and duration of each pulse.

Jet ventilators deliver gas pulses directly into the airway. These devices have the advantages of being simple to design and operate and are the only high-frequency ventilators capable of maintaining support in a sick adult (Carlon et al., 1981a,b). Humidification is a difficult problem particularly in small children where entrainment gas may be a negligible part of the total delivered volume. Tracheal erosion and obstruction have been reported in small animals, children, and adults, but this has been minimized by better humidification systems and lower flow velocities (Nordin et al., 1981, 1982; Pokora et al., 1983a,b; Meeuwis et al., 1983; Ophoven et al., 1983). Lung overdistention may be a major problem in infants on jet ventilators; it results in decreased cardiac output, pulmonary hypertension, and barotrauma (Nordin et al., 1981; Pokora et al., 1983b; Ophoven et al., 1983).

Flow interrupters are similar to jet ventilators except that the high-velocity gas jet enters a portion of the ventilator circuit proximal to the end of the endotracheal tube. This "set-back" configuration reduces peak flow velocity during inspiration. The use of synchronized valving in some of these devices also allows the creation of a "closed circuit" which facilitates larger tidal volume delivery to the distal airways. Although problems related to poor control of lung volume represent an area of difficulty, and maximum effective ventilatory rates are lower than those effective with HFOV, these devices have received the widest clinical use in infants to date.

V. Clinical Applications

A. Hyaline Membrane Disease

Marchak et al. (1981) laid the foundation for future attempts to use HFOV in hyaline membrane disease when they used a piston ventilator to support eight neonates with severe respiratory distress syndrome at frequencies from 8 to 20 Hz. These early results encouraged other investigators to study the effects of HFOV in humans and experimental animals with HMD (Kolton et al., 1982b; Kuehl et al., 1982, 1984; Marchak et al., 1981; James, 1983; Dorkin et al., 1983; Truog et al., 1083; Boyton et al., 1983; Ackerman et al., 1983, 1984a). Early publications on HFOV theorized that baroinjury might be lower when this technique was used in the treatment of premature infants with HMD (Marchak et al., 1981; Rossing, 1983). Short-term experiments in rabbits, baboons, and human premature infants suggested that ventilation with HFOV resulted in better oxygenation and ventilation than conventional ventilation, at lower mean airway pressure (Thompson et al., 1982; Marchak et al., 1981; Kuehl et al., 1982). Since it was presumed that peak downstream pressures would also be lower during HFOV, a great deal of enthusiasm developed for widespread clinical application.

Although premature baboons with HMD did well for short periods with HFOV alone, attempts to maintain them over longer intervals resulted in progressive alveolar collapse, hypercarbia, and hypoxemia (Ackerman et al., 1983, 1984a). Similar findings were observed in human neonates. The combination of HFOV with a carefully controlled "sigh" resulted in a more stable clinical course and prevented progressive atelectasis (Kuehl et al., 1984; Ackerman et al., 1983). Controlled clinical trials in the premature baboon, for periods of 24 and 96 hr, showed that animals treated with HFOV had more rapid saccular recruitment, resulting in lower oxygen requirements at lower mean airway pressure, compared to conventional ventilatory techniques. These differences were most marked in the first 12 hr; by 96 hr there were no clinical differences between the groups (Bell et al., 1984). At this time there is solid experimental evidence that the combination of HFOV and an intermittent sigh results in earlier saccular opening at a lower proximal mean airway pressure. Although FiO_2 can be decreased early, there is no evidence that ventilator-associated lung injuries are also decreased. Direct measurements of alveolar pressure during HFOV have shown that, under certain circumstances, they may be higher than proximal airway pressures (Allen et al., 1983). Therefore, final proof of the efficacy of HFOV in hyaline membrane disease will have to await animal studies of longer duration or controlled human trials.

B. Air Leak

Good clinical and experimental evidence supports the role of HFOV in infants and children with pulmonary interstitial emphysema (PIE) and bronchopleural fistulae. At the higher frequencies, intraluminal peak airway pressures fall and, if a patient can be adequately oxygenated and ventilated at these frequencies, the volume of air exiting from the airway should diminish. There is extensive clinical experience with high-frequency ventilation in infants with PIE, although most of the published data have not been with HFOV (Frantz et al., 1983; Ng and Easa, 1979; Harris, 1983). In theory, the higher the frequency, the less the volume of air leak and the more rapid the resorption of the interstitial air. Since oscillators are more efficient at the higher frequencies than other high-frequency ventilators, they should have particular applicability in these situations.

C. Pulmonary Hypoplasia

A number of infants with pulmonary hypoplasia have been successfully ventilated with HFOV. However, no controlled studies in animals or humans have been conducted. To date there is no evidence that long-term survival has improved in these infants.

D. Surgical Indications

At extremely high frequencies, transmission of pulmonary pressure is negligible. Thus, it is theoretically possible to operate in a virtually motionless field. This may ultimately prove to be advantageous in various forms of microsurgery.

E. Combinations of HFOV and Conventional Ventilation

The superimposition of an oscillatory waveform on a conventional respiratory cycle improves CO_2 elimination and lessens the requirement for positive-pressure ventilation (Boynton et al., 1983; El-Baz et al., 1983b; Harf et al., 1983). This combined technique has been used successfully to treat infants with HMD and other respiratory diseases. While it does reduce the requirement for conventional ventilation, there is no direct evidence that it reduces the incidence of ventilator-associated pulmonary injury.

VI. Complications

There are few long-term clinical or animal data on HFOV. Infant baboons with hyaline membrane disease ventilated for 96 hr with HFOV have been shown to have an unusual multilayered surfactant at necropsy (Ackerman et al., 1984b). The functional and clinical significance of this is unclear. The livers of these animals had fatty change and some hepatic venous engorgement (Coalson, personal communication, 1984). It is possible that the absence of physiological alveolar wall motion described during high-frequency oscillation of excised lungs may alter pressure receptors and some feedback mechanisms. Further long-term studies in suitable animal models will be needed to explore these and other possible issues of toxicity.

The ability of the clinician to choose optimum ventilatory settings during HFOV is complicated by the relative lack of chest-wall movement. The advantage of direct observation of the chest wall rising and falling, to help assess adequate gas exchange, is not available. It is possible therefore to err inadvertently on both the low and high sides of optimum lung volume. If too low a mean lung volume is chosen, progressive alveolar collapse may develop; in our experience this decrease in functional residual capacity may not be clinically apparent for several hours. Conversely, it is relatively easy to pick ventilatory settings that maintain the lung at large constant volumes. Decreased cardiac output and baroinjury can be expected at this end of the spectrum. We feel that one should continuously monitor pO_2 and pCO_2 in order to adjust ventilatory parameters adequately during HFOV. Devices that monitor mean lung volume continuously during HFOV will probably prove very valuable.

Pulmonary vasculature resistance is increased during lung expansion with PPV/PEEP. In patients with left-to-right cardiac shunts, such as infants with a patent ductus arteriosus (PDA), the use of conventional ventilatory techniques artificially elevates the pulmonary vascular resistance and reduces the left-to-right flow. This phenomenon is reduced or absent during HFOV where the lung is kept close to its mean volume. The presence of PDA in infants with HMD may prove to be a significant clinical problem during HFOV (Ackerman et al., 1984b).

Finally, the effect of low tidal volume breathing on respiratory centers and pulmonary stretch receptors is unknown. Consequences of long-term HFOV on the developing neural center of the premature are also unknown, although some investigators have observed the production of apnea during HFOV apparently related to neural mechanisms (Man et al., 1983; Thompson et al., 1981; Jonzon, 1977; England et al., 1984).

VII. Clinical Use in Adults

Nabil M. I. El-Baz

Adult respiratory distress syndrome (ARDS) describes complex pulmonary changes resulting from many different causes. ARDS is associated with widespread damage to alveoli, airways, and pulmonary capillaries. This causes inefficient gas exchange as a result of high airway resistance, low lung compliance, pulmonary edema, and alteration of pulmonary perfusion. The normal mechanics of breathing fail to provide adequate tidal volume, proper gas distribution, and efficient gas diffusion, precipitating progressive hypoxemia and hypercarbia.

Conventional intermittent positive-pressure ventilation (IPPV) was developed 30 years ago to duplicate the natural pattern of breathing by delivering a large tidal volume at a low respiratory rate (Kirby et al., 1975a; Downs et al., 1970; Lyager, 1970). Although this approach has proved safe and effective in the treatment of most forms of ARDS, the technique frequently fails to achieve adequate gas exchange in severe ARDS, despite the addition of high levels of positive end-expiratory pressure (PEEP).

Extracorporeal membrane oxygenators (ECMO) have been evaluated as an alternative approach. ECMO has been successful in providing adequate gas exchange in patients with severe ARDS, allowing time for the diseased lungs to heal. The complications associated with arterial and venous cannulation, systemic heparinization, and prolonged use of a perfusion pump have severely limited the value and applications of this technique for treatment of respiratory failure (Gallagher and Civetta, 1980; Qvist et al., 1975).

In an effort to provide adequate gas exchange in patients with severe ARDS, new techniques have been developed, generally defined as "high-frequency ventilation."

Many different modalities of high-frequency ventilation exist, and most of them are discussed and evaluated in this book. This section primarily discusses a method of combining two modalities of high-frequency ventilation to reap the benefits of both techniques, while minimizing their complications.

VIII. Treatment of Severe Respiratory Failure

HFOV was first used at our institution in five patients, aged 38-57 years, who had severe ARDS, as a result of various causes (postoperative pneumonia, septic shock, multiple trauma, chemotherapy lung toxicity). The patients developed progressive hypoxemia (PaO_2 below 45 mmHg) and death was imminent, despite maximal support with conventional mechanical ventilation (Table 1). HFV was used as an emergency life-saving measure; in two patients it was instituted during cardiac resuscitation.

HFV was initially delivered at a respiratory rate of 250 breaths/min, gas source pressure (driving pressure, DP) of 50 psi, and percentage insufflation time (IT%) of 50%. Respiratory rate was then progressively increased to 500, 1000, 2000, 3000, 4000, and 5000 breaths/min. Patients were maintained at each respiratory setting for 6-8 hr. HFV was delivered to these patients through a pneumatic ventilator, which is similar in design to HFOV unit of CHFV ventilator described in detail below.

Oxygenation significantly improved during HFV and was linearly related to the frequency used. PaO_2 was 53 ± 6 (SD) mmHg on 250 breaths/min, and progressively increased to 223 ± 57 mmHg at a respiratory rate of 5000 breaths/min. This significant improvement of oxygenation was probably the combined results of better gas distribution, greater gas diffusion, and enhanced ventilation/perfusion matching. The turbulent flow of HFOV provided efficient gas mixing and distribution at a low mean airway pressure, following the physical model discussed in Chapter 3 (Sec. VI). HFV was also associated with significant improvement of cardiovascular functions and cardiac output. Despite adequate oxygenation, CO_2 elimination was impaired and all patients developed severe respiratory acidosis. This complication was attributed to significant rebreathing during HFOV and unidirectional (downward) acceleration of gas diffusion. The hypercarbia of HFOV occurred after 24-48 hr in these

Table 1 Terminal Respiratory Failure Conventional Ventilation (IPPV)

PaO_2	
Tidal volume	20-30 ml/kg
Respiratory rate	20-40/min
PEEP	20-30 cm H_2O
FiO_2	1.0

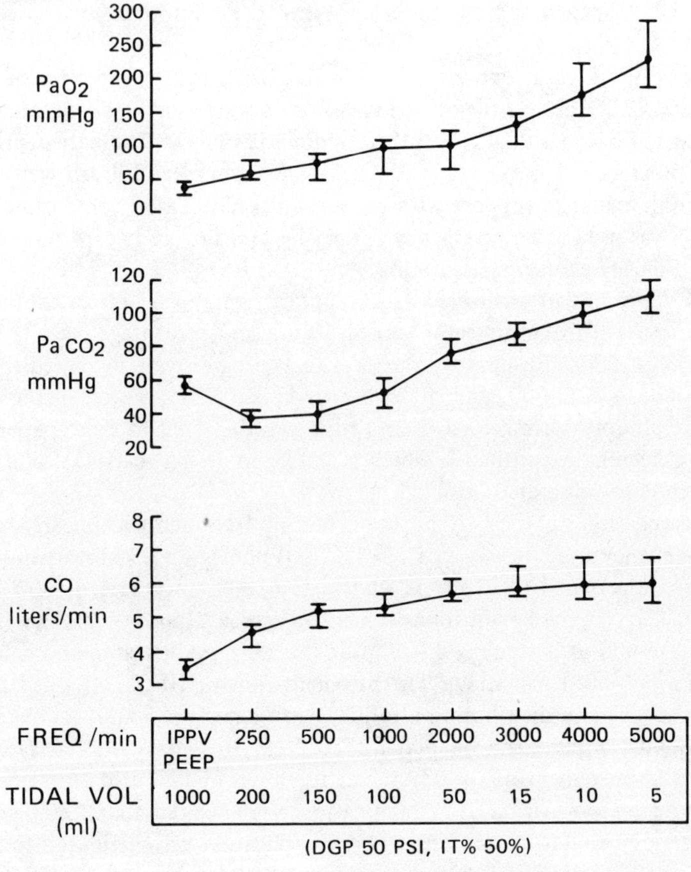

Figure 1 High-frequency ventilation for terminal respiratory failure.

patients. This delay is probably the result of the resumption of spontaneous breathing after discontinuation of muscle relaxants and sedatives which have provided a limited convective flow during HFOV. Figure 1 shows the PaO_2 and cardiac output obtained at various respiratory rates of IPPV and HFOV.

Attempts to deliver larger tidal volumes on HFOV (20-50 ml) in these patients, by increasing DP to 100 psi were associated with extensive barotrauma. Although CO_2 elimination was slightly improved, patients suddenly developed bilateral pneumothorax and pneumomediastinum. Despite immediate placement of chest tubes and reestablishment of IPPV and PEEP, all patients progressed to terminal respiratory failure and died within 6 hr.

The infusion of normal saline into the endotracheal tube, while patients were on HFV, to maintain mucosal humidification and prevent injury to the epithelial layer inadvertently caused mucosal damage. Continuous infusion of normal saline (0.9 sodium chloride) at 30 ml/hr delivered a worrisome amount of sodium (more than 6 g/day). Bronchoscopic examination, on the third day of HFOV, showed black discoloration and extensive crusting of the tracheobronchial mucosa, diagnosed as a chemical burn at autopsy in all patients.

IX. Combined High-Frequency Ventilation in Adults

The initial application of HFOV in patients with severe ARDS was associated with two major complications; inadequate humidification, and CO_2 accumulation with respiratory acidosis. The first problem was solved by incorporating a system to nebulize water; the second by developing a new technique defined as combined high-frequency ventilation (CHFV). This support method is based on the simultaneous administration of high-frequency positive-pressure ventilation (HFPPV) and high-frequency oscillatory ventilation (HFOV), each separately and independently controlled. The combined high-frequency ventilator is based on two pneumatic ventilators, each based on a multiple valve system, controlling a pneumatic solenoid. Rate of operation and duty cycle (percentage of a full cycle during which the valve remains open) can be independently adjusted. The solenoid valve interrupts the flow of gases under pressure, from the source to the patient. The driving gas pressure for each component of CHFV is manually regulated by a single-stage reducing valve. The two units share a common gas output and are synchronized (HFPPV turns off HFOV automatically). The system can generate a respiratory rate of 10-3000 breaths/min. The CHFV ventilator was designed and built in-house. A diagram of the system is shown in Figure 2.

CHFV was evaluated in 10 adult patients, aged 15-19 years, with ARDS of various origins (pneumonia, massive transfusion, aspiration pneumonitis, disseminated vasculitis, and necrotizing alveolitis). They developed terminal respiratory failure and severe progressive hypoxemia (PaO_2 below 50 mmHg), despite maximal respiratory support with IPPV and PEEP. Entry criteria in the HFOV study included a PaO_2 of 50 mmHg, FiO_2 = 1.0, tidal volume or 20 ml/kg, and PEEP of 15 cm H_2O. All patients were admitted and managed in our surgical intensive care unit (SICU) with continuous monitoring of systems and pulmonary pressures. Cardiac output based on by thermodilution and measurements of arterial and mixed venous blood gases measurements was obtained as clinically indicated. The patients required frequent administration of muscle relaxants (pancuronium) and sedatives (diazepam) to facilitate the administration of IPPV and PEEP. Continuous infusions of dopamine (10-20 μg/kg per

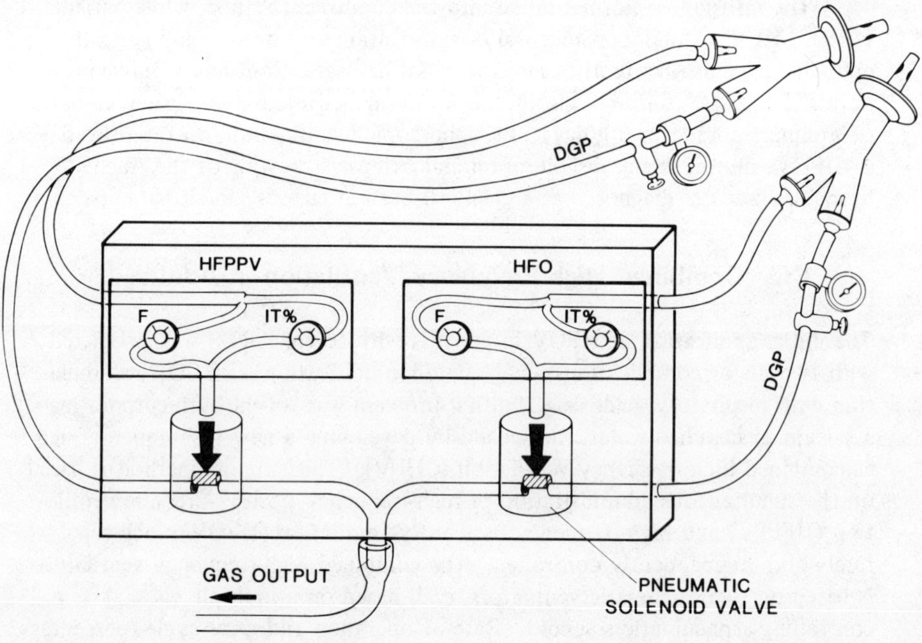

Figure 2 Combined high-frequency ventilator.

min) were also required by all patients, to maintain an acceptable cardiac output on IPPV.

CHFV was evaluated in these patients after they met the criteria of terminal respiratory failure and was compared to IPPV with PEEP, and independently administered HFPPV and HFOV. The three modalities of HFV were administered sequentially to each patient, always beginning with HFPPV, then HFOV, and finally CHFV. Each form of support was used for 24 hr. The same ventilation, tubing, and HFV endotracheal tube adaptor were used in each patient for all types of ventilation. Each patient served as his or her own control. Humidification was provided on HFV by nebulization of warm water. A continuous infusion of 30 ml/hr of distilled water, regulated by a volumetric pump (IMED), was introduced into the endotracheal tube adaptor and nebulized by jets of HFV gases (Fig. 3).

HFPPV was used at a rate of 250 breaths/min, DP psi, IT% 40%, and FiO_2 1.0. HFOV was used on the second day at a frequency of 2000 breaths/min, DP 35 psi, IT% 50%, and FiO_2 1.0. On the third day, CHFV was initiated and continued for 5-21 days. The HFPPV component of CHFV was adminis-

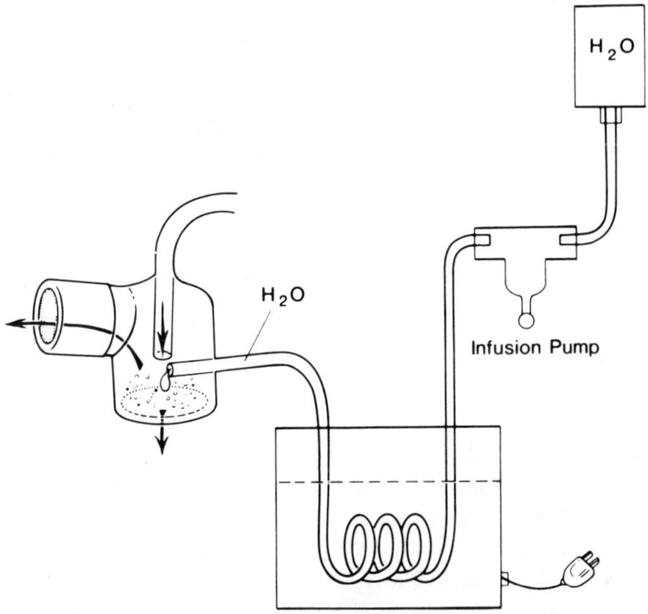

Figure 3 Humidification during combined high-frequency ventilation.

tered at 60 breaths/min, DGP 20 psi, IT% 40%, and FiO_2 1.0. The settings were chosen on the basis of previous experience with this system, and standardized for the purpose of this study.

Our criteria for reestablishment of conventional mechanical ventilation in patients receiving high-frequency ventilation were:

1. PaO_2 above 100 mmHg, with FiO_2 0.4, maintained on CHFV for at least 24 hr
2. Development of any complication directly related to any modality of HFV
3. Inability to improve oxygenation within a few hours of HFV

IPPV was resumed with a tidal volume of 10 ml/kg, respiratory rate 12 breaths/min, PEEP 10 cm H_2O, and FiO_2 0.4.

Initiation of HFV was associated with immediate improvement of oxygenation (Fig. 3). On the first day, HFPPV was associated with a slight improvement of oxygenation and CO_2 elimination was adequate ($PaCO_2$ 30-50 mmHg).

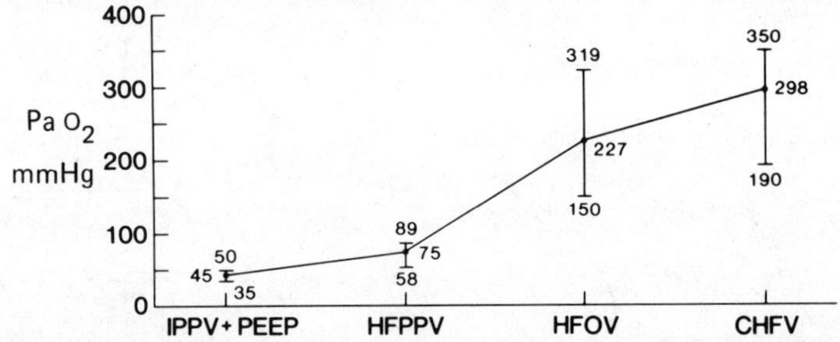

Figure 4 Administration of high-frequency oscillation resulted in a significant improvement in oxygenation.

The following day, administration of high-frequency oscillation was associated with a significant improvement in oxygenation (PaO_2 150-319 mmHg). Nonetheless, HFOV was associated with hypercarbia and respiratory acidosis ($PaCO_2$ 45-99 mmHg). On the third day, application of CHFV was also associated with efficient CO_2 elimination ($PaCO_2$ 24-42 mmHg) (Fig. 4).

Cardiac output (CO) improved significantly in all patients with each modality of HFV (Table 2). On IPPV and PEEP, CO was 4.1 ± 1.3 liters/min, with all patients receiving dopamine (10-20 μg/kg per min). HFPPV was associated with a significant increase of cardiac output (5.9 ± 1.4 liters/min) and CHFV (6 ± 2.1 liters/min). Dopamine was gradually withdrawn, in all patients, after establishment of HFV and was discontinued within 12-24 hr.

All three modalities of HFV were well tolerated by all patients. Muscle relaxation and heavy sedation were not required and all patients were able to

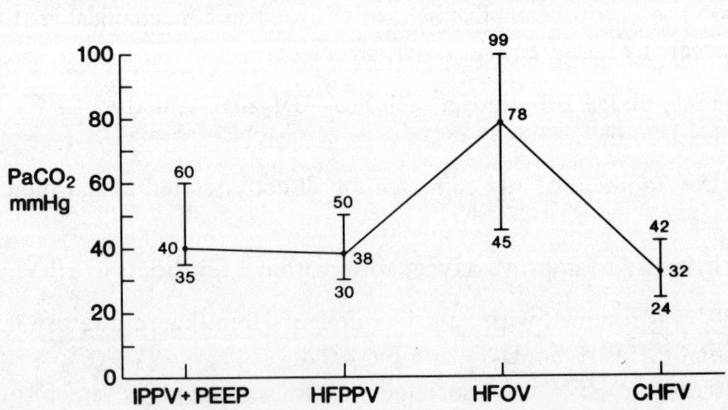

Figure 5 CO_2 elimination with combined high-frequency ventilation.

Table 2 Terminal Respiratory Failure Cardiac Output

IPPV + PEEP + dopamine	4 liters/min
HFPPV	5.9 liters/min
HFO	5.9 liters/min
CHFV	6 liters/min

breathe spontaneously through an open inspiratory circuit. Consciousness was reestablished in all patients, who were able to communicate with their families and the nursing staff. Patients used writing pads, and deflation of the endotracheal tube cuff allowed some vocalization. Improved communication probably provided a psychological gain to patients, families, and ICU staff.

Despite significant improvements in respiratory and cardiac function, eight patients (80%) died as a result of multisystem failure. They received CHFV for 5-21 days. Postmortem lung examination showed extensive consolidation, lack of aeration, and disseminated necrotizing alveolitis. The other two patients continued to improve. They received CHFV for 5 days, then successfully met the criteria for reestablishment of conventional ventilation. One of them required repeated abdominal surgical procedures, while receiving IPPV and PEEP, and he developed peritonitis followed by hepatic and renal failure, and died 3 months after the application of CHFV. The other patient progressively improved, was successfully weaned and extubated, and left the hospital alive. Table 3 summarizes respiratory and cardiac variables of these two patients during the last hour of CHFV and after reestablishment of conventional ventilation. FiO_2 was 0.4.

This study showed that CHFV successfully reversed the intractable hypoxemia of terminal respiratory failure, which had not responded to conventional IPPV and PEEP. Although the mechanism by which HFV provided effective gas exchange is not known with certainty, clearly CHFV offers a new approach for pulmonary gas exchange and management of severe respiratory failure (El-Baz et al., 1983a).

CHFV provides two different gas kinetics for O_2 and CO_2. Oxygenation is achieved by acceleration of gas diffusion through the HFOV component of CHFV, as suggested by the difference between PaO_2 values observed on IPPB and HFPPV compared to that during HFOV and CHFV. CO_2 elimination is achieved independently, by convection, through the HFPPV component, as suggested by the significant difference in $PaCO_2$ between HFOV and CHFV. Although PaO_2 and $PaCO_2$ are controlled independently by the component of CHFV, the associated increase in PaO_2 during CHFV, compared to HFOV might be the result of an improvement of gas distribution, gas diffusion, and recruitment of alveoli. The convective flow of HFPPV causes an intermittent increase in peak airway pressure, which may recruit additional alveoli to gas exchange.

Table 3 CHFV Survivals

	CHFV	IPPV + PEEP
PaO_2 (mmHg)	139 ± 14	78 ± 12
PaCO (mmHg)	39 ± 4	41 ± 5
CO (liters/min)	5.3 ± 0.3	4.3 ± 0.7
Q_s/Q_t (%)	12 ± 2	23 ± 7

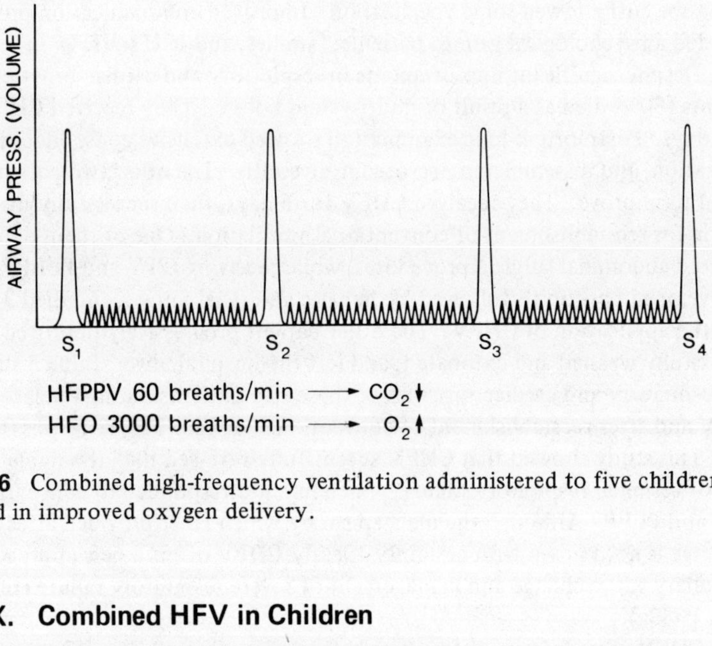

Figure 6 Combined high-frequency ventilation administered to five children resulted in improved oxygen delivery.

X. Combined HFV in Children

CHFV was also evaluated for respiratory support in five children, ages 2 months to 4 years. These patients developed terminal respiratory failure as a result of IRDS, fulminating pneumonia, or multiple trauma. They developed progressive hypoxemia, despite the use of IPPV at respiratory rates between 40 and 60 breaths/min, tidal volumes between 20 and 35 ml/kg, and PEEP between 15 and 25 cm H_2O. PaO_2 was 28-41 mmHg, FiO_2 1.0, and $PaCO_2$ 38-61 mmHg.

These five children received CHFV when death appeared imminent as a result of severe progressive hypoxemia. The HFPPV component of CHFV was administered at a frequency between 40 and 60 breaths/min, driving pressure be-

Table 4 Terminal Respiratory Failure in Pediatric Patients

	IPPV + PEEP		CHFV	
PaO_2 mmHg	32	(28-41)	112	(86-193)
$PaCO_2$ mmHg	43	(38-61	39	(23-41)
CI (liters/min)	1.2	(0.9-1.4)	1.94	(1.2-2.1)

tween 5 and 15 psi, inspiratory time of 0.1 sec. Synchronous HFOV was at a frequency between 1000 and 3000 breaths/min, DP between 10 and 20 psi, IT% 50%. FiO_2 was 1.0.

CHFV achieved adequate oxygenation and alveolar ventilation in all patients (Table 4). PaO_2 during the first 6 hr of CHFV was 86-198 mmHg. CHFV was also associated with significant improvement of cardiac index (Table 4). Despite the improvement of oxygen delivery during CHFV, three patients developed multisystem failure and died within 2-5 days. The other two patients had progressive hypoxemia, despite maximal support with CHFV for 3 and 5 days. Conventional IPPV and PEEP were reestablished in these two young patients after the failure of CHFV to maintain adequate oxygenation. This was associated with further deterioration of oxygenation, cardiorespiratory failure, and both died within 1 hr after reinstitution of IPPV and PEEP.

CHFV achieved adequate gas exchange in all patients, after the failure of conventional methods of ventilation to maintain acceptable oxygenation. Although its application in preterminal patients could not prevent a high mortality rate, results were equal to or better than those achieved with a membrane oxygenator. CHFV accomplished efficient gas exchange, both for oxygenation and CO_2 elimination. This new approach to mechanical ventilation deserves further investigation in different forms of respiratory failure.

References

Ackerman, N. B., Kuehl, T. J., Coalson, J. J., Escobedo, M. B., Stoddard, R. A., Minnick, L., Null, D. M., Robotham, J. L., and deLemos, R. A. (1983). Distal airway rupture during high frequency ventilation (HFV) in the premature baboon with hyaline membrane disease (abstract). *Crit. Care Med.* **11**:223.

Ackerman, N. B., Jr., Coalson, J. J., Kuehl, T. J., Stoddard, R., Minnick, L., Null, D. M., Escobedo, M. B., Robotham, J. L., and deLemos, R. A. (1984a). Pulmonary interstitial emphysema in the premature baboon with hyaline membrane disease. *Crit. Care Med.* **12**(6):512.

Ackerman, N., Jr., Kuehl, T., Mack, J., Stoddard, R., Minnick, L., Yoder, B., Bell, R., Null, D., Jr., Escobedo, M., Robotham, J., and deLemos, R. (1984b). Cardiovascular interactions with high frequency ventilation: preliminary observations in premature baboons with hyaline membrane disease. *Crit. Care Med.* **12**(3):338.

Allen, J. L., Keefe, D. H., Fredberg, J. J., Glass, G. M., and Frantz, I. D. (1983). Alveolar pressure and pulmonary impedance during high frequency oscillation. *Pediatr. Res.* **17**:370A.

Bell, R. E., Kuehl, T. J., Coalson, J. J., Ackerman, N. B., Jr., Null, D. M., Jr., Escobedo, M. B., Yoder, B. A., Cornish, J. D., Nalle, L., Skarin, R. M., Montes, M., Cipriani, C. A., Robotham, J. L., and deLemos, R. A. (1984). High frequency ventilation compared to conventional ventilation in treatment of hyaline membrane disease in primates. *Crit. Care Med.* (in press).

Boynton, B. R., Friederichsen, G., Kopotic, R., and Mannino, F. L. (1983). Combined high frequency oscillatory ventilation and conventional ventilation in neonates. *Crit. Care Med.* **11**:223.

Brusasco, V., Knopp, T. J., Schmid, E. R., and Rehder, K. (1984). Ventilation-perfusion relationship during high frequency ventilation. *J. Appl. Physiol.* **56**:454.

Butler, W. J., Bohn, D. J., Bryan, A. C., and Froese, A. B. (1980). Ventilation by high frequency oscillation in humans. *Anesth. Analg.* **59**:577.

Carolon, G. C., Kahn, R. C., Howland, W. S., Ray, C., and Trunbull, A. D. (1981a). Clinical experience with high frequency jet ventilation. *Crit. Care Med.* **9**:1.

Carlon, G. C., Miodownik, S., Ray, C., and Kahn, R. C. (1981b). Technical aspects and clinical implications of high frequency jet ventilation with a solenoid valve. *Crit. Care Med.* **9**:47.

Dorkin, H. L., Stark, A. R., Werthammer, J. W., Strieder, D. J., Fredberg, J. J., and Frantz, I. D., III. (1983). Respiratory system impotence from 4 to 40 Hz in paralyzed infants with respiratory distress. *J. Clin. Invest.* **72**:903.

Downs, J. B., Klein, E. F., Jr., and Modell, J. H. (1983). The effect of incremental PEEP on PaO_2 in patients with respiratory failure. *Anesth. Analg.* **52**:210.

El-Baz, N., Faber, L. P., and Doolas, A. (1983a). Combined high-frequency ventilation for treatment of terminal respiratory failure; a new technique. *Anesth. Analg.* **62**:39.

El-Baz, N., Penfield, F., and Doolas, A. (1983b). Combined high-frequency ventilation for management of terminal respiratory failure. *Anesth. Analg.* **62**:39.

England, S. J., Onayemi, A., and Bryan, A. C. (1984). Neuromuscular blockade enhances phrenic nerve activity during high-frequency ventilation. *J. Appl. Physiol.* **56**:31.

Frantz, I. D., Werthammer, J., and Stark, A. R. (1983). High frequency ventilation in premature infants with lung disease. Adequate gas exchange at low tracheal pressure. *Pediatrics* **71**:438.

Fredberg, J. J. (1980). Augmented diffusion in the airway can support pulmonary gas exchange. *J. Appl. Physiol.* **49**:232.

Gallagher, J., and Civetta, J. B. (1980). Goal-directed therapy of acute respiratory failure. *Anesth. Analg.* **59**:813.

Goldstein, D., Slutsky, A. S., Ingram, R. H., Westerman, P., Venegas, J., and Drazen, J. (1981). CO_2 elimination by high frequency ventilation (4 to 10 Hz) in normal subjects. *Am. Rev. Respir. Dis.* **123**:151.

Harf, A., Legall, R., and Chang, H. K. (1983). Mechanical ventilation with superimposed high frequency oscillation (abstract). *Am. Rev. Respir. Dis.* **127**: 253.

Harris, T. R. (1983). High frequency jet ventilation treatment of neonates with life-threatening restrictive lung disease. *Pediatr. Res.* **17**:316A.

James, L. S. (1983). *Pediatrics* **71**:280.

Jonzon, A. (1977). Phrenic and vagal nerve activities during spontaneous respiration and positive pressure ventilation. *Acta Anaesthesiol. Scand. Suppl.* **64**:29.

Kirby, R. R. (1979). Ventilatory support and pulmonary barotrauma. *Anesthesiology* **50**:181.

Kirby, R. R. (1980). High-frequency positive-pressure ventilation (HFPPV): What role in ventilatory insufficiency? *Anesthesiology* **52**:109.

Kirby, R. R., Downs, J. B., Civetta, J. B., Modell, J. H., Dannemiller, J. H., Klein, E. F., and Hodges, M. (1975a). High level positive end expiratory pressure (PEEP) in acute respiratory insufficiency. *Chest* **67**:156.

Kirby, R. R., Pery, J. C., Calderwood, H. W., Ruiz, B. C., and Lederman, D. S. (1975b). Cardiorespiratory effect of high positive end-expiratory pressure. *Anesthesiology* **43**:533.

Kolton, M., Cattran, C. B., and Kent, G. (1982a). Oxygenation during high-frequency ventilation compared with conventional mechanical ventilation in two models of lung injury. *Anesth. Analg.* **6**:323.

Kolton, M., Cattran, C. B., Kent, G., Volgrest, G., Eng, P., Froese, A. E., and Bryan, A. C. (1982). Oxygenation during high frequency ventilation compared with conventional mechanical ventilation in two models of lung injury. *Anesth. Analg.* **61**:323.

Kuehl, T., Meredith, K., Ackerman, N., Minnick, L., Stoddard, R., Hilliard, L., Escobedo, M., Coalson, J., Null, D., Robotham, J., and de Lemos, R. (1982). High vs. low frequency ventilation in the premature baboon with RDS. *Pediatr. Res.* 195A.

Kuehl, T. J., Coalson, J. J., Ackerman, N. B., Jr., Escobedo, M. B., Bell, R., Yoder,

B., Minnick, L., Stoddard, R., Meredith, K., Hilliard, J. L., Smith, F. S., Cipriani, C., Null, D. M., Robotham, J. S., and deLemos, R. (1984). High frequency ventilation in the treatment of hyaline membrane disease: the use of a baboon model to determine an acceptable ventilatory strategy. *Pediatrics* (in press).

Kumar, A., Pontoppidan, H., Falke, K. H., Wilson, R. S., and Laver, M. B. (1973). Pulmonary barotrauma during mechanical ventilation. *Crit. Care Med.* **1**: 181.

Lunkenheimer, P. S., Frank, I., Ising, H., Keller, H., and Dickhuth, H. H. (1973). Intrapulmoner Gaswechsel unter simultaner Apnoe durch transtrachealen, periodischen intrathorakalen Druckwechiel. *Anaesthetist* **22**:232.

Lyager, S. (1970). Ventilation/perfusion ratio during intermittent positive-pressure ventilation. *Acta Anaesthesiol. Scand.* **14**:211.

Mammel, M. C., Gordon, M. J., Connett, J. E., and Boros, S. J. (1983). Comparison of high-frequency jet ventilation and conventional mechanical in a meconium aspiration model. *J. Pediatr.* **103**:630.

Man, G. C. W., Man, S. F. P., and Kappagoda, C. T. (1983). Effects of high frequency oscillatory ventilation on vagal and phrenic nerve activities. *J. Appl. Physiol.* **54**:502.

Marchak, B. E., Thompson, W. K., Duffy, P., Miyaki, T., Bryan, M. H., Bryan, A. C., and Froese, A. B. (1981). Treatment of RDS by high frequency oscillatory ventilation: a preliminary report. *J. Pediatr.* **99**:287.

Meeuwis, H., Vaes, L., and Klain, M. (1983). High frequency jet ventilation in a 3-year-old child. *Crit. Care Med.* **11**:309.

Ng, K. P. K., and Easa, D. (1979). Management of interstitial emphysema by high frequency low positive pressure hand ventilation in the neonate. *J. Pediatr.* **95**:117.

Ngeow, Y. K., and Mitzner, W. (1982). A new system for ventilating with high frequency oscillation. *J. Appl. Physiol.* **53**:1638.

Nordin, U., Keszler, H., and Klain, M. (1981). How does high frequency ventilation affect the mucociliary transport. *Crit. Care Med.* **9**:160.

Nordin, U., Klain, M., and Keszler, H. (1982). Electron microscopic studies of tracheal mucosa after high frequency jet ventilation (abstract). *Crit. Care Med.* **10**:211.

Ophoven, J. P., Mammel, M. C., Gordon, M. J., and Boros, S. J. (1983). High frequency jet ventilation: tracheobronchial histopathology (abstract). *Pediatr. Res.* **17**:386A.

Pokora, T. J., Bing, D. R., and Boros, S. J. (1983a). Neonatal high frequency jet ventilation. *Pediatr. Res.* 359A.

Pokora, T., Bing, D., Mammel, M., and Boros, S. (1983b). Neonatal high frequency jet ventilation. *Pediatrics* **72**:27.

Qvist, J., Pontopiddan, H., Wilson, R., Lowenstein, E., and Laver, M. D. (1975). Hemodynamic response to mechanical ventilation with PEEP: The effect of hypervolemia. *Anesthesiology* **42**:45.

Ratliff, I. L., Hill, J. D., Fallat, R. J., Parrot, J., and Tucker, H. J. (1975). Complications associated with membrane lung support by venoarterial perfusion. *Ann. Thorac. Surg.* **19**:537.

Rieke, H., Hook, C., and Meyer, M. (1983). Pulmonary gas exchange during high frequency ventilation in dogs. *Respir. Physiol.* **54**:1.

Rossing, T. H. (1983). Fresh gas bias flow during high frequency ventilation. (abstract). Proceeding of International Symposium on High Frequency Ventilation. Edited by G. C. Carlon.

Rossing, T. H., Slutsky, A. S., Lehr, J., Drinker, P. A., Kamm, R., and Drazen, J. M. (1981). Tidal volume and frequency dependence of carbon dioxide elimination by high frequency ventilation. *N. Engl. J. Med.* **305**:1375.

Rossing, T. H., Solway, J., Saari, A. F., Gauriely, N., Slutsky, A. S., Lehr, J. L., and Drazen, J. M. (1983). Fresh gas bias flow during high frequency ventilation—effects of position on carbon dioxide elimination in humans. *Clin. Res.* **31**:259A.

Saari, A. F., Rossing, T. H., Solway, J., and Drazen, J. M. (1984). Lung inflation during high-frequency ventilation. *Am. Rev. Respir. Dis.* **129**:333.

Saramiento, A., Bryan, C., Jobe, A. H., Ikegami, M., and Jacobs, H. C. (1983). High frequency oscillations vs. conventional ventilation of premature lambs. *Pediatr. Res.* **17**:333A.

Scotter, D. R., Thurtell, G. W., Raats, P. A. C. (1967). Dispersion resulting from sinusoidal gas flow in porous materials. *Soil Sci.* **104**:306.

Sjöstrand, U. (1980). High-frequency positive-pressure ventilation (HFPPV): A review. *Crit. Care Med.* **8**:345.

Sjöstrand, J. U., and Eriksson, I. A. (1980). High rates and low volumes in mechanical ventilation—not just a matter of ventilatory frequency. *Anesth. Analg.* **59**:567.

Slutsky, A. S., Drazen, J. M., Ingram, R. H., Kamm, R. D., Shapiro, A. H., Fredberg, J. J., Loring, S. H., and Lehr, J. (1980). Effective pulmonary ventilation with small volume oscillation at high frequency. *Science* **209**:609.

Slutsky, A. S., Kamm, R. D., Rossing, T. H., Loring, S. H., Lehr, J., Shapiro, A. H., Ingram, R. H., Jr., and Drazen, J. M. (1981). Effects of high frequency tidal volume and lung volume on CO_2 elimination in dogs by high frequency (2-30 Hz) low tidal volume ventilation. *J. Clin. Invest.* **68**:1475.

Thompson, W. K., Marchak, B. E., Froese, A. B., and Bryan, A. C. (1981). Vagotomy reverses apnea induced by high frequency oscillatory ventilation. *J. Appl. Physiol.* **51**:1484.

Thompson, W. K., Marchak, B. E., Froese, A. B., and Bryan, A. C. (1982). High frequency oscillation compared with standard ventilation in pulmonary injury model. *J. Appl. Physiol.* **52**:543.

Truog, W. E., Standaert, T. A., Murphy, J., Palmer, S., Woodrum, D. E., Hodson, W. A. (1983). Effect of high-frequency oscillation on gas exchange and pulmonary phospholipids in experimental hyaline membrane disease. *Am. Rev. Respir. Dis.* **127**:585.

Zapol, W. M., Snider, M. T., and Schneider, R. C. (1977). Extracorporeal membrane oxygenation for acute respiratory failure. *Anesthesiology* **46**:272.

AUTHOR INDEX

Italic numbers give the page on which the complete reference is listed.

C

D

E

H

I

J

K

L

M

N

S

T

SUBJECT INDEX

H

I

J

L

BOY[illegible]

N. 5

B00/8 11+